Instructor's Resource Manual and Test Bank

to accompany

POTTER * PERRY
Fundamentals of Nursing

evolve

The Latest *Evolution* in Learnin

Evolve provides online access to free learning resources and activitie
designed specifically for the textbook you are using in your class.
The resources will provide you with information that enhances the
material covered in the book and much more.

Visit the Web address listed below to start your learning evolution tod

▶▶ LOGIN: *http://evolve.elsevier.com/Potter/fundamenta*

Evolve Instructor Resources for Potter/Perry: Fundamentals of Nursing
6th edition offers the following features:

- ### Instructor's Resource Manual
  A guide for the instructor to be used in the development of class presentations,
  clinical experiences, and evaluations of student learning. Included in this manua
  are: Classroom Discussions, Interactive Exercises, Clinical Skills/Techniques,
  Client Care Experiences, Resources for Student Activities, and Critical Thinking
  Exercises and Answers

- ### Test Bank
  Exam View computerized test bank includes NCLEX-style questions for each
  chapter with answers, rationales, and page references, organized by chapter.

- ### Power Point Slides
  Lecture slides for each chapter, to download for visual enhancement of class
  lectures and discussions.

- ### Image Collections
  Search, view, and download the selection of approximately 400 images from the
  textbook.

- ### Checklists
  Checklists for all of the nursing skills from the textbook

- ### WebLinks
  An exciting resource that lets you link to hundreds of websites carefully chosen
  supplement the content of the textbook. The WebLinks are regularly updated,
  with new ones added as they develop.

Think outside the book... *evolve*

Instructor's Resource Manual and Test Bank

to accompany
POTTER * PERRY
Fundamentals of Nursing

Patricia A. Castaldi, RN, MSN, RN
Director
Practical Nursing Program
Union County College
Plainfield, New Jersey

Test Bank rationales prepared by
Barbara Caton, RN, MSN
Assistant Professor
Southwest Missouri State University–West Plains
West Plains, Missouri

6th Edition

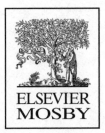

ELSEVIER
MOSBY

11830 Westline Industrial Drive
St. Louis, MO 63146

INSTRUCTOR'S MANUAL AND TEST BANK TO ACCOMPANY
FUNDAMENTALS OF NURSING, 6TH EDITION   0-323-03245-1
Copyright 2005, by Mosby, Inc. All rights reserved.

Notice

Nursing is an ever-changing field. Standard safety precautions must be followed, but as new research and clinical experience broaden our knowledge, changes in treatment and drug therapy may become necessary or appropriate. Readers are advised to check the most current product information provided by the manufacturer of each drug to be administered to verify the recommended dose, the method and duration of administration, and contraindications. It is the responsibility of the treating physician, relying on experience and knowledge of the patient, to determine dosages and the best treatment for each individual patient. Neither the Publisher nor the author assumes any liability for any injury and/or damage to persons or property arising from this publication.

The Publisher

International Standard Book Number: 0-323-03245-1

Executive Editor: Susan R. Epstein
Senior Developmental Editor: Maria Broeker
Publishing Services Manager: Gayle May

Printed in the United States of America

Last digit is the print number: 9   8   7   6   5   4   3   2

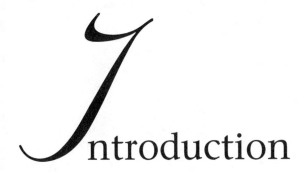ntroduction

This Instructor's Resource Manual and Test Bank to accompany the sixth edition of Potter and Perry's Fundamentals of Nursing has been developed to assist in the preparation of classroom, laboratory, and clinical educational activities for fundamentals of nursing courses. Although there are differences in curricula and teaching styles, this manual should be able to assist in class preparation by highlighting chapter information, thus saving valuable time and effort.

This manual includes two sections. In Section I, suggestions for classroom discussions, interactive exercises, clinical skills, and clinical activities are provided for each chapter in the text. Resources for Student Activities are available to reproduce and assign to students for use individually or in a group. Teaching strategies in the manual correspond with the emphasis of the content in the text. In addition, the Critical Thinking Exercises from the text and suggested answers are provided.

Section II of the manual is a revised test bank that includes over 700 questions and answers including rationales. Page numbers indicate where the content is covered in the text.

The primary intent of this Instructor's Manual and Test Bank is to be a quick reference and resource for you, the instructor, to use with your students. Your suggestions for future editions are welcomed.

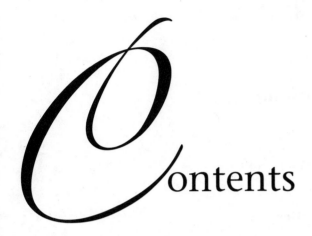

Contents

1

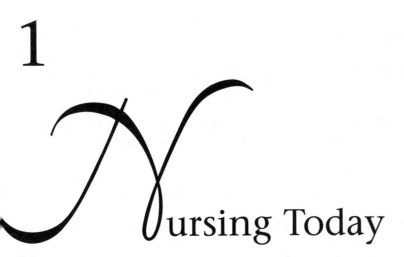

Nursing Today

Instructor Media Resources

Instructor's Resource CD
evolve Instructor's Resources

Instructor's Manual
ExamView Test Bank
Image Collection
Power Point Slides
Weblinks

Student Media Resources

CD COMPANION

- Review Questions
- Glossary

evolve WEBSITE

- Review Questions
- Student Learning Activities
- Glossary

Classroom Discussion

1. Review and discuss the historical evolution of the nursing profession within the context of the society of the era. Provide students with a chronologic outline to facilitate discussion and note taking.

2. By using a selected nursing journal as a reference, present a broad overview of the development of nursing practice through the 20th century by highlighting the changes in the focus of articles, advertisements, etc.

3. Discuss definitions of nursing. Ask students about their own philosophies of nursing.

4. Review the different pathways to becoming a registered nurse (see Resources for Student Activities).

5. Discuss the legal concepts associated with nursing practice, including licensure, standards of practice, and nurse practice acts.

7. Ask students to identify the goal of graduate nursing education in the preparation of professional nurses. Discuss the health care settings or situations in which a nurse would require this level (Master's or Doctoral) of nursing education.

8. Review the differences between continuing and in-service education programs. Ask students to identify possible topic areas that may be presented in both types of programs.

9. Ask students to determine what a career ladder program may look like in the following health care settings: acute care, long-term care, and home care.

10. Ask students to provide examples of actual activities associated with the varied roles of the nurse (see Resources for Student Activities). Use available educational media that portray nurses in various roles and settings.

11. Ask students to share their individual nursing career goals/interests and discuss the education and experience required for those particular career avenues.

12. Invite an advanced practice nurse and/or nurse working in a nontraditional area (sports medicine, sales, etc.) to discuss his or her role, educational preparation, and experience.

13. Discuss the collaborative role of the nurse with other members of the health team

14. Review the characteristics of a profession, and ask students to determine how nursing fulfills each one.

15. Review the development and purposes of professional nursing organizations.

16. Discuss the political influence of nursing and on nursing. Ask students to identify the skills that are necessary in the political process, and how nurses may be involved in reform.

17. Invite a nurse who has been elected to public office to speak to the class about nursing power and politics.

18. Stimulate a class discussion on current and future trends in nursing

*I*nteractive Exercises

1. Assign students to write and/or report about a major historic figure or event that helped to shape the profession of nursing.

2. Assign students, individually or in small groups, to review a specific year's publication of a nursing journal, and report verbally, or in writing, on the types of articles, advertisements, and job opportunities presented at the time.

3. Assign students to visit different agencies where nurses are employed and to observe the roles they have assumed in the agency.

4. Assign students to attend, if available, a multidisciplinary client care conference at an affiliating agency.

5. Have students attend a meeting or convention (especially the Student Nurses Association) to observe activities.

6. Have students bring in examples from the media (e.g., Internet, newspaper, magazines) that reflect current changes or trends in practice or societal influences on nursing.

7. Based on a current issue affecting nursing or health care, have students determine the mechanism by which policy or reform may be initiated. Ask students to follow through on those mechanisms, such as writing to a legislator about his or her views.

8. Provide students with case studies, and have students identify the various roles that are assumed by the nurse.

9. Have students investigate educational programs that are available locally and on-line for their ongoing nursing education (AD or Diploma to BSN, BSN to MSN).

10. Ask students to develop a recruitment plan to encourage people to enter the nursing profession.

$\mathcal{R}$esources for Student Activities

Comparative Chart of Nursing Education
Nursing Roles Chart

Comparative Chart of Nursing Education

	Diploma	Associate	Baccalaureate	Master's	Doctorate
Average Time Needed to Complete the Program					
Degree or Credential Received					
Primary Focus/ Preparation of the Graduate					
Preparation for RN Licensure?					
Specialized or Generalized Study					
Usual Setting					

Nursing Roles

	Actual Clinical Examples
Care Giver	
Advocate	
Manager	
Communicator	
Educator	

Critical Thinking Exercises (from text page 24)

1. Observe various levels of nursing practice, such as a staff nurse, advanced practice nurse, and nurse educator. Identify similarities and differences in their roles and educational preparation.

2. Outline some career objectives for yourself over the next 5-year period. Obviously the first would be to complete your nursing program, but decide what you want to do as a professional nurse, and then outline strategies to achieve these goals.

3. Part of your education includes experiences in different types of health care settings. How would your role in the primary care setting be different from your role in the acute care setting?

Suggested Answers

1. Answers will vary among students, but the whole idea of this exercise it to get them to think of nursing as a career and life-long learning.

2. Common: professional nursing background, client-centered care, life-long learning Differences: Primary practice role may be different (e.g., acute care vs. primary care vs. educational setting). Level of education (e.g., staff nurse may need initial educational preparation, but advanced practice nurse needs Master's degree). Educator may need Master's degree or doctorate.

3. The nurse in the acute care setting focuses on providing care that will help the acutely ill client improve his or her current state of health and return home. The primary care nurse focuses on helping the client maintain his or her level and promote an ongoing healthy lifestyle. Although nurses in both settings have responsibilty for providing the client and family with education about the illness and self-care, the perspective and focus of their care differ considerably.

2

*H*ealth Care Delivery System

Classroom Discussion

1. Discuss the current status of the health care system and how it will influence both nurses and consumers. Review regulatory or government interventions, including certificates of need, professional standards review organizations, and prospective payment systems.

2. Discuss methods of financing health care services, including eligibility and coverage, with managed care, government plans, private insurance, etc.

3. Discuss the differences in availability/access to health care for clients from different socioeconomic backgrounds and geographic locations.

4. Ask students to provide examples of how finances and politics may influence health care delivery.

5. Invite an advanced practice nurse to discuss his or her educational preparation and role in a managed care environment.

6. Discuss the ethical issues surrounding restricted access to health care.

7. Review the levels of care, the wide variety of health care agencies available, and the types of client services that may be offered at each.

8. Discuss the current issues in health care delivery:
   a. Competency of providers
   b. Population-based care
   c. Acute care re-design
   d. Quality health care
   e. Continuum of care

9. Review The Five Rights of Delegation. Ask students for specific examples of what care may be delegated to unlicensed assistive personnel.

10. Discuss Nursing's Agenda for Health Care Reform and how it may conform to or clash with current overall health care reform measures.

11. Ask students to identify possible discharge-planning concerns for the following client examples. A client who is:
    a. Newly diagnosed with diabetes mellitus
    b. Paralyzed on the left side after a stroke (cerebrovascular accident; CVA)
    c. Recovering from a heart attack (myocardial infarction; MI)
    d. Using oxygen continuously
    e. Receiving long-term intravenous (IV) therapy and medications.

12. Review the concept of the multidisciplinary health team approach and the use of critical pathways.

Interactive Exercises

1. Organize a debate on the issue: Is health care a right or a privilege?

2. Assign students to attend workshops/information sessions on new health care funding. Stimulate a debate on whether health care costs are justified.

3. Arrange for students to visit a variety of health care–delivery agencies and report, orally or in writing, on the following (see Resources for Student Activities):
   a. Entry into and exit from the system
   b. Environment
   c. Types of clients
   d. Nurse's role
   e. Payment structure
   f. Services offered
   g. Availability to clients (hours of operation, insurance accepted, etc.)

4. Have students, working in small groups, participate in a simulated work re-design project by using, if possible, a true-life situation from an acute or long-term care facility.

5. Assign students to obtain a journal article or news item on trends or funding in health care from the Internet or another current media source.

6. Have students develop an outline for a teaching plan specific to the health promotion, disease protection, and/or health protection/safety needs of the following clients:
   a. School-aged children at summer camp
   b. Senior citizens at a community center
   c. Middle adults in a work setting

7. Have students obtain actual insurance claim forms and brochures for discussion. Have students practice completing these forms according to the instructions.

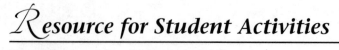

Resource for Student Activities

Health Agency Assessment Form

Student: _____

Name of Facility:

Location:

Hours of Operation/Availability:

Transportation Available to the Site:

Services Provided on Site:

Restrictions/Requirements (Insurance, etc.):

Costs:

Staffing and Responsibilities:

Role of the Nurse(s):

Affiliations (hospitals, etc.):

Response of Clients:

Student Comments:

Critical Thinking Exercises (from text page 44)

1. Mr. Giesler is an 82-year-old man who underwent surgery for a total knee replacement. He is alert and oriented and has been able to give good feedback when asked to explain activity restrictions at home. He will be taking a pain medication for his knee along with his regular antihypertensive medication and vitamins. Mr. Giesler will continue to go to rehabilitation even after discharge. His doctor has recommended use of a walker and gait training and muscle strengthening. To what health care service might you refer Mr. Giesler, and what is your rationale?

2. When entering Mrs. Saguchi's room, the nurse notices that the client seems anxious to speak. Mrs. Saguchi explains, "I am worried about going home. My doctor wants me to go home today. My daughter is coming in from out of town but will not be here until 3 days from now. I live by myself, and I would like to stay here at least until my daughter arrives. The hospital is making money off of my surgery. Can't I stay 1 more day?" Is Mrs. Saguchi's request reasonable? What would be your response as the nurse?

3. Spend time observing a nurse who works on one of the clinical areas on which you are assigned. Ask if you can follow him or her during client rounds. Then ask the nurse what he or she knows about one of his or her clients. Ask the nurse to explain how this knowledge will affect how he or she plans care for that client.

Suggested Answers

1. Mr Giesler would be a good candidate for a home care referral as a result of his knee replacement and need for an assistive device (the walker). The home care nurse will assess Mr. Giesler's home environment to determine whether safety hazards exist. His medication regimen is not an issue and should not be considered as a reason for referral. He will likely need physical therapy to strengthen the knee and use the walker properly. This service can be provided through home care or through a community outpatient rehabilitation facility.

2. You might explain, "Mrs. Saguchi, I understand your concern. I want to go over with you the things that you will need to do to take care of yourself at home. Are there any other family members or neighbors perhaps who could look in on you until your daughter arrives? We can determine if the home care agency can visit you in your home. I know it is difficult to understand, but the hospital receives a standard payment regardless of the number of days you spend with us. The hospital does not make more money if you stay with us for a longer period. Would you like to have me call your doctor to inform her of your concerns?"

3. Spend time observing a nurse who works in one of the clinical areas to which you are assigned. Ask if you can follow her or him during client rounds. Then ask the nurse what she or he knows about one of the clients. Ask the nurse to explain how the knowledge will affect the plan of care for that client.

3

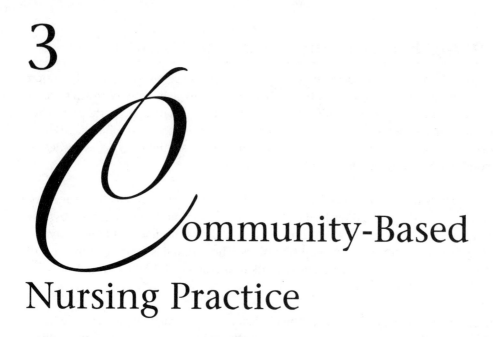

Community-Based Nursing Practice

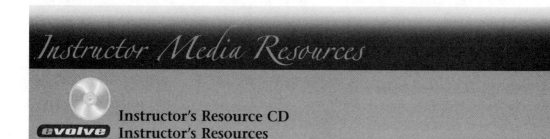

Instructor Media Resources

Instructor's Resource CD
evolve **Instructor's Resources**

Instructor's Manual
ExamView Test Bank
Image Collection
Power Point Slides
Weblinks

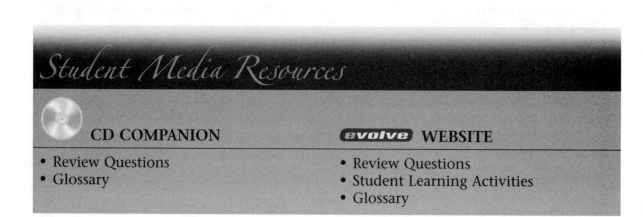

Student Media Resources

CD COMPANION

- Review Questions
- Glossary

evolve **WEBSITE**

- Review Questions
- Student Learning Activities
- Glossary

Classroom Discussion

1. Discuss the differences between public health and community nursing. Ask students to identify how nursing practice may also be different.

2. Ask students to identify the types of clients who may require community health care, and the special needs that may be seen with different age groups.

3. Invite a nurse and/or case manager from a public health or home health agency to speak to the class about his or her educational background, experience, and role.

4. Discuss the difference in approach and case management in the community. Have students problem solve how nursing procedures may need to be adapted.

5. Discuss the roles of the nurse, and other professionals and paraprofessionals, in community health care settings.

6. Discuss the type of care that may be delegated to ancillary personnel in public health or home care settings.

7. Review the continuum of care as it extends into the home, focusing on discharge planning within the acute and restorative care settings.

8. Guide students in the development of a care plan/pathway for a client requiring home care.

9. Review reimbursement mechanisms for home care.

10. Discuss the competencies recommended by the Pew Commission for community health nurses: (a) case manager, (b) collaborator, (c) educator, (d) counselor, (e) advocate, and (f) change agent. Ask students for specific examples of nursing activities related to each competency.

11. Compare and contrast the implementation of Quality Improvement in the acute care and community health environments.

Interactive Exercises

1. Have students role play a case-study situation for a client requiring home care, with a focus on a case-management approach.

2. Assign students to observe nurses at a community agency. Have students report, orally or in writing, on their observations, including the types of clients seen, services offered, and reimbursement structure.

3. Obtain a sample public health or home care nurse's caseload and ask students to determine a schedule for visiting, along with necessary referrals or equipment.

4. Have students report, orally or in writing, on the changes that have occurred in community-based health care over the past decade, or on current issues and trends.

5. Assign students to complete a community assessment and report orally and/or in writing about its population/demographics, services, and possible health care concerns.

Resource for Student Activities

Vulnerable Populations in the Community

Population	Health Concerns	Nursing Interventions
Poor		
Homeless		
Abused		
Substance Abusers		
Severely Mentally Ill		
Older Adults		

Critical Thinking Exercises (from text page 58)

1. As a nurse managing a severely disabled child, you learn that there is an absence of respite services to provide parental support and limited educational resources in your community. What role of the community-based nurse would be important to establish a special education day-care service, operated by volunteer educators?

2. Mr. Crowder is a 42-year-old man with diabetes mellitus and visual impairment. Your assessment reveals that he is homeless and that he currently spends nights in a shelter two blocks away. He has

been unable to acquire medications or proper diet to control his blood sugar. What factors might you consider in attempting to improve Mr. Crowder's adherence to medication administration?

3. Conduct a community assessment of an area that you have visited infrequently. Observe the community locale by driving through the more populated area. Look for the following services: hospital, clinic, drugstore, grocery, schools, park or playground, and police and fire departments.

Suggested Answers

1. Determine what the needs are in the community regarding respite care services. Are they the same type of respite care (e.g., after-school care for children of special needs, or after-school care to assist with some education regarding life skills). Second, the community nurse needs to know what, if any, resources are available to meet some of these needs. Do any foundations in the area provide financial support for special education teachers' aids to work in this type of program? Who in the special school system can help establish, maintain, and evaluate this program?

2. Show him ways to pick appropriate foods from nutrition programs (e.g., meals at homeless shelters). Investigate medical services for medically underserved people in the community. Investigate any vocational rehabilitation resources to assist with job skills or job placement. Determine availability of jobs that may trade room and meals for janitorial or maintenance activities.

3. Write down where health care resources are located. Determine their accessibility. Locate senior citizen centers that may provide some meals and health-screening activities. Look at the number, location, and hours of service for local drugstores, clinics, grocery stores. Are the neighborhoods of these services safe with adequate lighting?

4

*T*heoretical Foundations of Nursing Practice

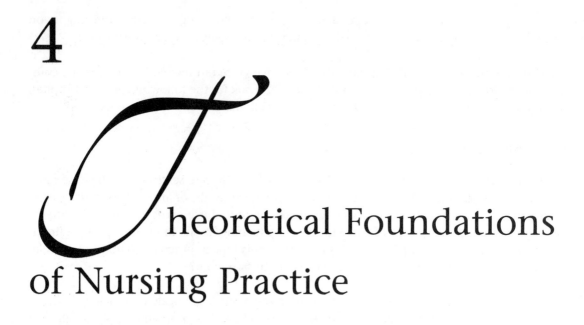

Instructor Media Resources

Instructor's Resource CD
evolve **Instructor's Resources**

Instructor's Manual
ExamView Test Bank
Image Collection
Power Point Slides
Weblinks

Student Media Resources

CD COMPANION

• Review Questions
• Glossary

evolve **WEBSITE**

• Review Questions
• Student Learning Activities
• Glossary

Classroom Discussion

1. Define and identify the need for theories in nursing practice.

2. Identify the components of a theory, including concepts, definition, and assumptions.

3. Describe the different types of theories, and ask students to provide examples of how they may be applied in nursing. Ask students what purpose or value theoretical development has for nursing practice.

4. Describe the components of nursing theoretical models: domain and paradigm. Specify the aspects of the nursing paradigm.

5. Ask students to identify how nursing theories relate to the nursing process.

6. Have students provide examples of interdisciplinary theories and how they may be applied in nursing situations.

7. Discuss the similarities and differences of the various conceptual models/nursing theories. Guide students in the application of one or more of the models/theories to an actual or simulated case-study example.

Interactive Exercise

1. Assign students to investigate articles in current nursing journals to see if nursing theories are used as the basis for nursing practice and/or research.

Resource For Student Activity

Nursing Paradigm Chart

Linkages	Description	Specific Theory Example
Person		
Health		
Environment Situation		
Nursing		

Critical Thinking Exercises (from text page 71)

1. Part of your education includes experiences in different types of health care settings. Take a theory and explain how it might apply in different health care settings.

2. What differences would you expect between the application of the theory in a hospital, a skilled care facility, and a community-based facility? Would you expect any commonalities?

3. From the following, identify those questions you think are theory-generating or theory-testing research. Would you expect that some of these are related to one another, and, if so, how?
    a. Do clients who receive a prescribed exercise program wean more quickly from the mechanical ventilator?
    b. What are the perspectives of family members in making end-of-life care decisions for a loved one?
    c. How does a family of divorce perceive their family hardiness?
    d. Do family members who know about their loved ones' advance directives have an easier time with end-of-life care?
    e. What are the perceptions of clients who wean from mechanical ventilation?
    f. How does a family member in a divorced family measure his or her own level of hardiness?
    g. Do family members who know about their loved ones' advance directives implement these directives during end-of-life care?

Suggested Answers

1. Outpatient setting, may use Orem's self-care theory, whereas in an acute care setting, Roy's adaptation model may be more appropriate. Working in a health promotion environment and behavior modification areas, King's theory of goal attainment may assist the client in modifying behaviors. Last, Swanson's theory of caring may be used to redesign the nursing care of a particular agency.

2. Differences are based on the types of clients and services of the agency. A hospice organization may use a combination of Jean Watson and Orem's theory to provide care to client and family and client. A community-based setting may use a community organization perspective. Last, when providing health promotion in a children's day-care facility, a framework for practice may be based on developmental theories.

3. Some of these questions may be related to an overall area of research, but the theory-generating questions should be addressed first. Then the investigator can then test elements of the generated theory.
    a. Theory generating
        i. What are the perspectives of family members in making end-of-life care decisions for a loved one?
        ii. How does a family of divorce perceive their family hardiness?
        iii. What are the perceptions of clients who wean from mechanical ventilation?
        iv. How do first-time fathers view their initial parenting skills?
    b. Theory testing
        i. Do family members who know their loved ones' advanced directives have an easier time with end-of-life care?
        ii. Do family members who know their loved ones' advance directives implement these directives during end-of-life care?

18   Chapter 4: Theoretical Foundations of Nursing Practice

iii. How does a family member in a divorced family measure his or her own level of hardiness?

iv. Do clients who receive a prescribed exercise program wean more quickly from the mechanical ventilator?

v. Do first-time fathers feel more comfortable with their parenting skills after a parenting class designed specifically for first-time fathers?

5

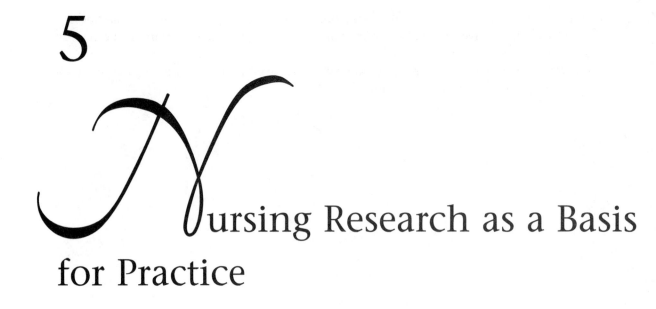

Nursing Research as a Basis for Practice

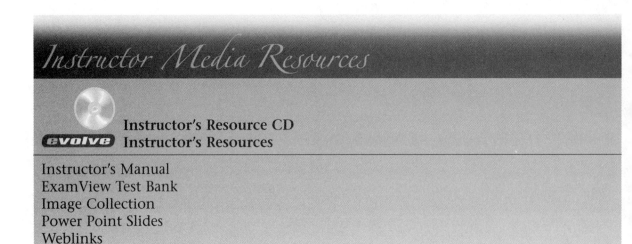

Instructor Media Resources

Instructor's Resource CD
evolve **Instructor's Resources**

Instructor's Manual
ExamView Test Bank
Image Collection
Power Point Slides
Weblinks

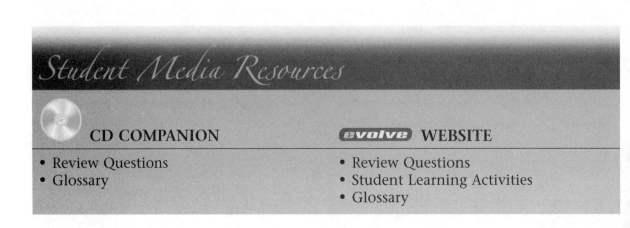

Student Media Resources

CD COMPANION

- Review Questions
- Glossary

evolve **WEBSITE**

- Review Questions
- Student Learning Activities
- Glossary

Classroom Discussion

1. Discuss the historical background and role of research in nursing.

2. Explain how scientific and nursing research are used to acquire knowledge and predict phenomena.

3. Ask students to identify how nursing research relates to the determination of the effectiveness of client care.

4. Discuss and provide examples of the different types of research that may be conducted.

5. Identify the role of nurses prepared at different educational levels in the research process.

6. Discuss how nursing research and the nursing process are interrelated.

7. Ask students to identify how nurses, including students, may participate in data collection for and the care of clients participating in research studies.

8. Discuss the ethical considerations associated with the research process, including informed consent, confidentiality, and anonymity.

9. Invite a nurse researcher to speak to the class about his or her role, educational preparation, and experience.

10. Discuss how the development of questions regarding clinical nursing problems may stimulate nursing research studies.

11. Provide examples of the ways in which nursing research has been used to enhance and improve nursing practice.

Interactive Exercises

1. Have students investigate and report on how nursing research may coordinate with Quality Improvement (QI) studies within an agency.

2. If possible, have students attend an IRB (Institutional Review Board) meeting to observe topic areas and procedures.

3. Assign students individually, or in small groups, to select an area for nursing research. Have them determine how and where the research will be conducted, who the researchers and participants will be, what resources may be needed, and how the findings may be applied to nursing practice.

4. Provide students with a nursing research article, and have students identify the type of information that is presented by the author(s). Assign students to obtain their own research articles on an area of interest and report the following on an index card: topic area, methods used, ethical considerations, results, and application to practice (see Resource for Student Activity).

Client Care Experience

1. If possible, have students participate in limited data collection for an actual clinical study in an affiliating agency.

Resource for Student Activity

Nursing Research Article Worksheet

Topic Area	Methodology	Ethical Considerations	Results	Application to Practice

Critical Thinking Exercises (from text page 86)

1. The nurse is concerned about learning to clean a pressure ulcer properly. Explain the benefits to the client if the nurse learns how to clean the sore by the scientific method versus trial and error.

2. If you wished to determine the best method for cleaning a pressure ulcer, how would you approach this problem?

3. You have noticed an increase in client falls. What method would you use to determine the exact number of falls in a specific time period? How would you determine which clients are falling? How could you use nursing research to implement an intervention for fall prevention? How would you determine the success or failure of the intervention?

Suggested Answers

1. The client receives interventions that have been proven successful. Measures are more cost effective and time efficient. The client receives the most current type of care.

2. Experimental design with treatment group(s) and a control group. We currently have a controlled/comparison study to determine a method of cleaning a pressure ulcer. I also want students to use literature to implement a research utilization method. Both are acceptable answers.

3. Falls
   a. Determine the number of falls: Can be done either with a medical record review or incident review
   b. Determine which clients are falling: Do frequency counts on the number of falls encountered by clients with fractured hips, hip replacements, taking hypertensive medications, with impaired immobility, prolonged bed rest, etc.
   c. Test a new intervention (e.g., specific method of getting client to dangle before getting out of bed vs. traditional method)
   d. Determine the change in number of falls after the interventions. This number can be a total number of falls for a particular unit or the number of falls can be broken down by client type, as in item b.

6

$\mathcal{H}$ealth and Wellness

Classroom Discussion

1. Discuss how the *Healthy People 2010* approach differs from the current U.S. practices. Ask students to write and/or talk about how the goals of *Healthy People 2010* could be specifically addressed in their own community.

2. Discuss the concept of health and the variables that affect health. Have students identify their beliefs about what "being healthy" means to them.

3. Compare the different health/illness models by applying them to the same case-study situation.

4. Explain the levels of prevention, and provide examples of nursing interventions for each one.

5. Discuss illness and how clients may demonstrate illness behaviors. Ask students to share their own and/or their family's illness experiences and behaviors.

6. Have students identify and give examples of internal and external variables and risk factors that may influence health. Review the stages of health behavior change and nursing interventions.

7. Discuss how the following illnesses may affect the roles and behaviors of a family:
   a. Chronic (chronic obstructive pulmonary disease [COPD], diabetes)
   b. Acute (myocardial infarction [MI], trauma)]
   c. Terminal (cancer)
   d. Physically deforming (burns, mastectomy)
   e. Neurologic impairment

8. Discuss how health care and the role of the nurse may change in accordance with the levels of prevention.

Interactive Exercises

1. Have students interview each other to determine the:
   a. Types of health promotion activities in which they engage to maintain wellness
   b. Risk factors present in themselves/family members

2. Assign students to interview a "client" (family member or friend) who has experienced an acute or chronic illness. Have the students present the assessment findings to the class and stimulate discussions on different client responses and nursing interventions for these individuals.

Resources for Student Activities

Comparison Chart for Review of Health/Illness Models
Levels of Prevention Study Chart

Health/Illness Models

	Key Concepts	Meaning of Health	Meaning of Illness	Client's View/Role	Nurse's Role
Health/ Illness Continuum					
Health Belief					
Health Promotion					
Basic Human Needs					
Holistic Health					

Levels of Prevention Chart

Level of Prevention	Focus	Role of the Nurse	Examples
Primary			
Secondary			
Tertiary			

Critical Thinking Exercises (from text page 104)

1. Identify two people you know—one whom you consider "healthy" and the other whom you consider "unhealthy." What are the differences between these individuals? What characteristics did you use to determine health status?

2. How would you describe your current state of health: excellent, good, fair, or poor? What definition of health did you use to make this judgment? List the current health-promotion, wellness, and illness-prevention activities that you regularly engage in. Should any areas be improved or changed? What will influence your ability to adopt any needed changes?

3. Assess the lifestyle patterns of someone you know. Identify risk factors that increase this person's vulnerability to illness or susceptibility to disease. Could the risk factors present be modified?

4. With this same individual, how could you approach the subject of risk-factor modification? What influences exist that will assist the individual in making a change? What barriers exist that may prevent maintenance of a change in health behavior? What resources are available to you and to this individual that may assist in the change process?

5. Have you witnessed illness behavior of yourself or someone you know? Did you (or they) respond differently to an acute versus a chronic illness? Evaluate the different responses you remember. Explore how the various internal and external variables influenced your reactions and behaviors. Was there an impact on the individual's self-concept or on family roles and dynamics?

Suggested Answers

1. Students should identify two people, one they consider healthy, and one they consider to be unhealthy. Differences between the two should be listed, including a discussion of the characteristics of these differences that are considered healthy and unhealthy.

2. Students should examine their health status and describe it in terms of excellent, good, fair, or poor. They should include their definition of health, and list the current health-promotional, wellness, or illness-prevention activities in which they engage. Students should discuss the areas that need to be improved or changed and what factors will influence their ability to adopt these changes.

3. Students should identify risk factors that increase vulnerability to disease for someone they know. Modifiable risk factors should be identified.

4. Students could describe a discussion of risk-factor modification with the individual from question 3. Barriers to health-behavior change should be identified. Resources also should be addressed.

5. Students should identify components of illness behavior, particularly an acute versus a chronic illness. Internal and external variables that may have influenced illness behavior should be included.

7

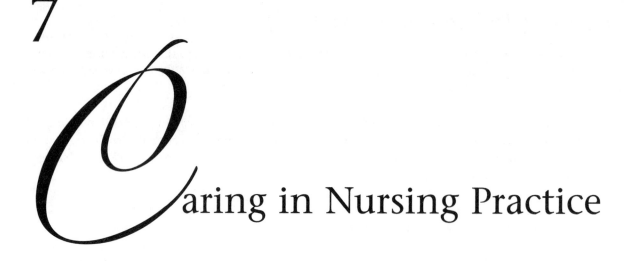

Caring in Nursing Practice

Instructor Media Resources

Instructor's Resource CD
evolve **Instructor's Resources**

Instructor's Manual
ExamView Test Bank
Image Collection
Power Point Slides
Weblinks

Student Media Resources

CD COMPANION

- Review Questions
- Glossary

evolve **WEBSITE**

- Review Questions
- Student Learning Activities
- Glossary

Classroom Discussion

1. Discuss the definitions of caring and how caring may be demonstrated.

2. Ask students to identify their own definitions and perceptions of caring.

3. Compare and contrast the theoretical views regarding caring, including those of Benner, Leininger, Watson, and Swanson.

4. Discuss the findings regarding clients' perceptions of nurses' caring behaviors.

5. Review what is meant by an "ethic of care."

6. Ask students to describe how the advocacy role in nursing relates to caring.

7. Discuss how nurses may implement caring behaviors for their peers in clinical practice.

Interactive Exercise

1. Arrange role-playing situations of nurse/client interactions that demonstrate caring or noncaring behaviors. Ask students to identify how the noncaring behaviors may be changed.

Caring Behaviors in Nursing

Nursing Behaviors	Specific Examples
Providing Presence	
Touch	
Listening	
Knowing the Client	
Spiritual Caring	
Family Care	

Critical Thinking Exercises (from text page 115)

1. Lindsey is a senior nursing student assigned to care for Mrs. Lowe, a 62-year-old client being treated for lymphoma (cancer of the lymph nodes). Mrs. Lowe is to receive an injection for her pain. In what way can Lindsay show caring in the way she administers the injection to Mrs. Lowe?

2. Mr. Leonard is a 42-year-old man who is married and has two teenage daughters. He underwent surgery this morning for an angioplasty to correct obstruction of his coronary arteries. The recovery room nurse calls the nursing division and tells you that Mr. Leonard has arrived, is stable, and will likely be there for 2 to 3 hours. His doctor will be up to the division shortly. What can you do to demonstrate caring for Mr. Leonard?

3. During your next clinical practicum, select a client to talk with for at least 15 to 20 minutes. Ask the client to tell you about his or her illness. Review the skills of listening in this chapter and in Chapter 23. Immediately after your discussion, reflect on the discussion with the client, and answer the following questions:
   a. What do you believe the client was trying to tell you about his or her illness?
   b. Why was it important for the client to share his or her story?
   c. What did you do that made it easy or difficult for the client to talk with you?
   d. Would you rate yourself a good listener? If not, why not? If so, explain.
   e. The next time you are assigned to a clinical agency, ask to read their philosophy and standards of care documents. Does the language in the documents represent a caring ethic?

Suggested Answers

1. Lindsey can begin by explaining to Mrs. Lowe what the injection is for and the anticipated time it will take to help relieve her discomfort. Lindsey should use eye contact while she talks with Mrs. Lowe. If Mrs. Lowe is receptive, Lindsey might hold her hand or gently rub her back as she offers her explanation. This can also be a time to listen to any concerns or fears that Mrs. Lowe might have. The manner in which Lindsey positions Mrs. Lowe for the injection also can convey caring, helping her to turn with minimal discomfort. Finally, the way Lindsey handles the syringe and administers the injection quickly and safely also conveys caring.

2. Caring for the family is an important aspect of your care for Mr. Leonard. Let the family know about the message from the recovery room. Have the family remain in the waiting area so that they can easily be found by the physician. Ask if they have any questions about the care Mr. Leonard will receive once he returns from surgery.

3. Exercises to be completed with students at your site. Answers will vary.

8

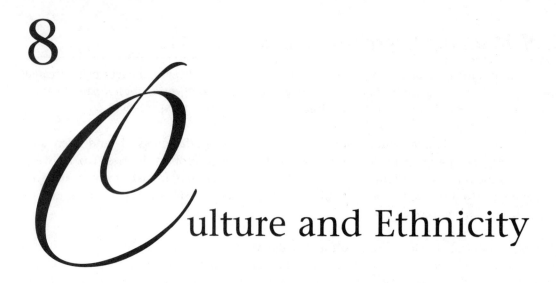

Culture and Ethnicity

Classroom Discussion

1. Discuss the concepts of culture, ethnicity, and religion.

2. Review cultural processes: enculturation, acculturation, assimilation, and biculturalism.

3. Discuss the concept of transcultural nursing and culturally competent care, including the recognition of the cultural identity of both the client and the nurse.

4. Review cultural healing modalities. Ask students to provide additional examples of each type of health care practice and the effects on nursing practice.

5. Review Leininger's Culture Care Theory and Sunrise Model and its application in nursing.

6. Discuss the cultural contexts of health and illness, comparing Western with non-Western cultural practices.

7. Review the current demographics of the local community and larger society, and their influence on overall health care needs.

8. Ask students to share personal experiences in regard to traditional health beliefs and practices.

9. Compare and contrast the health beliefs (illness cause and prevention and remedies) of Asian Americans, African Americans, Native Americans, Hispanic-Americans, and European Americans. Ask students from these diverse groups to add or correct information in the group discussion.

10. Discuss specific cultural health practices related to the following critical life events:
    a. Pregnancy
    b. Childbirth
    c. Newborn care
    d. Postpartum
    e. Grief and loss

11. Ask students to integrate examples of religious and spiritual practices into the discussion on cultural care.

12. Invite a nurse who works in a community setting with clients from diverse sociocultural backgrounds to discuss cultural competence.

13. Describe the components of a cultural assessment.

Interactive Exercises

1. Assign students to investigate the resources that are available in an affiliating agency for promoting communication and education for clients with language differences (i.e., interpreters, multilingual information packets).

2. Have students bring in examples, from the media and/or Internet, of health problems/needs specific to one or more sociocultural group(s).

3. Have students role play one or more of the following, or similar transcultural situations:
   a. Teaching a client with a language difference to give an injection
   b. Explaining to a client how home remedies are interacting with her prescribed medication
   c. Adapting acute or home care routines to avoid conflicts with religious practices
   d. Completing a health history with the client's entire family "camping out" and monopolizing the conversation
   e. Preparing a client, who has always worn a special amulet around her neck, for surgery
   f. Preparing an Islamic woman for a pelvic examination

4. Assign students to research the health practices of a specific cultural group. Organize a "cultural awareness" class in which students share their information on the specific culture with the group. Interest may be stimulated with the inclusion of traditional foods, music, etc.

5. Assign students to review the demographics of their own communities and begin to determine specific health care practices and needs.

Client Care Experiences

1. Conduct pre- and/or postclinical conferences for discussion of cultural adaptations that may have been implemented for clients of diverse backgrounds. Ask students to share information on possible barriers to and/or resources for transcultural nursing.

2. Working individually, or in small groups, have students identify the following, specific to sociocultural needs/adaptation, for an assigned client and/or a case-study situation:
   a. Nursing diagnoses
   b. Long-/short-term goals and desired client outcomes
   c. Nursing interventions
   d. Evaluation criteria/measures

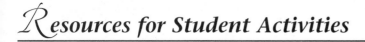

Resources for Student Activities

Cultural Assessment Components

Components	Examples
Ethnic heritage/ethnohistory	
Biocultural history/risk factors	
Social organization/socioeconomic	
Religious or spiritual practices	
Communication patterns	
Time orientation	
Caring beliefs and practices	
Experience with the health care system	

Critical Thinking Exercises (from text page 135)

1. You were about to begin giving a male Arabic Muslim his morning care when he stated, "I don't want a bath now." He got annoyed when you tried explaining that you have to do it at this time. Before you left the room, he asked you to leave a basin of water and towel by his bedside. He also asked you to get his small rug from his closet.
   a. How would you respond to the client?
   b. What might be the reasons for his refusal and annoyance?

2. A 50-year-old Chinese woman is hospitalized with a respiratory condition. She insisted that you give her warm water and rub her back with Tiger balm liniment. When her lunch came, consisting of a turkey sandwich, tossed salad, and milk, she asked that you take it back.
   a. How would you respond to the client's requests?
   b. What is the significance of her requests?
   c. Why did she refuse her lunch?

3. You are assigned to a 60-year-old Indian Hindu widow who is admitted with chest pain and shortness of breath. The client had recently arrived from India to visit her son and pregnant daughter-in-law. She can speak only Gujarati and understands very little English. She is accompanied by her son.
   a. What areas would you include in your focused cultural assessment?
   b. How would you communicate with the client?
   c. Identify ways to preserve and/or accommodate the client's culture.
   d. What aspects of the client's life way may need repatterning?

Suggested Answers

1.
    a. Ask the client how he wants his AM care done. Accommodate his preference.

    b. Muslim males generally expect gender-congruent care. If the nurse is a young female, he may not want to be in close contact with an unrelated female, as it is not allowed in his culture. The client is getting ready to pray and wanted to do his ritualistic washing before he prays. Muslims pray five times daily and wash their face, ears, hands, arms, and feet before praying. They pray on a rug.

2.
    a. Give her the warm water. You can ask her to tell you what the liniment is and request for the doctor to order it.

    b. The Chinese believe in restoring balance between yin and yang to restore health. Respiratory conditions are considered yin illnesses (caused by too much cold and dampness). Tiger balm is a counterirritant that produces local heat and vasodilation. Drinking cold and iced drinks is believed to create further imbalance.

    c. The Chinese are generally lactose intolerant. Diet is a pathway to restore balance between yin and yang.

3.
    a. Meaning of pain, desire for pain medication, diet, communication, family hierarchy, family support

    b. Request a trained interpreter to explain her medical condition. Expect her son to be consulted for decision making.

    c.
        - Provide privacy and gender-congruent care, as modesty is valued.
        - Show respect, as older women are treated with dignity by younger ones.
        - Allow client to consult her son, as it is a male-dominant society.
        - Provide vegetarian diet (no beef) and accommodate home-cooked meals with some adjustments. They prefer highly spicy foods.
        - Allow consistent presence of family members and friends at bedside.
        - Offer pain meds and observe for nonverbal and somatic complaints (difficulty sleeping, loss of appetite) of pain or no complaints at all.

    d.
        - Diet: use of unsaturated oils.
        - Expression of pain and need for pain relief: pain is seen as a consequence of past deeds (*karma*) that must be borne to improve one's rebirth. Hindus believe in *moksha* (reincarnation of the soul).
        - Hesitance of females to make decisions on their own. Male members generally make decisions and speak for females.

9

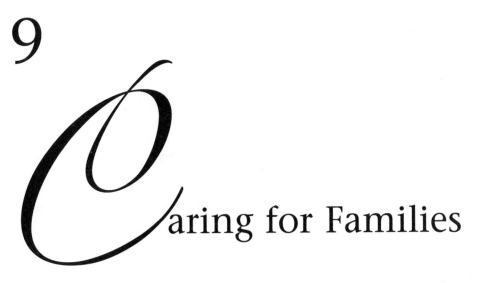

$\mathcal{C}$aring for Families

Instructor Media Resources

Instructor's Resource CD
evolve **Instructor's Resources**

Instructor's Manual
ExamView Test Bank
Image Collection
Power Point Slides
Weblinks

Student Media Resources

CD COMPANION

- Review Questions
- Glossary

evolve **WEBSITE**

- Review Questions
- Student Learning Activities
- Glossary

Classroom Discussion

1. Review the definition of and the different forms of families.

2. Stimulate a discussion on current trends and alternative lifestyles associated with families, and their influence on nursing and health care.

3. Describe the theoretical approaches to viewing the family, including the application of systems and developmental theories.

4. Discuss the structure and function of the family and the roles that may be assumed by family members.

5. Review the developmental stages of the family.

6. Explain the concepts of family nursing: family as context, family as client, and family as system. Provide examples that demonstrate the difference in these approaches.

7. Ask students to identify what should be included in an assessment of a family.

8. Discuss health promotion activities that may be implemented for families. Ask students to provide examples of specific interventions or teaching/learning plans that focus on family needs and cultural practices.

9. Invite a family practice nurse/counselor to speak to the class about his or her role, educational background, and experiences.

10. Ask students to identify how the following situations may influence the family unit:
    a. A single father has a heart attack (myocardial infarction; MI) and is no longer able to continue in his current job.
    b. A mother of three young children is in an auto accident, is paraplegic, and must use a wheelchair.
    c. An adolescent in an extended family demonstrates schizophrenic behavior.
    d. A child in a blended family is having difficulty at school.
    e. A newborn has a severe neurologic impairment, and four other siblings are in the home.
    f. The primary wage earner in the family is recently unemployed.

11. Guide students in the application of the nursing process by using an actual or simulated family case study.

Interactive Exercises

1. Have students bring in an example from the media and/or Internet on changes in the family, and/or assign students to investigate a current trend or issue in family life (i.e., single parenting, domestic violence).

2. Have students obtain an article from a nursing journal that discusses family-centered nursing care.

3. Assign students to report, orally or in writing, on the support systems/resources that are available to the family within the affiliating agency or local community.

Client Care Experience

1. Working individually or in small groups, have students identify the following, specific for an assigned family situation and/or case-study example:
   a. Nursing diagnoses
   b. Long-/short-term goals and desired client outcomes.
   c. Nursing interventions
   d. Evaluation criteria/measures

Critical Thinking Exercises

1. Kathy is a parish nurse and is working with a family in her church. This is a family of four: Carol, a 45-year-old single mother; her two adolescent sons, Matt and Kent; and Sara, her 76-year-old mother, who is in the last stages of terminal breast cancer. This family has lived together for 10 years, and Sara was a great support to Carol when her husband died 11 years ago. She helped Carol to parent Matt and Kent. This family has decided to care for Sara in the home until the end. Kathy is going to help the family achieve this goal.
   a. What assessments are important?
   b. How will Kathy help the family achieve this goal?
   c. How will Kathy help the family determine their strengths, weaknesses, and resources?

2. Dan has been divorced from Kim for 7 years. Neither has remarried, and they have three girls: Annie, Angela, and Abby, ages 10 to 14 years. At the time of the divorce, Dan was human immunodeficiency virus (HIV) positive. He has had active disease for 5 years, has not responded to therapy, and is in the end stages of the disease. Kim has had repeated tests and remains HIV negative. They have shared all parenting responsibilities and maintain a friendly relationship. Dan and Kim have decided that it might be easier for this family of five to live together again. This decision is so that Dan can be active in his girls' lives without placing caregiver demands on Kim when the family visits Dan overnight. Kim also wants to care for her former husband.
   a. What challenges will this family face as they reunite?
   b. How will the nurse determine what support services are needed by the family?

3. Mr. and Mrs. Baillargeron, both in their early 50s, are the youngest members of large Catholic French-Canadian family. They are employed full time and have two teenage children of their own. Both sets of their parents are in their 80s and have chronic health problems. All of their brothers and sisters are geographically farther away. How can you assist Mr. and Mrs. Baillargeron in developing extended resources to aid in caring for their parents and at the same time maintain the responsibilities of their own family unit?

Suggested Answers

1.
   a. Assess the changing state of Sara's health. Ask and observe how the family functions, interacts, solves problems, and determines workload. Assess Carol, Matt, and Kent's feeling/fears about Sara's impending death.

b. Identify specifically what the family's goals are. Determine their plans to achieve this goal.

c. Ask the family what they view as strengths and weaknesses. Observe the family, and share what the nurse views as strengths and weakness and how to improve on the weaknesses. The determination of needed resources should be an ongoing assessment. These needs will change over time, and the nurse must collaborate with the family to (1) determine need, (2) obtain new resources, and (3) identify friends, family, etc., who can assist.

2.

a. As this family begins to live in the same household, challenges will occur regarding division of work, decision making, and co-parenting. In addition, they will confront the issue of dealing with the death of a parent, from an illness that may have some social stigma issues with some people. The girls are approaching adolescence or are adolescents.

b. Assess the family regarding their perceived needs. Assess family needs and point out nonperceived needs. Determine strength and weaknesses.

3. Mr. and Mrs. Baillargeron are "sandwiched" between elder parents and teenage children, while trying to meet the demands and expectations of their full-time jobs and other outside commitments. The nurse can aid this family in finding outside resources for their elder parents. Ideas include the following: Have the teenagers post a web page and maintain it for the distant family members regarding the parents'/grandparents' needs, concerns, and information. Ask the extended family to send money to help support the inexpensive, community-based, gerontologic day care with activities, meals, games, health lectures, and socialization, or pay CNAs at night as their health demands increase. Have the family sign up for rotating weekends to stay with the grandparents (e.g., one weekend per month). The family members who live farther way may send more money or cards, letters, pictures, or e-mails. Additional support may be available through the church and community center. Any of these efforts would help relieve the responsibilities of total caretaking by any one person, which creates caregiver role strain and decreased ability to function. These efforts also remind the elders that they are still part of their community and decreases the potential for depression and elder abuse (which is all too common when elders have been isolated from their peers).

10

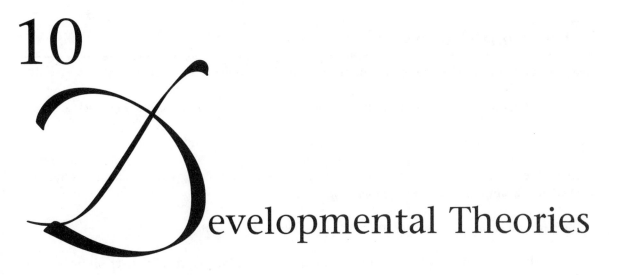

Developmental Theories

Instructor Media Resources

Instructor's Resource CD
evolve **Instructor's Resources**

Instructor's Manual
ExamView Test Bank
Image Collection
Power Point Slides
Weblinks

Student Media Resources

CD COMPANION

- Review Questions
- Glossary

evolve **WEBSITE**

- Review Questions
- Student Learning Activities
- Glossary

Classroom Discussion

1. Explain the relevant terminology, including growth, development, and maturation.

2. Describe the role of human-development theories and their application to nursing practice.

3. Discuss and provide specific examples of the principles of growth and development.

4. Review the four major areas of theory development: (a) biophysical, (b) psychoanalytic/psychosocial, (c) cognitive, and (d) moral development.

5. Compare and contrast the various theories of human development.

6. Ask the students to identify how the nurse may apply developmental theories to client interactions. Have students provide examples of situations that the nurse may encounter with clients of different ages.

7. With actual or simulated case studies, guide students in the application of selected developmental theories in the assessment of clients and determination of nurse/client interactions.

Client Care Experiences

1. Have students identify the developmental level and requirements of their assigned clients, and discuss, orally or in writing, how the nurse/client interactions may be adapted to meet their client's needs. Review the application of developmental theories to client assignments in clinical postcare conferences.

Critical Thinking Exercises (from text page 169)

1. A 76-year-old woman has just been diagnosed with breast cancer. She also has severe cardiovascular disease that limits her choices of treatment. Her oncologist has recommended a series of chemotherapy that her cardiologist believes would be fatal. Her family is urging her to do all that is recommended. The client, who is in good spirits despite her diagnosis, chooses palliative care. Based on her developmental stage, how can you help the family adjust to her choice?

2. A 50-year-old woman expresses dismay that her children, ages 20 and 23 years, are no longer living at home. Her husband is still working full time but looking to retire in a couple of years. She is concerned that she is not needed and is bored with her life. Identify the developmental task of Erickson's theory that best fits this woman's situation. How will the nurse assist this client in changing her lifestyle while understanding her developmental tasks?

3. Parents of an 18-month-old toddler describe to the nurse during their routine visit to the pediatrician that their child is walking and getting into everything. By using your knowledge of Erikson's developmental theories, at what stage is this child, and what approach would be helpful for these parents?

4. Two 11-year-old girls are spending the day together at the mall. They exit one store, and one of the girls shows her friend a small purse that she stole from the store. Her friend is upset and wonders how she should respond. What moral advice would you want to discuss with this young girl?

Suggested Answers

1. Based on this woman's developmental stage, she should be allowed to make informed choices about her health treatment plan. Her family needs to understand that she has been informed of all choices and options available, and that she has made a decision that she is most comfortable with for her stage.

2. This client is struggling with Erikson's developmental task of generativity versus stagnation. The nurse can assist the client in determining what activities are pleasurable for her to pursue during this stage. Activities such as volunteer work, or community or civic work will help her feel productive and benefit the community at large.

3. According to Erikson, an 18-month-old toddler is struggling with his newfound independence. The best approach for these parents would be for them to recognize that this is a normal response of their toddler to explore the environment. Caregivers must allow this exploration while providing supervision and taking safety precautions.

4. This young girl would need to discuss what her friend had done and what action she should take in response. She could tell her friend that what she had done is wrong and that she can't go to the mall with her under these circumstances. She should be advised to discuss this incident with her parents as well.

11

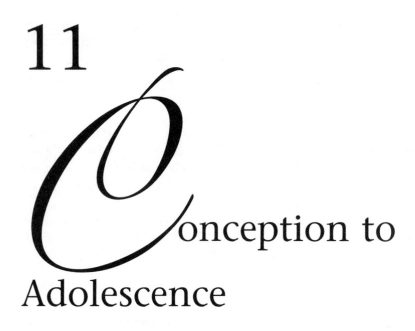

Conception to Adolescence

Instructor's Resource CD
evolve **Instructor's Resources**

Instructor's Manual
ExamView Test Bank
Image Collection
Power Point Slides
Weblinks

Student Media Resources

CD COMPANION

- Review Questions
- Glossary

evolve **WEBSITE**

- Review Questions
- Student Learning Activities
- Glossary

Classroom Discussion

1. Review conception, intrauterine life, and the transition to extrauterine life. Identify or ask students to identify the following for each trimester of pregnancy and childbirth:
   a. Characteristics of physical, cognitive, and psychosocial development
   b. Specific health concerns, risks, and health promotion/safety activities

2. Review growth and development of the neonate, infant, toddler, preschool child, school-age child, and adolescent. Identify or ask students to identify the following for the neonate, infant, toddler, school-age child, and adolescent:
   a. Characteristics (milestones) of physical, cognitive, and psychosocial development
   b. Language development and communication patterns
   c. Specific health concerns, risks, and health promotion/safety activities

3. Discuss how perceptions of health and illness are developed in young children.

4. Discuss the effect of hospitalization on children and parents/caretakers. Ask students to provide examples of possible behavior patterns based on the developmental level of the child.

5. Discuss and ask students to provide additional examples of implementation strategies for the hospitalized child in relation to minimizing separation anxiety, establishing trust, reducing fear, minimizing physical discomfort, fostering normal growth and development, and incorporating play and diversional activity into daily care.

6. Provide examples of childhood behaviors, and have students apply the developmental theories of Piaget, Erikson, Freud, and Kohlberg to each scenario.

7. Invite a maternal/child nurse and/or pediatric nurse practitioner to speak to the class about his or her role, educational background, and experiences.

Interactive Exercises

1. Assign students to report, orally or in writing, on the support systems/resources that are available within an affiliating agency or local community for pregnant families, neonates, infants, toddlers, preschoolers, school-age children, adolescents, and parents.

2. Have students, working individually or in small groups, design a teaching plan for parents of infants, toddlers, preschool children, school-age children, and/or adolescents based on a specific health need or concern of this age group, incorporating cultural practices as appropriate. Have the students present the teaching plan to the class and/or to the target group of parents within an agency or community setting (i.e., school group).

3. Have students obtain an article from a nursing journal that focuses on a specific health need or concern associated with prenatal clients and/or children of this age group (i.e., home safety, nutrition). Assign students to complete an oral and/or written report on an identified health need or concern for neonates, infants, toddlers, preschool children, school-age children, or adolescents.

4. Have students design activities and/or identify age-appropriate toys for infants, toddlers, preschool children, school-age children, and adolescents. (Piaget's stages of development may be used as a framework).

5. Organize a role-playing activity in which students simulate interactions with parents of newborns and infants, toddlers, preschool children, school-age children, and/or adolescents. Use the following or similar situations:
   a. A 3 year old having surgery tomorrow
   b. A 6-month-old infant requiring numerous diagnostic tests
   c. A 5 year old who will be having a series of injections
   d. A 2 year old who has never been away from home and is hospitalized for an indefinite period
   e. A 9 year old who has leukemia
   f. A 15 year old newly diagnosed with diabetes mellitus
   g. An 18 year old who has extensive burns

Client Care Activities

1. Have students assess and report on the developmental status/activities of clients in one or more of the following settings: prenatal clinic, obstetrician's/pediatrician's office, day-care center, preschool, well-baby clinic, elementary or high school.

2. Assign students to observe and/or participate in the nursing care of prenatal clients, newborns, infants, toddlers, preschool children, school-age children, and adolescents in an acute care or community health setting. Discuss the experience with the group, focusing on the specific nursing interventions implemented for these clients/families.

3. Guide students in the application of the nursing process for prenatal clients, neonates, infants, toddlers, preschool children, school-age children, and/or adolescents. Working individually or in small groups, have students complete a care plan or clinical pathway for a client from this age group.

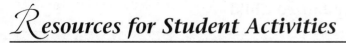

Resources for Student Activities

Comparative Assessment: Neonate to Adolescent
Assessment of Hospitalized Child

Comparison Chart: Neonate to Adolescent

Assessment Area	Neonate	Infant	Toddler	Preschool Child	School-age Child	Adolescent
Physical Development						
Cognitive Development						
Psychosocial Aspects						
Health Concerns						
Health Promotion Activities						

Hospitalized Child

	Assessment Data
Developmental Stage	
Response to Hospitalization	
History of Prior Illness, Hospitalization, Separation	
Medical History	
Perception of Illness (If Able to Obtain)	
Available Support Systems	

Critical Thinking Exercises (from text page 214)

1. Mrs. Wong is attending the antepartum clinic for the first visit. A major area for focus is health promotion. What areas should the nurse present at this time? Mrs. Wong asks whether it is better to breast-feed or bottle-feed.

2. The parents of 2-year-old Tyrese are concerned because he cries and fusses when his parents leave him at the day-care center and go to work. Identify nursing measures that will minimize separation anxiety for Tyrese.

3. What measure can parents and teacher use to help the school-age child accomplish Erikson's task for this stage of development?

4. Twelve-year-old Elizabeth is brought to the pediatric clinic for a physical examination. She is concerned about her lack of physical development compared with her peers. Discuss ways to educate Elizabeth about puberty and the variations that occur.

5. Seventeen-year-old Ricardo wants very much to belong and be accepted by his peers. He expresses concern when his peers begin to plan a party with alcohol and girls. What should be discussed to help support his feelings and need to belong?

Suggested Answers

1. The nurse should present a review of a well-balanced diet, emphasizing the need for folic acid intake during her pregnancy. A usual weight gain of 25 to 30 pounds is considered acceptable. She should be instructed to avoid dieting and skipping meals. She should try to avoid stressful situations and to avoid the use of any drugs or home remedies. The nurse should explain the importance of continuing with regular daily exercise during her pregnancy.

    The nurse should assess the client's knowledge and feelings regarding infant feedings. The client should be given the advantages of both methods of feeding and supported on her decision.

2. Tyrese's parents should be made aware that separation anxiety is normal for this stage of development. To help this child build on the trust established earlier and the skills of autonomy, the parents should give simple, concrete explanations regarding when they will return. Time should be tied into an activity or reference that he can relate to at this age (meals or bedtime).

3. Parents and teachers should recognize that the developmental struggle of the school-age child, according to Erikson, is to master industry. These adults can best foster the children by offering them new learning skills within their developmental scope. Children should be guided and encouraged with their struggle to accomplish each new task. Praise and support should be given to the child to encourage efforts and reward successes.

4. The nurse at the pediatric clinic has the opportunity to review with Elizabeth her perceptions and knowledge of puberty. The nurse can inform her of the individualized rates for the onset of puberty. Open discussions along with pamphlets and written information can guide this teen toward a better understanding of the developmental changes of this stage.

5. Ricardo should be given an opportunity to discuss his concerns about his peers and his desire to belong to the group. Adolescents need to fit in and be part of a group. Although this need is important, he should be guided to express his own moral code and be comfortable saying "no" when he feels that it's right to do so.

12

Young to Middle Adult

Classroom Discussion

1. Discuss the theories related to young and middle adulthood and how the nurse may apply them to clinical situations.

2. Ask students to identify how young and middle adults demonstrate their cultural backgrounds and practices.

3. Review the developmental tasks and health perceptions that may be associated with young and middle adults.

4. Review growth and development of the young and middle adult. Identify or ask students to identify the following for the young and middle adult:
   a. Characteristics of physical, cognitive, and psychosocial development
   b. Specific health and psychosocial concerns
   c. Risk factors and health promotion/safety activities

5. Discuss tasks/concerns associated with the young adult, including career, finances, marriage, parenthood, establishment of a family, and care of older parents.

6. Provide an overview of pregnancy and the development of the childbearing family.
   Identify and/or ask students to identify specific health needs and concerns for the childbearing family.

7. Stimulate a discussion on different lifestyles of the young adult family, such as single parenting, homosexual relationships/parenting, dual-income families, etc.

8. Discuss the specific health risks associated with the young and middle adult.

9. Invite an adult nurse practitioner to speak to the class about his or her role, educational background, and experiences dealing with this age group and their specific health needs.

10. Ask students to discuss the concept of a "midlife crisis" and how it may affect an individual.

11. Ask students from this age group to share their own experiences in dealing with families, children, employment, school, and other lifestyle decisions/responsibilities.

Interactive Exercises

1. Assign students to report, orally or in writing, on selected support services/resources that are available within an affiliating agency or community for young and middle adults.

2. Have students obtain examples from the Internet, other media resources, or articles from nursing journals related to the stressors that may be prevalent in the lives of young and middle adults, such as industry downsizing and unemployment, two parents working and managing child care, etc.

3. Assign students to complete an oral and/or written report on an identified health need or risk factor associated with young and middle adulthood (i.e., need for breast and testicular self-examination).

4. Arrange for students to observe young or middle adults at a health screening, clinic, childbirth class, or community activity (i.e., PTA meeting) and report on the type of interactions and communication patterns that were demonstrated.

5. Working individually or in small groups, have the students design and present a teaching plan based on a specific health need of this age group.

Client Care Experiences

1. Assign students to observe and/or participate in the nursing care of young and middle adult clients in an acute care, rehabilitation, or community health setting. Discuss the experience with the group, focusing on the specific nursing interventions implemented for these clients.

2. Guide students in the application of the nursing process for young and middle adult clients. Working individually or in small groups, have students complete a care plan or clinical pathway that is specific for an actual young or middle adult client and/or case-study situation (incorporating cultural practices, as appropriate).

Resource For Student Activities

General Assessment Young to Middle Adult

Age: Height:

Sex: Weight:

	Description/Comparison with Norms
Physiological Development	
Cognitive Development	
Psychosocial Development	
Career/Job-related Activities	
Health Concerns/ Health Promotion Activities	
Leisure Activities	

Critical Thinking Exercises (from text page 232)

1. Joan K. is a 24-year-old woman who smokes two packs of cigarettes per day. She began smoking when she was 14 years old. Joan complains to the nurse at the clinic, "I just can't seem to kick the habit, no matter how hard I try." What information does the nurse need to know to assist Joan in quitting smoking?

2. James D., age 48 years, married, and the father of 13- and 16-year-old sons, has recently had to assume the responsibility of caring for his 78-year-old mother after she had a stroke. Describe the nurse's role in assisting James in caring for his mother.

Suggested Answers

1.
- Joan's motivation to quit smoking
- Techniques that Joan has used in the past to try to quit smoking
- Type of support that Joan has to quit smoking
- Barriers for Joan to quit smoking, real or perceived
- Joan's health status and any effects that her longevity in smoking may already have had on her health status

2. Assessment of James' mother's functional status to determine specific needs that will have to be addressed or planned for.
- Assisting James to determine what type of care will be necessary to meet his mother's need and where those needs will best be met. The nurse will need to assist James to determine whether his mother can be cared for in his home or whether his mother needs long-term care in a health care agency.
- Assessing James' support systems in caring for his mother
- Supporting James in developing a plan to provide care for his mother
- Referring James to the appropriate services, such as home care agencies, social services, and financial services, that will be needed to care for his mother
- Ongoing evaluation of the care James' mother will receive and assisting James to revise their plan of care as needed

13

*O*lder Adult

Classroom Discussion

1. Discuss the demographics of the aging population and their relation to health care delivery.

2. Review myths and stereotypes associated with the older adult and the aging process.
   Have students bring in media examples of how these are perpetuated in society.

3. Discuss the biologic and psychosocial theories of aging.

4. Ask students to identify the developmental tasks and psychosocial changes specific to the older adult life stage (i.e., retirement, isolation, death).

5. Review growth and development for the older adult.
   Identify and/or ask students to identify the following:
   a. Characteristics of physical, cognitive, and psychosocial development
   b. Specific health and psychosocial concerns
   c. Risk factors, perceptions of health, and health promotion/safety activities

6. Discuss the differences between normal physiologic aging and pathologic changes.

7. Invite a gerontologic nurse practitioner to speak to the class about his or her role, educational background, and experiences with older adults.
   Invite a senior citizen to speak to the class about societal changes and health care concerns. Discuss the experience with the group, focusing on the perceptions of the individual(s) from this age group.

8. Stimulate a discussion on the societal influences that currently affect older adults, including changes in the work force, health care coverage (Medicare), housing, and access to the community and its resources.

9. Discuss the following specific nursing interventions that may be implemented for older adults, including:
   a. Therapeutic communication
   b. Touch
   c. Reality orientation
   d. Validation
   e. Reminiscence
   f. Body-image therapy

Interactive Exercises

1. Assign students to report, orally or in writing, on the support systems/resources and health care services that are available in the affiliating agency or community for the older adult.

2. Working individually or in small groups, have students design a teaching plan for a group of older adults based on a specific health need or concern.
   Have the students present the teaching plan to the class and/or to the target group within an agency or community setting.

3. Assign students to complete a brief oral and/or written report on an identified health need or psychosocial change associated with older adults.

4. Organize an "empathetic experience" for the students to simulate some of the physiologic/pathologic changes associated with aging. Use the following, or other similar ideas:
   • Place pebbles in the shoes and bind the hands and feet to simulate arthritis
   • Rub vaseline on eyeglasses to simulate cataracts
   • Limit mobility with the use of a cane, walker, or other assistive devices
   • Apply earmuffs to reduce auditory input, and put gloves on the hands to reduce tactile sensation

5. Have students observe and report on the activities and interactions of older clients in a community setting, such as a senior citizen center or housing complex, health screening, or day-care agency.

Client Care Experiences

1. Assign students to observe and/or participate in the nursing care of older adults in an acute care, extended care/nursing home, rehabilitation, or community setting.

2. Guide students in the application of the nursing process for older adult clients, incorporating cultural practices as appropriate. Working individually or in small groups, have students complete a care plan/clinical pathway specific for an older adult client and/or case-study example.

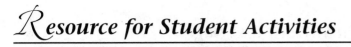

Resource for Student Activities

Specific Interventions for the Older Adult

	Interventions
Home Safety	
Nutrition	
Medication Administration	
Exercise	
Socialization	
Access to Resources	

Critical Thinking Exercises (from text page 257)

1. Mr. Brown, age 73 years, has come to the clinic for a routine check of his blood pressure. It is normal (130/80 mm Hg). He tells you that he wants to do everything he can to stay healthy. What advice can you give him on health promotion and disease prevention?

2. Mrs. Shephard's daughter has come with her to the clinic. She is concerned about her mother's memory. She tells you that although her mother's memory is usually excellent with only occasional forgetting of names or the location of keys, this has suddenly changed. Two days ago, Mrs. Shephard phoned her daughter 6 times in 2 hours asking where her husband (the late Mr. Shephard) was, and when told of his death 4 years ago, denied this fact. When her daughter arrived at her house to check on her, she found that Mrs. Shephard had emptied the contents of all the closets onto the floor and accused her daughter of theft. Mrs. Shephard has spent the last 2 nights at her daughter's house because her daughter is concerned about her safety. From Mrs. Shephard's daughter's report, you suspect delirium (acute confusional state). What questions should you ask and what areas should you assess to identify the possible causes of Mrs. Shepard's confusion?

3. You and your colleague, Jane Doe, RN, are having lunch together. She tells you that she does not know very much about assessing older adults and asks for some pointers on how to do a good, thorough assessment. What advice can you give her on the process of geriatric assessment?

Suggested Answers

1.
- Regular exercise
- Balanced diet (limiting fat and salt)
- Weight reduction if overweight
- Smoking cessation
- Immunization for influenza, pneumococcal pneumonia, and tetanus
- Monitoring of cholesterol (treatment of hyperlipidemia)
- Continued monitoring of blood pressure (even though his pressure is normal today)
- Stress reduction
- Screening for early detection of cancer

2.
- Is Mrs. Shephard taking any new medications, or have there been any changes in her usual medications? (Ask about prescription and over-the-counter medications.)
- What has been Mrs. Shephard's nutritional and fluid intake recently?
- Has she has any problems with urination suggestive of urinary tract infection?
- Has she has any shortness of breath or cough?
- Has she had any signs of other infections?
- Has Mrs. Shephard fallen recently or sustained any injuries?
- Is Mrs. Shephard in pain?

3.
- Allow extra time
- Don't rush
- Offer the older adult a rest period, or complete the assessment in several sessions

58   Chapter 13: Older Adult

- Compensate for visual impairment
- Compensate for hearing impairment
- Compensate for memory impairment by getting extra information from a family member, but only with the consent of the older adult
- Ask about strengths and resources as well as limitations

14

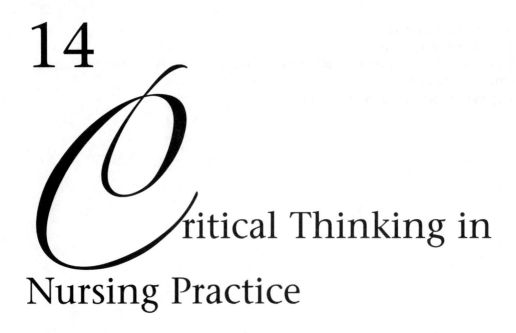

Critical Thinking in Nursing Practice

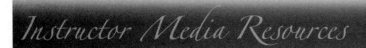

Instructor Media Resources

Instructor's Resource CD
evolve **Instructor's Resources**

Instructor's Manual
ExamView Test Bank
Image Collection
Power Point Slides
Weblinks

Student Media Resources

CD COMPANION

- Review Questions
- Glossary

evolve **WEBSITE**

- Review Questions
- Student Learning Activities
- Glossary

Classroom Discussion

1. Provide a definition for critical thinking, including the inherent skills, aspects (reflection, language, and intuition), and levels (basic, complex, commitment).

2. Discuss the components and concepts of the critical thinking model presented:
   a. Specific knowledge base
   b. Experience
   c. Competencies
   d. Attitudes
   e. Standards

   Have students give examples of actual activities that may occur with each phase.

3. Share with students personal nursing situations in which inferences were made about the client, and actions taken based on professional knowledge and experience.

4. Taking a case study or actual client situation, have students discuss how they would adapt the environment and nursing care to meet the client's specific individual needs.

5. With one or more of the following examples, have students identify what the nurse may expect to find and what questions should be answered for a client experiencing:
   a. Acute pain
   b. Incontinence
   c. Dyspnea
   d. A reddened skin area
   e. Presbycusis
   f. Hypotension
   g. Presbyopia
   h. Arthritis

6. Stimulate a discussion on what resources could be used in health care settings if an emergency situation (i.e., hurricane) existed and no running water or power was available, and supplies were dwindling.

7. Discuss how critical thinking and the nursing process "mesh" together. Guide students through the steps of the nursing process, providing examples of critical thinking throughout. Demonstrate how the use of clinical inferences and accurate diagnostic reasoning leads to successful clinical decision making.

   NOTE: The critical thinking model is used throughout the text, in coordination with the nursing process, as a basis for client care experiences. Practice in its application may help to enhance future learning and clinical problem solving.

Interactive Exercises

1. Have students complete a flow sheet that follows a common decision-making process, such as buying a car (see Resources for Student Activities).

2. Have students write about or present the concept of creativity in nursing care by using the following or a similar situation: A client with frequent memory lapses requires numerous oral medications at home and does not have the financial resources to purchase commercially available assistive devices.

3. Arrange an individual or group exercise for students to use critical thinking skills. Set up stations in classrooms or skill laboratories where the students encounter one of the following or similar client situations:
   a. The "client" (student volunteer or mannequin) is found lying on the floor beside the bed.
   b. Discrepancies are noted in the medication orders and the available supplies.
   c. An incorrect intravenous (IV) solution is hanging, running at the wrong rate, dripping, and/or infusing into an area with phlebitis or infiltration.
   d. The client states a difficulty: discomfort, difficulty breathing, dizziness.

   Have students identify, orally or in writing, what the nursing actions should be in these situations. Discuss the activity in a "debriefing" session.

Client Care Experience

1. Provide the students with an example of a multiple client assignment in an acute, long-term, or home care setting. Have students prioritize the assignment and discuss the rationale for their decisions.

2. Ask students to identify priorities and alternative methods of care for an assigned client.

Resources for Student Activities

Flow Chart
Decision-making Process

Critical Thinking Flow Chart

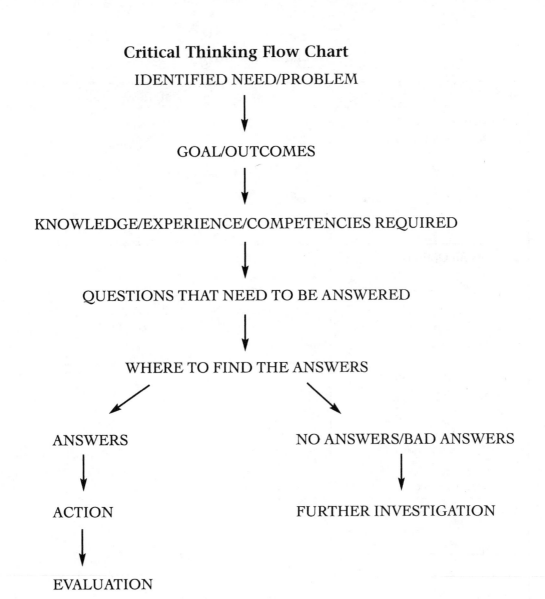

IDENTIFIED NEED/PROBLEM

GOAL/OUTCOMES

KNOWLEDGE/EXPERIENCE/COMPETENCIES REQUIRED

QUESTIONS THAT NEED TO BE ANSWERED

WHERE TO FIND THE ANSWERS

ANSWERS

ACTION

EVALUATION

NO ANSWERS/BAD ANSWERS

FURTHER INVESTIGATION

*OUTSIDE INFLUENCES: TIME, MONEY, RESOURCES, PEOPLE INVOLVED, ENVIRONMENT

Decision-making Process

Steps	Application Examples
1. Recognize and Define the Problem or Situation	
2. Assess All Options	
3. Weigh Each Option versus Criteria	
4. Test Possible Options	
5. Consider the Consequences of the Decision	
6. Make the Final Decision	

Critical Thinking Exercises (from text page 274)

1. Select a day, and write a journal entry describing any one of the following experiences that stimulated your thinking: an interaction you had with a client, an interaction you had with your spouse or one of your children, or an interaction you had with someone you were trying to help. For the entry, discuss each of the following:
   a. Describe, as thoroughly as you can, what you thought and what you did.
   b. Describe your decision-making process.
   c. Describe what you would do differently when a similar incident occurs.
   d. Describe your strengths and weaknesses in dealing with the situation. Identify your thoughts, perceptions, and feelings.

2. The following nurse's note was entered for Mrs. Simmons, a client who visited the general medicine clinic.

   Mrs. Simmons visited the general medicine clinic with a 7-day bout of blurred vision and dizziness. Client reports vision is blurred or distorted, preventing her from performing routine activities such as preparing meals, writing checks, and some mornings, performing her own hygiene and grooming. She has the most difficulty seeing close objects, although her distant vision also is blurred. Blurring is present with and without use of glasses. On examination, pupils are equal and reactive to light and accommodation. Visual fields are normal. She was unable to read newsprint in the newspaper or read the instructions on the nutrition information chart on the wall. She is active in her local church activities, but this has declined recently. Mrs. Simmons denies having a headache but also has noticed some dizziness. She is currently taking estrogen, a calcium supplement, and propranolol (Inderal).

   Evaluate the nurse's note with regard to the use of intellectual standards. What is complete and significant in the note versus superficial or trivial? What is relevant versus irrelevant? What is clear versus unclear?

3. Consider the following statements, and describe which is an example of an inference, problem solving, or clinical decision making. Support your answer with a rationale.
   a. As the nurse enters a client's room, she observes that the intravenous (IV) line is not infusing at the ordered rate. The nurse checks the flow regulator on the tubing, looks to see if the client is lying on the tubing, checks the point of connection between the tubing and the IV catheter, and then checks the condition of the site where the IV catheter enters the client's skin.
   b. The client is turning frequently in bed, holds his abdomen with his left hand, and tells the nurse, "My stomach is killing me." The nurse examines the client's abdomen, inspects the incision made during surgery 24 hours ago, and asks the client to rate the discomfort on a scale of 0 to 10. The client rates the pain a 9, compared with a 4 just 3 hours ago. The nurse concludes that the pain is related to incisional trauma and administers a prescribed analgesic. The nurse checks the client 30 minutes later and finds that the client is more relaxed and the pain is at a 5.
   c. The nurse reviews a client's medical record and finds that the client has ingested only 600 ml of fluids over the last 24-hour period. The client also has a low urinary output. The nurse conducts an assessment and finds the client to have poor skin turgor and difficulty concentrating when asked questions about his medical history. The nurse exits the client's room and tells the physician that the client is likely becoming dehydrated.

4. Mr. Spicer is a terminally ill client. His wife and son are asking you about the type of pain control he is receiving. Mrs. Spicer is asking that the physician increase her husband's medication, even if it means he will not be responsive. She does not want her husband to suffer. The son is vehemently opposed to too much narcotic, feeling that his father is still able to make decisions for himself. Mr. Spicer remains alert much of the time and is able to talk with you about his feelings regarding death. He seems to appreciate your availability in talking with him. How might you apply the critical thinking attitudes of fairness, responsibility, and creativity in this case study?

Suggested Answers

1. Exercises to be completed with students at your site. Answers will vary.

2. When the nurse considered Mrs. Simmons' problem, it was important to apply intellectual standards in her data collection so that ultimately good clinical decisions could be made. A portion of her note shows completeness and significance. This includes the description of the visual alteration, such as the duration, its effect on activities of daily living, and the extent of visual change. The data reported are significant, as they will help the nurse determine what to recommend in assisting Mrs. Simmons with daily activities. The nurse's description of the client's dizziness was incomplete and failed to describe the manner or extent to which the dizziness affected her ability to function. The note about Mrs. Simmon's church activities at this point is irrelevant until more information can be added. Has her participation at church declined because of her visual disturbance or dizziness? That is unclear. The description of Mrs. Simmons' medications also was incomplete. The nurse should have included dosages and the purpose for each medication prescribed.

3. A is an example of problem solving. The nurse collects data in an attempt to solve the problem of the reduced IV infusion rate. The nurse explores all possible factors very methodically to find the cause, which will then provide a solution.

   B is an example of clinical decision making. The nurse explores the nature and extent of the client's pain, determines the origin to be the surgical incision, and chooses an intervention (analgesic) to relieve the pain.

   C is an example of an inference. The data regarding the condition of the client's fluid balance allow the nurse to draw a conclusion that dehydration is developing.

4. As the nurse, you are responsible for determining Mr. Spicer's values and beliefs and for allowing him to make decisions about his ultimate care. Take time to talk with Mr. Spicer on a one-to-one basis at length. Listen carefully to what he has to say. Do not let your own biases influence how you think Mr. Spicer's pain should be managed. Look at Mr. Spicer's situation objectively: is he having unnecessary discomfort? Has he received his prescribed medications on time? Can his pain be better managed while still maintaining his level of alertness? The nurse can be creative by recommending a family conference. Mr. Spicer would have to agree, but the conference would bring together all parties to discuss their concerns and to hear from a nurse and physician how Mr. Spicer's pain can best be managed.

15

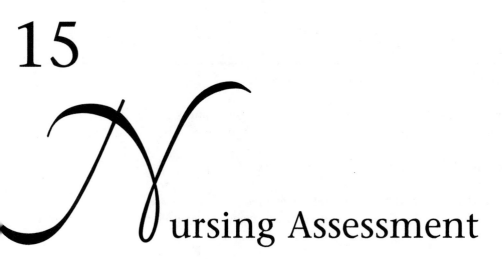

$\mathcal{N}$ursing Assessment

Instructor Media Resources

Instructor's Resource CD
evolve Instructor's Resources

Instructor's Manual
ExamView Test Bank
Image Collection
Power Point Slides
Weblinks

Student Media Resources

CD COMPANION

- Review Questions
- Glossary

evolve WEBSITE

- Review Questions
- Student Learning Activities
- Glossary

Classroom Discussion

1. Review the process and methodology of client assessment.

2. With the critical thinking approach, ask students to think about and identify what follow-up/questions are necessary when a client states that he or she has a problem (e.g., pain, difficulty sleeping).

3. Discuss the difference between subjective and objective data.

4. Review the potential sources of data for accurate assessments.
   Ask students to determine the advantages and disadvantages of the different types of data and data sources.

5. Share personal experiences and techniques with the students about data collection and assessment in the clinical area.

6. Review the components of a nursing history.

7. Discuss the client interview, phases, and techniques. Provide examples of what information may be best obtained with problem-seeking, direct, and open-ended questions. Identify possible barriers and facilitators when conducting an interview.

8. Discuss the purpose of and the findings from a physical examination.

9. By using pictures and/or videos of client situations/specific problems (i.e., decubitus ulcers, peripheral edema), ask students to make preliminary inferences and determine how the situations may be further investigated. Ask students how they would validate and interpret the data obtained.

Interactive Exercises

1. By using a student "actor" portraying a variety of possible client situations (i.e., abdominal pain, limping, emotional upset), have students quickly assess what they observe. Provide students with a listing of possible client data, and have them write or verbally identify which are objective and subjective.

2. Videotape or audiotape students conducting interviews with their peers. Individually, or in a group, critique the techniques used. Focus on areas that may have required additional clarification and/or barriers to the communication process. (Save tapes of student interviews for review as they proceed through the educational program)

3. For the following diagnostic test results (or other selected examples), have students write and/or report as to whether they are within normal limits and, if not, what the values may indicate:
WBC, 35,000/mm^3
RBC, 3.5 million/mm^3
Hematocrit, 32/100 ml
Hemoglobin, 11.5 gm/100 ml
Platelets, 70,000/mm^3
BUN, 25 mg/100 ml
Uric acid, 9 mg/100 ml
Potassium, 4.2 mEq/L
Urine specific gravity, 1.032

4. Have students work individually or in small groups to complete a written assessment on a student peer or from a case-study situation. An assessment tool specific to a nursing framework/theorist or health care facility may be used. (See Resources for Student Activities.)
Have students :
a. Identify objective and subjective data
b. Cluster the data collected

Case Study:

A 72-year-old woman has been admitted to the medical center with a diagnosis of congestive heart failure. She states that she came to this country with her son 5 years ago. She lives alone in a second-floor apartment. Her son lives about 10 miles away and visits as often as possible, but "he works very hard and has a family of his own." The client has been independent up to this point, but indicated that she becomes tired quickly after cleaning and shopping. Sometimes the client feels as if her heart is "skipping." She also has been getting up in the middle of the night to urinate. The client speaks and understands both English (somewhat limited) and Spanish (fluent in speech, reading, and writing). The physician has prescribed digoxin (Lanoxin), 125 mg qd, and furosemide (Lasix), 40 mg bid, and a 2-gram sodium diet. The client becomes slightly short of breath on exertion, experiences occasional memory lapses, and has 2+ edema of both lower extremities. Her vital signs are as follows: BP, 150/94; T, 98.4; P, 68; R, 18.

Client Care Experiences

1. With Gordon's Functional Health Patterns or another nursing framework, have students complete a focused assessment of a particular system or problem for an assigned client.

2. Assign students to do a brief interview with an actual client (with or without an assessment tool), and have them return to discuss their findings and feelings as a group. Focus on verbal and nonverbal communication patterns.

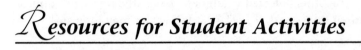

Assessment According to Gordon's Functional Health Patterns

Health Pattern	Client Status
Health Perception/ Health Management	
Nutritional/Metabolic	
Elimination	
Activity/Exercise	
Cognitive/Perceptual	
Sleep/Rest	
Self-perception/Self-concept	
Role/Relationship	
Sexuality/Reproductive	
Coping/Stress/Tolerance	
Value/Belief	

Nursing Health History

BIOGRAPHICAL INFORMATION

Name _____ Sex _____ Date _____

Address _____

Family member or significant other name _____

Address/phone number _____

Marital Status_____ Religious preference/practices _____

Occupation _____

Length of occupation _____

Health care provider _____

Insurance _____

Reason for seeking health care _____

PRESENT ILLNESS

Onset _____ Sudden or gradual _____

Duration _____

Symptoms _____

Precipitating factors _____

Relief measures _____

Expectations of health care providers _____

PAST HISTORY

Illnesses: Childhood _____

          Illnesses & hospitalizations _____

          Operations _____

          Major illnesses _____

Allergies: Type _____

          Reaction _____

          Treatment _____

Immunizations _____

Habits: Ethanol _____ Smoking _____ Drugs _____

        Duration _____

Medications: Prescribed _____

             Self-medicated _____

Sleep patterns _____

Exercise patterns _____

Nutritional patterns _____

Work patterns _____

FAMILY HISTORY

Health of parents, siblings, spouse, children _____

Risk factor analysis: cancer, heart disease, diabetes mellitus, kidney disease, hypertension, mental disorders

_____

Nursing Health History—Cont'd

ENVIRONMENTAL HISTORY

Cleanliness _____

Hazards _____

Pollutants _____

PSYCHOSOCIAL/CULTURAL HISTORY

Primary language _____

Cultural activities/social group _____

Community resources _____

Mood _____

Developmental stage _____

REVIEW OF SYSTEMS

Head: Headaches _____   Dizziness _____

Vision: Last eye exam _____

                   Glasses _____   Contacts _____ (hard, soft, long wearing)

                   Blurring _____   Double vision _____

                   Pain _____   Inflammation _____

Hearing: Impairment _____   Type of hearing aid _____

                                             Date of new batteries _____

                   Discharge/pain _____

Nose: Allergic rhinitis _____   Type of allergen _____

                                                  Relief measures _____

                   Frequency of colds/year _____

                   History of polyps, fracture, surgery _____

                   Sinuses _____

                   Nose bleeds _____

Throat & mouth: Last dental exam _____

                   Dentures _____

                   Pain/bleeding _____

                   Speech disorders _____

                   Swallowing problems _____

Respiratory: Cough _____   Sputum/hemoptysis _____

                   Dyspnea _____   Dyspnea on exertion _____

                   Pain _____

                   Activity tolerance _____

                   Last chest x-ray _____

Circulatory: Pain _____   Palpitations _____

                   Edema _____   Numbness _____   Tingling _____

                   Changes in color/hair of extremities _____

                   Syncope _____   Dizziness _____

Nursing Health History—Cont'd

Nutritional:	Appetite _____	
	Nausea _____	Vomiting _____
	Weight loss/gain _____	
Elimination:		
Bowel:	Pattern _____	Use of laxatives _____
	Constipation/diarrhea _____	
	Bleeding _____	Ostomy _____
Urine:	Pattern _____	Medications _____
	Incontinence _____	Infections _____
	Hematuria _____	Catheter _____
Reproductive:	Pregnancies _____	Children _____
	Last Pap test _____	Results _____ LMP _____
	Bleeding/discharge _____	
	Self-breast/testicular exam _____	
Neurological:	Orientation _____	Convulsions _____
	Paralysis/paresthesia ____	Weakness _____
	Incoordination _____	Headaches _____
Musculoskeletal:	Pain _____	Stiffness _____
	Deformity _____	
	Exercise patterns _____	
Integument:	Color _____	Turgor _____
	Texture _____	Temperature _____
	Rashes/lesions _____	
Vital Signs:	Temperature _____	Pulse _____
	Respirations _____	BP _____

*C*ritical Thinking Exercises (from text page 297)

1. Consider the following scenario:

   "Mr. Williams, I am your nurse, Sarah Mason. I am going to be asking some questions about your health so that we can do a good job planning your nursing care. Before we begin, do you have any questions?" (Patient has none.) "OK, let's begin by my asking you what has brought you to the hospital?" (Patient has had recurrent chest pain for 3 days.) "Is the pain sharp? Dull? Tell me what causes you to have the pain." (Pain begins with exercise.) "Is there anything else that causes you to have pain?"

   Critique this scenario by answering the following questions:
   a. During the interaction, what questions did Sara use that were open ended?
   b. Did Sarah probe to exhaustion? If so, what was the purpose?
   c. Critique Sarah's introduction.
   d. What is the advantage of open-ended questions over closed-ended questions?

2. Mrs. Lewis comes to the well-baby clinic for her infant's 1-month examination. She tells her nurse, Ethan, that the baby has not been sleeping well during the night. In addition, Mrs. Lewis has noted a rash on the baby's abdomen. Write three questions that Ethan might ask to assess the two potential problems Mrs. Lewis has presented. What assessment technique might the nurse apply to assess the rash that would not be used to assess the baby's sleep pattern?

3. Dallas Hanson is waiting to have surgery this morning for a cancerous tumor of the larynx. He tells the nurse, "I am afraid I will not be able to speak again." The nurse asks, "What has your physician explained about the possible outcomes of surgery?" Mr. Hanson states, "He thinks he can save my voice but will not know until he gets inside and sees the tumor." The nurse asks, "Are you having any discomfort right now?" "No," replies Mr. Hanson. The nurse takes a set of vital signs while preparing Mr. Hanson for transport to the operating room. The nurse also examines Mr. Hanson's intravenous (IV) site, looking for any inflammation around the insertion area. She notes that the site is clear, without inflammation or tenderness.

Describe the subjective and objective data gathered in this scenario.

Suggested Answers

1. Sarah used the open-ended questions, "What has brought you to the hospital?" and "Tell me what causes you to have pain?" Sarah probed to exhaustion when assessing the patient's perception of what causes his pain. Sarah asked, "Is there anything else that causes you to have pain?" Sarah's introduction appropriately included her name and the purpose of the interview. She did not give her status or job position. She also could have explained the estimated time it would take to conduct the interview. Open-ended questions have the advantage over close-ended questions, in that they allow clients to explain their problems or concerns in depth. Close-ended questions limit a client's response to a question.

2. Ethan might use several questions to assess the infant's health status fully. For example, "Tell me what you normally do to prepare the baby for sleep." "Tell me what you mean by not sleeping well." "What do you think might be causing the problem?"
   As for the infant's rash, Ethan might ask, "How long have you noted the rash?" "Have you changed what the baby is eating, or have you changed what you use to bathe the baby?" "When did the baby begin not to sleep well, and do you believe it was related to the rash in any way?"
   Ethan would use physical examination techniques to assess the condition of the rash.

3. Objective data included Mr. Hanson's vital signs and the appearance and condition of the IV site. Subjective data include Mr. Hanson's fear regarding the loss of speech and the absence of pain.

16

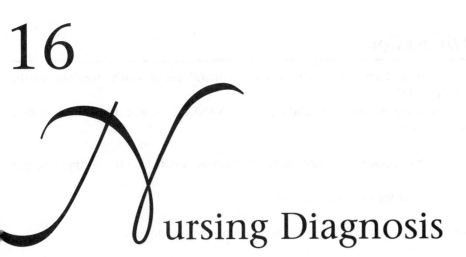

Nursing Diagnosis

Classroom Discussion

1. Discuss the evolution of nursing diagnosis and the development and role of North American Nursing Diagnosis Association (NANDA).

   Review how nursing diagnoses are developed/added to the NANDA listing and how those general diagnoses may be used with clients.

2. Present the process by which the collection, clustering, and analysis of data lead to nursing diagnosis.

3. Demonstrate the correct format for nursing diagnoses.

4. Ask students to identify the difference between medical and nursing diagnoses.

5. Identify possible sources of diagnostic error and ways in which the nurse may avoid or correct those errors.

6. Have students identify possible assessment data and related factors for sample nursing diagnoses.

Interactive Exercises

1. Provide examples of properly and improperly formulated nursing diagnoses, and have students critique and, if indicated, correct the statements.

2. Working individually or in small groups, have students formulate nursing diagnoses based on an assessment of a student peer, assigned client, and/or case-study situation (see Chapter 15). Have students record/select the nursing diagnoses on actual health care agency documentation forms.

Client Care Experience

1. For an assigned client, have students complete an assessment and identify one or more nursing diagnoses. Discuss the assessment findings and diagnoses in the postclinical conference.

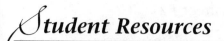
Nursing Diagnosis Worksheet #1

Assessment Data	Nursing Diagnosis	Related Factors
	Samples: Deficient Fluid Volume Imbalanced Nutrition: Less Than or More Than Body Requirements Deficient Knowledge Impaired Skin Integrity Constipation Chronic Pain	

Chapter 16: Nursing Diagnosis   77

Nursing Diagnosis Client Worksheet #2

Assessment Data	Diagnostic Label	Related Factors

Critical Thinking Exercises (from text page 315)

1. Mrs. Spezio has a pressure ulcer over the coccyx that is 5 cm in diameter and approximately 1 cm deep. The tissue surrounding the ulcer is inflamed and tender to touch. Mrs. Spezio is a transfer from a nursing home where she had resided for 6 months after a massive stroke. She is unable to move independently in bed and does not sense pressure or discomfort over her coccyx or hips. Given this clinical situation, identify the defining characteristics and related factors for the nursing diagnosis *Impaired skin integrity*.

2. Examine the following two sets of data. Identify normal standards with which to compare the data, and then make a reasoned conclusion about the client need or problem the data tend to support.

   Data Set I   *Data Set II*
   Poor oral intake   Awakens 2 to 3 times during night
   Low white blood cell (WBC) count   Takes about 1 hour to fall asleep
   Has a surgical wound   Reports becoming tired easily at work
                                        Worried about job security

3. Identify nursing diagnoses that might apply to the data sets in question 2.

4. Review the following nursing diagnoses and identify those that are stated correctly and those that are stated incorrectly:
   Anxiety related to fear of dying
   Self-care deficit: toileting related to incontinence
   Fatigue related to chronic emphysema
   Need for mouth care related to inflamed mucosa

Suggested Answers

1. The defining characteristics are the destruction of skin layers as described by pressure ulcer 2 inches in diameter and 1 cm deep. Additional defining characteristics include disruption of skin surface described as tissue inflamed and tender to touch. Two related factors exist in this client's situation: the client's physical immobilization and reduced sensation.

2. For the data set of poor oral intake, low white blood cell count, and presence of surgical wound, normal standards would include normal intake of approximately 2000 calories per day with a fluid intake of 2500 ml per day, normal WBC count of 5000 to 10,000, and absence of break in skin. A reasoned conclusion for this data set is "prone to infection."

   For the data set of awakens 2 to 3 times a night, takes an hour to fall asleep, reports feeling tired at work, and worried about job security, normal standards would include awakens once a night, falls asleep within 30 minutes or less, and reports able to do work without fatigue. A reasoned conclusion for this data set is "difficulty sleeping."

3. Answer: The diagnosis of *Risk for infection* applies to the first data set.
   The diagnosis of *Disturbed sleep pattern* applies to the second data set.

4. *Anxiety related to fear of dying* is a correctly stated diagnosis.

Self-care deficit: toileting related to incontinence is incorrect because the etiology is a clinical symptom. The diagnosis would be accurate if it were to read: *Self-care deficit: toileting related to cognitive impairment.*

Fatigue related to chronic emphysema is incorrect because the etiology is a medical diagnosis.

Need for mouth care related to inflamed mucosa is incorrect because the label is an intervention.

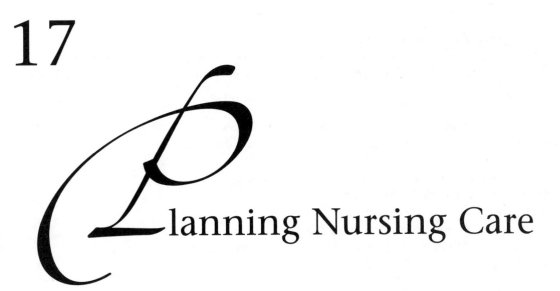

17

Planning Nursing Care

Instructor Media Resources

 Instructor's Resource CD
evolve **Instructor's Resources**

Instructor's Manual
ExamView Test Bank
Image Collection
Power Point Slides
Weblinks

Student Media Resources

CD COMPANION

- Review Questions
- Glossary

evolve **WEBSITE**

- Review Questions
- Student Learning Activities
- Glossary

Classroom Discussion

1. Discuss how planning follows from assessment and nursing diagnosis and what is incorporated in the planning stage of the process.

2. Discuss assigning priorities and its importance. Have students assign priorities to a series of client situations/nursing diagnoses according to Maslow's hierarchy of needs.

3. Present information on client-centered goals and outcomes:
   a. Involvement of client and family
   b. Focus in different health care settings
   c. Difference between long- and short-term goals
   d. Difference and relation between goals and expected outcomes
   e. Format for documenting goals and outcomes

4. Discuss what difficulties may be encountered in developing client goals/outcomes.

5. Explain and then provide examples of nurse-initiated, physician-initiated, and collaborative interventions.

6. Discuss how the Nursing Interventions Classification (NIC) is related to nursing diagnosis, and how it may be used in nursing education, practice, research, and costing.

7. Ask students to explain the purpose of the care plan. Review the different formats for documenting nursing process, including nursing care plans and critical pathways. Discuss the differences and similarities that may be found in varied health care settings.

8. Guide students, by using overheads, blackboard, or handouts, through the process of assessment, nursing diagnosis, and planning with an actual or case-study client situation. Focus on the factors involved in the selection of nursing interventions.

9. Discuss the role of consultation and the use of a consultant as part of the nursing process. Invite an actual or potential nursing consultant (i.e., ostomy nurse, pediatric nurse specialist) to speak to the class about his or her role.

Interactive Exercises

1. Provide students with properly and improperly written client goals and outcomes and have them critique and correct them, if indicated.

2. Have students identify types of interventions (nurse-initiated, physician-initiated, or collaborative) from a list that includes examples of each type.

3. Organize a debate or discussion on the advantages and disadvantages of standardized forms and care plans.

4. Assign students to attend a workshop, program, or demonstration of a computerized nursing care–plan documentation system, as available.

5. Provide students with properly and improperly written nursing interventions, and have the students critique and correct them, as indicated.

6. Have students, working individually or in small groups, identify long- and short-term client-centered goals, expected outcomes, and nursing interventions based on the nursing diagnoses that were formulated for a student peer assessment and/or case-study situation.

Client Care Experience

1. Have students identify long- and short-term client-centered goals, expected outcomes, and nursing interventions based on the nursing diagnoses that were formulated for the client assignment.

Resources for Student Activities

Critical Pathway Sample Form
Kardex Care Plan Format
Refer to Chapters 15 to 16 for additional tools

Multidisciplinary Critical Pathway

Medical Diagnosis (Code):   **Expected length of stay:**

Nursing Diagnosis/Client Need:

Expected Outcomes:

Interventions	1st Day (Date)	2nd Day (Date)	3rd Day (Date)
Nursing			
Treatments			
Medications			
Diagnostic Tests			
Diet Therapy			
Consults/Referrals			
Teaching/ Discharge Needs			

Kardex Care Plan

Nursing Diagnosis/ Client Problem	Expected Outcomes	Nursing Interventions

Critical Thinking Exercises (from text page 337)

1. Write a goal and expected outcome for each of the following clinical scenarios:
   a. Mr. Jacko has recently been diagnosed with asthma and is to be discharged tomorrow. His physician has ordered a metered-dose inhaler for Mr. Jacko to use daily. The client has not used an inhaler before. He asks the nurse, "What do I do at home if I have trouble using this thing?" The nursing diagnosis for Mr. Jacko is *Deficient knowledge regarding use of a metered-dose inhaler related to inexperience.*
   b. Ms. Snow has had a high fever for several days. She is diaphoretic and very fatigued. She has difficulty turning herself in bed because she has little energy and she is overweight. The skin over her bony prominences is intact at this time, with some redness appearing over the coccyx area. Reddened area blanches with fingertip pressure. The nursing diagnosis for Ms. Snow is *Risk for impaired skin integrity related to moisture and impaired mobility.*

2. Mrs. Drew is a 68-year-old woman with a diagnosis of congestive heart failure. Her heart does not have the strength to contract as strongly as normal and thus is unable to pump blood efficiently through the circulation. As a result, she is experiencing fatigue, shortness of breath, especially following light exertion, edema of the lower extremities, cough, and occasional palpitations. She complains of feeling weak and tired when ambulating down the hall. She tends to have more palpitations after walking only about 10 to 20 feet. Mrs. Drew lives alone, and she expresses concerns as to how she will care for herself. When asked if her neighbors can assist, she says she would rather not have to depend on them. The nurse talks with her at length and finds that Mrs. Drew has difficulty finding ways she can minimize her exertion when performing routine activities at home.

   Identify three nursing diagnoses for Mrs. Drew, and order those diagnoses by high, intermediate, or low priority.

3. Which of the following are errors in writing a nursing intervention?
   a. Suction client nasotracheally.
   b. Assigned RN will assist client with active range-of-motion (ROM) exercises at 0800, 1200, 1600, 1900.
   c. Assigned RN will instruct client in medication administration 11/10 and 11/11.

Suggested Answers

1. An appropriate goal for Mr. Jacko would be: Client will self-administer metered-dose inhaler correctly by 10/12. Appropriate outcomes would include: Client will manipulate metered-dose inhaler correctly; Client will identify frequency of inhaled doses; Client will deliver dose through inhalation.

   An appropriate goal for Ms Snow is Skin will remain intact and free of signs of pressure by 10/12. Appropriate outcomes would include: Skin will remain dry; Coccyx area will show no redness.

2. Mrs. Drew's priorities are Decreased cardiac output, Activity intolerance, and Ineffective coping, in that order of priority.

3. Answer b is a correctly stated intervention, including the person to perform the action, the precise action, and time. Answers a and c are incorrect. Answer a does not include the person to perform action or time. Answer c does not include specifics about type of medication or aspects of the administration process to be taught.

18

*I*mplementing Nursing Care

Classroom Discussion

1. Discuss what is included in the implementation phase of the nursing process.

2. Review protocols and standing orders. Discuss the differences between the two and how they may be implemented in acute, long-term, and outpatient/home care settings.

3. Discuss the role of reassessment in the nursing process and the revision of the care plan/pathway, including the:
   a. Introduction of new data
   b. Alteration/addition/deletion of nursing diagnoses
   c. Adaptation/alteration of nursing interventions
   d. Selection of evaluation methods

4. Share situations in which assessment of the situation indicated the need for assistance from another nurse or ancillary personnel. Ask students if they can think of other instances in which assistance may be required.

5. Discuss what should be done when the nurse is not familiar with treatments, medications, or other agency policies and procedures.

6. Ask students to think about the knowledge and skills that are necessary for the implementation of nursing care.

7. Discuss delegation from a nursing perspective. Ask students to share how they feel about delegating certain activities to other paraprofessionals (i.e., medication administration, catheterization).

8. In the following situations (or other examples), have students identify what information is required before carrying out the intervention:
   a. Clients with medication orders for laxatives, antihypertensives, diuretics
   b. An older client who has had a stroke and is scheduled to ambulate

9. Discuss the differences and relations between cognitive, interpersonal, and psychomotor nursing skills.

Interactive Exercises

1. Have students identify, orally or in writing, specific nursing interventions required in the following areas:
   a. Assistance in performance of activities of daily living (ADLs)
   b. Counseling
   c. Teaching
   d. Physical care techniques
   e. Controlling adverse reactions
   f. Preventive measures

2. Have students work in small groups to determine what adaptations may be made in nursing care for clients (of different ages) with:
   a. Visual or hearing impairments
   b. Strong cultural ties: rituals and practices
   c. Language barriers
   d. Altered perceptions: memory lapses, loss of contact with reality

3. Assign students to research and report on an article from a nursing journal that supports a specific nursing intervention.

4. Have students, working individually or in small groups, adapt/revise the plan of care for the student peer, assigned client, and/or case-study situation. Provide possible changes in status that would require the revision.
   For the case study in Chapter 15, revise the plan of care based on the following information:
   a. Increasing edema in the client's lower extremities
   b. Loss of appetite and desire for personally prepared foods
   c. Increased dyspnea on exertion
   d. Son's recent unemployment and loss of income

Client Care Experiences

1. Assign students to observe or participate in communicating nursing activities at a change-of-shift report, conference, or staff meeting.

2. Have students adapt or revise the plan of care for an assigned client. Discuss the changes in status that required the revision in the clinical postcare conference. Focus on the use of the critical thinking model in client interactions.

Resources for Student Activities

Student Care Plan Format
Refer to Chapters 15 to 17 for additional tools

Student Care Plan

Supporting Data	Nursing Diagnosis	Goals/ Outcomes	Nursing Intervention	Scientific Rational	Evaluation Measures

Critical Thinking Exercises (from text page 352)

1. Sue is a junior nursing student. She is to care for Mr. Nelson, a 56-year-old client who underwent a total knee replacement yesterday. Sue was able to talk with Mr. Nelson briefly after surgery and reviewed his complete medical record. In preparing for clinical today (postoperative day 1), Sue has identified acute pain and impaired physical immobility as his primary nursing diagnoses. Sue has developed a plan of care with interventions to relieve pain and promote mobility; including use of patient-controlled analgesia (PCA), safe positioning techniques, use of guided imagery, and support of the use of ROM exercises on a continuous passive motion (CPM) machine. As Sue prepares to implement her plan of care, what should she specifically do initially? What complications might she anticipate and prevent?

2. Brad is assigned to care for Ms. Reznick, who has been diagnosed to have Crohn's disease, an inflammatory condition of the bowel. Ms. Reznick has had considerable abdominal pain, accompanied by cramping and frequent diarrheal stools. Her nursing history shows that she has lost 15 pounds over the last 2-month period. Her appetite has been poor. One of the many nursing diagnoses for Ms. Reznick is *Imbalanced nutrition: less than body requirements related to decreased nutrient intake and increased nutrient loss through diarrhea.* What factors should Brad consider in selecting interventions for Ms. Reznick?

3. You are assigned to ambulate Mr. Clay, who had abdominal surgery 24 hours ago. Mr. Clay weighs 270 pounds and is 6 feet tall. He has a PCA system for pain control. His intravenous (IV) fluids are running at 100 ml/hr, and he has two IV antibiotics scheduled to run every 6 hours. What questions do you need to answer before you attempt to ambulate this client?

Suggested Answers

1. Sue must first reassess the client. In Mr. Nelson's case, Sue should reassess his pain and determine whether the ordered PCA is providing relief or if a new form of analgesia is being given. She should further assess Mr. Nelson's receptivity to guided imagery. Sue's assessment also should include measurement of Mr. Nelson's ROM in his affected knee and determine whether today's medical orders have implications for planned nursing therapies. Sue will use this information to determine if revision to her plan of care is necessary.

   Mr. Nelson is young and likely mobile. Nonetheless, depending on pain control and success of surgery, he may be prone to restricting movement. Immobilization, even in the short term, can affect joint ROM, elimination, pulmonary ventilation, and skin circulation. Sue must anticipate and consider ways to prevent complications (e.g., turning and positioning frequently, encouraging deep breathing exercises, and promoting a diet of fluids and fiber, if allowed).

2. First, Brad should consider the expected outcome for Ms. Reznick's nutritional problem. Likely the outcome will be to improve Ms Reznick's nutritional intake; thus Brad will consider ways to improve the client's appetite and introduce ways to increase intake of nutrients. Brad should focus on the defining characteristics of the nursing diagnosis; are their options to control the diarrhea and increase intake? Perhaps the physician has already ordered medication for the diarrhea; if not, Brad might consult with the physician. Brad also should refer to the nursing literature. Most clients with severe Crohn's disease will receive total parenteral nutrition (TPN). Brad should review this therapy and know the nursing implications. In addition, he should determine whether the literature suggests useful ways to improve the client's appetite. In reviewing ways to intervene, Brad should consider

whether any chosen interventions are feasible. What are the dietitians planning for this client? Is the client allowed to eat orally, and if so, might some foods aggravate the inflammation of the bowel rather than improve intake? Brad should review with the client any planned interventions to be sure they are acceptable to Ms. Reznick. Finally, any interventions must be those that Brad is competent to perform. Administration of TPN may require IV skills that Brad has not yet applied.

3. The nurse should consider what resources (e.g., equipment or personnel) are available to assist the client with ambulation. Because of the client's weight and the fact that the client is having pain, the nurse will likely need another colleague to assist Mr. Clay safely out of bed and to ambulate. The nurse should consider when the antibiotics are due to be infused so that ambulation can be planned after the infusion. This eliminates additional tubing and IV bags to be carried as the client walks down the hall. The nurse also should consider the PCA pump and IV system and how they operate. Usually the client can ambulate with both in place.

19

$\mathcal{E}$valuation

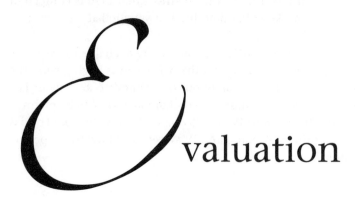

Classroom Discussion

1. Discuss the Nursing Outcomes Classification (NOC) project.

2. Review the relation between client goals, expected outcomes, and evaluative measures.

3. Present the steps of the evaluation process. Discuss observations that must be made and questions that must be asked and answered to determine attainment of goals.

4. Discuss examples of specific evaluation measures in relation to expected outcomes. Relate the discussion to continuity of care, discharge planning, and documentation. Provide examples of how evaluative measures may vary in different health care settings.

5. Discuss the process and aspects of evaluation in respect to client focus and health care delivery.

6. Ask students to identify the process that occurs when client goals are met neither partially nor completely.

7. Review the process/components of Quality Improvement (QI) in health care settings. Relate QI to the evaluation component of the nursing process rationale for the selection of evaluation measures, criteria, and standards.

8. Stimulate a discussion on how the nursing process is realistically used in a managed care environment with earlier discharges.

9. Have students determine possible evaluative measures for the following client goals:
   a. Client will maintain a low-fat diet.
   b. Client will self-inject insulin.
   c. Client will have a diminished amount of pain (less than 3 on 1 to 10 scale).
   d. Client will remain free of infection at surgical incision site.
   e. Client will evidence decreased anxiety and greater attention span.

Interactive Exercises

1. Have students, working individually or in small groups, document client responses and evaluate attainment of goals for a student peer and/or case-study situation care plan. For simulated situations, have students decide the client outcomes and whether goals were met. Ask students to identify how the plan of care may be revised to assist the client to attain goals.

2. From the following situation, have students identify assessment versus evaluation measures/data:
   The nurse is preparing to document on a client who had abdominal surgery this morning. Vital signs were within acceptable limits. The surgical incision was intact, with no drainage noted. Coughing and deep breathing were done according to schedule.
   The client experienced a moderate degree of pain at the incision site, which was relieved after administering the prescribed analgesic. Family members have expressed an interest in learning client care activities.

Client Care Experiences

1. Have students document client responses and evaluate attainment of goals for an assigned client. Ask students whether the client outcomes and goals were met. Ask students to identify how the plan of care may be revised to assist the client to attain goals.

2. For an assigned client, have students develop and submit an entire plan of care for at least one nursing diagnosis.

Resources for Student Activities

Agency Care Plan Sample Format
Steps in the Evaluation Process
Refer to Chapters 15 to 18 for additional tools.

Agency Care Plan Sample

Client Name:

Date/Initials	Nursing Diagnosis	Short-term Goals/Outcomes	Resolved/Revised (Date/Initials)	Nursing Actions/Orders

Discharge Planning:

Steps in the Evaluation Process

Steps	Examples
Identify Evaluative Criteria and Standards	
Collect Data to Determine Whether Criteria or Standards Are Met	
Interpret and Summarize Findings	
Document Findings and Any Clinical Judgment	
Terminate, Continue, or Revise Care Plan	

Critical Thinking Exercises (from text page 367)

1. Mr. Vicar has been visiting the clinic for more than a month. He visits weekly for follow-up care for a chronic venous stasis ulcer of the left leg. The nurse's note at the time of his first visit contained the following information: "Ulcer with irregular margins, 4 cm wide by 5 cm long, approximately 0.5 cm deep, with foul-smelling purulent yellowish drainage. Only subcutaneous tissue visible. Skin around ulcer, brownish rust in color. Zinc oxide and calamine gauze applied to ulcer; elastic wrap bandage applied to gauze. Client instructed to return in 1 week." As the nurse who is caring for the client on the follow-up visit, what expected outcomes would you anticipate for the goal of "Wound will demonstrate healing within 4 weeks"? What evaluative measures would you use to determine whether the wound was healing?

2. The nursing staff on the general medicine unit are discussing a number of issues during their monthly staff meeting. Two additional RNs have been hired to work the night shift. Staff nurses have not been conducting routine reviews of clients' discharge plans. The nurse manager has announced that discharge-planning conferences will be held at 1:30 PM each weekday. A new safety syringe is being introduced and will require staff to attend in-service training sessions. Over the last 3-month period, a 10% incidence rate for pressure ulcers was observed. That is an increase when compared with the last 6 months. The wound-care nurse specialist will be consulting on the floor.
   a. Of all the nursing unit issues, which one would you identify as a professional outcome?
   b. Which one would you identify as a client outcome?

3. Mr. Becker is a 78-year-old man who has been diagnosed with terminal lung cancer. He reports a loss of appetite and a 6-pound weight loss over the last 1-month period (152 pounds to 146 pounds). He is able to chew and swallow food without difficulty. Mr. Becker denies feeling nauseated but states, "I just have no interest in food." His wife reports that he eats only a portion of what is served, "He gets full so quickly." Mrs. Becker also reports that her husband is less active around the house, sleeps poorly, and is unable to talk about his diagnosis. The nurse develops a nursing diagnosis of *Imbalanced nutrition, less than body requirements, related to a decline in food intake.*
   a. What would be an appropriate goal for Mr. Becker's plan of care?
   b. Identify expected outcomes to use in measuring success of the care plan.
   c. What evaluative measures would the nurse use to determine Mr. Becker's progress?

4. Mr. Becker returns to the physician's office 2 weeks later. Mrs. Becker has been serving smaller and more frequent meals as recommended by the nurse. She has also worked hard to select a menu that is appealing to Mr. Becker. He continues to deny feeling nauseated. Mrs. Becker reports, "Some days he seems to eat better, but other days he just won't eat much. I think the smaller portions help." Mr. Becker's weight is now 145 pounds. His food diary shows that in some meals, he has eaten most of his food, but in other meals, intake is minimal. He tells the nurse, "I know I should try to eat more, but what is the use?"
   a. How would you interpret Mr. Becker's progress?
   b. How would you revise the plan of care?

Suggested Answers

1. Anticipated outcomes would include: size of ulcer will decrease, drainage will clear, drainage will be free of odor, skin around ulcer will clear without inflammation.

   Evaluative measures would include: measurement of the size of wound by using a centimeter ruler, measurement of the depth of the wound by using a sterile cotton-tipped applicator, observation of appearance of wound and surrounding skin, detection of odor from drainage.

2. The failure of nurses to review clients' discharge plans is a professional outcome. The increased incidence of pressure ulcers is a client outcome.

3. An appropriate goal for Mr. Becker's plan of care would be "Client will maintain or increase weight in next 2 weeks." With a diagnosis of terminal cancer, weight maintenance is likely more realistic than is weight gain.

   Appropriate expected outcomes would include: Client will maintain weight of 146 pounds over next 2 weeks, client will eat 75% of meals, and client will report improvement in appetite.

   The nurse would use evaluative measures such as: weighing the client, asking the client to describe appetite, having wife maintain a food diary to record actual food intake.

4.
   a. His weight loss has slowed, but it continues. The smaller meals may have helped improve intake.
   b. Continue the interventions aimed at food intake; however, consider further assessment of Mr. Becker's emotional status. Is depression or grief over his diagnosis altering his interest in eating? Interventions aimed at his psychological comfort may prove beneficial in improving his intake. The nursing diagnosis might be revised to *Imbalanced nutrition, less than body requirements due to grief response to illness.*

20

$\mathcal{M}$anaging Client Care

Classroom Discussion

1. Discuss the competencies of an entry-level nurse.

2. Discuss the nursing care–delivery models:
   a. Functional nursing
   b. Team nursing
   c. Total patient care
   d. Primary nursing
   e. Case management.

   Ask students to identify where and in what situations each of the models may be best used. Have students identify the advantages and disadvantages associated with each model.

3. Discuss the current leadership and management roles in nursing. Ask students to identify the leadership opportunities available to student nurses and the skills necessary to assume leadership roles.

4. Invite a nurse executive or manager to speak to the class about his or her role, educational preparation, and experience.

5. Review team communication and the Five Rights (requirements) of Delegation.

6. Discuss the process/components of Quality Improvement (QI) in health care settings, including the different approaches that may be taken with the process.

7. Invite a nurse, preferably the QI nurse director, to speak to the class about his or her role in relation to the health care–delivery process in the agency.

8. Review actual QI projects from an affiliating agency, if possible, and discuss possible rationale for the selection of evaluation measures, criteria, and standards.

9. Review centralized, decentralized, and matrix management structures. Have students identify the advantages and disadvantages of each type of structure.

10. Discuss the key elements in the decision-making process:
    a. Responsibility
    b. Autonomy
    c. Authority
    d. Accountability
    e. Staff involvement

Interactive Exercises

1. Have students, working individually or in small groups, provide information on the number and qualifications of staff and the types of clients, and have students develop a staffing pattern and client assignment for an acute care or long-term care unit, or home care agency. Have them incorporate aspects of time management and prioritization.

2. Assign students to attend a QI meeting in a health care agency, or attend a workshop on the subject, and complete an oral or written report on their experience.

3. Assign a small group of students to develop a QI project specific to one area of client care or nursing education. Have students use the models for QI as a guide (i.e., Focus PDCA).

Client Care Experiences

1. Assign students in the clinical area to observe/work with the coordinator, team leader, or regional supervisor and document the leadership characteristics that are demonstrated Have them share their observations and experiences in a postclinical discussion.

2. Discuss the aspects of care provided by the students that may be delegated to a nursing assistant.

Critical Thinking Exercises (from text page 386)

1. John, an RN, is working with Tammy, a nursing assistant, to manage care for five clients. John has completed morning assessments and rounds on the assigned clients and is giving Tammy directions for what she should do in the next hour. John says to Tammy, "Why don't you go to room 415 and see what Mr. Thomas needs and go to room 418 to check whether Mrs. Landry is doing all right." Based on what you know about delegation, were these appropriate or inappropriate directions for the nursing assistant? Provide a rationale for your answer.

2. The unit in which you are working has identified a problem: clients are receiving initial doses of newly ordered medications 6 to 8 hours after the order is written. Your manager asks you to be the head of a QI team to investigate this problem. Who would you want to be on your team? What would your first priority be? What data would you want to collect related to this problem?

3. You have just received morning shift report on your clients. You have been assigned the following clients:
   - A 52-year-old man who was admitted yesterday with a diagnosis of angina. He is scheduled for a cardiac stress test at 9:00 AM.
   - A 60-year-old woman who was transferred out of intensive care at 6:30 AM today. She had uncomplicated coronary bypass surgery yesterday.
   - A 45-year-old man who experienced a myocardial infarction 3 days ago and is complaining of pain rated as 5 on a scale of 0 to 10.
   - A 76-year-old woman who had a permanent pacemaker inserted yesterday and is complaining of incision pain rated as a 7 on a scale of 0 to 10.
   Which one these clients do you need to see first? Explain your answer.

Suggested Answers

1. The directions given by John to Tammy were inappropriate. John did not communicate clear directions to Tammy regarding what specifically should be done for the two clients. John violated the principle that tasks are delegated, not clients. He also did not apply what he learned from his assessments during his rounds. John did not provide clear directions to Tammy about what tasks to perform. When delegating, the RN should see the client first and determine what tasks need to be delegated. Next John needed to consider if it was appropriate to delegate these tasks. John must also

consider whether Tammy is qualified to perform the tasks delegated. It is important in delegation to assess the knowledge and skills of the person you are delegating to. After completing these steps, John should then provide Tammy with a clear set of directions as to what tasks she needs to complete for each client.

2. It would be important to include on the QI team persons who are involved in the process. The team should be made up of an RN from the unit, a physician, a pharmacist, and a unit secretary from the unit. The first priority is to identify the steps in the process from the initial written order to the delivery of the medication to the client. The process needs to be analyzed for improvement. Data to collect should include the number of steps in the process; the number of people involved in the process; types of medications typically ordered; the time it takes for each step to occur; length of time for each step related to type of medication ordered; how is the delivery of medication to the unit made; and how is the RN notified of the arrival of the medication on the unit.

3. As the RN, you need to see the 45-year-old client who experienced a myocardial infarction 3 days ago who is currently complaining of 5/10 chest pain. Chest pain in a myocardial infarction is an indication of a serious physiological problem that is an immediate threat to the client's survival and safety and therefore is a first-order priority. The client with the pacemaker insertion who is complaining of incision pain is demonstrating a second-order priority in asking for pain-relief measures. The client who is scheduled for the cardiac stress test has third-order priority needs related to teaching for the scheduled cardiac test. The client who had bypass surgery and is stable has fourth-order priority needs that are actual or potential problems that she will need help with in the future. Currently, she is not showing any higher priority needs.

21

$\mathcal{E}$thics and Values

Classroom Discussion

1. Discuss the definition of ethics.

2. Discuss ethical terms and provide examples of each within a nursing context.

3. Discuss the Codes of Ethics as they relate to nursing practice and accountability.

4. Have students identify what the role of the ethics committee is in ethical decision making and how the nurse may be involved in the process.

5. Discuss the definition of values and value systems from a nurse and a client perspective.

6. Discuss individual perceptions regarding values and how they are learned and changed.

7. Review the formation of values, including the advantages and disadvantages of different modes of value transmission, and sociocultural influences.

8. Ask students to discuss how the nurse incorporates values into his or her personal and professional practice.

9. Stimulate a discussion on client advocacy and the promotion of individual values.

10. Discuss the values-clarification process, incorporating the concept of being nonjudgmental, with no right or wrong answers.

11. Provide students with the following, or other actual or simulated situations in which values clarification may be implemented. Ask them for their responses and how their own values may coincide or conflict with those of the client.
    a. A client who elects not to continue with possible life-saving therapy
    b. A client who elects to have an abortion, or who chooses to give the child up for adoption
    c. An adult who places his or her parent in a nursing home

12. Ask the students to share their thoughts about the relation between values and ethics.

13. Review the concept of caring in respect to values and ethics in nursing practice.

14. Review and provide examples for the philosophical constructions of deontology, utilitarianism/teleology, feminist ethics, and the ethics of care.

15. Discuss ethical principles.

16. Ask students to speak about how financial resources may have an impact on ethical decision making. Have them identify areas that they believe are most at issue in various health care settings and/or specialties.

17. Discuss the legal and ethical implications associated with informed consent and advance directives.

18. Use an actual or simulated client experience as a stimulus for a discussion on ethics in practice. Guide students in the application of the methodology for ethical decision making to an actual or simulated client situation.

19. Ask students to verbalize about how ethics/ethical principles are interwoven in the nursing research process.

20. Review contemporary issues in bioethics.

Interactive Exercises

1. Have students complete a Cultural Values Exercise (Chapter 21, Box 21-6) or select their own 10 values and assign priorities to the list.

2. Organize a debate on one of the following issues (or a similar topic):
   a. Withholding care from a client with religious beliefs that forbid the treatment versus overriding his or her wishes through a court order
   b. Placing only clients who can afford transplants on a waiting list versus placing all clients in need on the list
   c. A Do Not Resuscitate (DNR) order versus a "slow code" versus a full code
   d. A nurse who refuses to care for certain clients [i.e., acquired immunodeficiency syndrome (AIDS), abortions] versus the agency's needs and the client's right to health care

4. Provide students with actual or simulated client situations and ask them to identify, orally or in writing, where ethical principles are applied appropriately (e.g., providing client dignity during procedures) or not applied (e.g., calling a client "sweetie").

5. Assign students to attend an ethics committee meeting, if possible, to observe the functions and procedures, or invite a representative to speak to the class about the role of the committee.

6. Have students bring in examples from the media of actual or possible ethical dilemmas for health care providers.

Client Care Experiences

1. Have students identify possible ethical concerns for assigned clients in pre- or postclinical conferences. Ask students to determine what resources are available within the agency or community to assist in working through an ethical dilemma.

2. Have students determine the client's values and identify how they compare with their own value systems.

Resources for Student Activity

Cultural Values Exercise (Box 21-6, p. 395 of the text)
Ethical Decision Making Worksheet

Ethical Decision-Making Worksheet

Is this an ethical dilemma?

Relevant information:

Examination of own values:

Identification of the problem:

Courses of action:

Negotiation of the outcome:

Evaluation of the action:

104   Chapter 21: Ethics and Values

C ritical Thinking Exercises (from text page 402)

1. Complete the "cultural values" exercise (see Box 21-6 of the text, p. 395) with your classmates or with members of another class of professionals. Compare the answers and discuss the differences.

2. You are caring for a 17-year-old client who has been admitted for treatment of sickle cell crisis. She needs fluid management and comfort management. Even though she is receiving narcotics around the clock, she continues to complain of pain. She also complains about her roommate, the food, and the intravenous line. She comes from a community far from the hospital, and her mother cannot visit every day. She has an older brother who has been convicted of possession of illegal drugs. Discuss your approach to this client. Rank her needs. What is your priority action, based on what you know so far? Examine and describe your opinions about pain, pain management, and addiction.

3. You are a clinic nurse in a small community clinic. A 45-year-old male client has been coming to the clinic for several years for treatment and support of his acquired immunodeficiency syndrome (AIDS). During recent months, he has lost his long-term companion to AIDS. In addition, both his parents died many years ago. His clinical condition has deteriorated. His vision is failing, his nutritional status is difficult to maintain, and he has been hospitalized 3 times in the past 3 months for pneumonia. He asks for your help in planning his suicide. Discuss your response to his request. Begin by an examination of your personal feelings about suicide. Include a discussion about your understanding of AIDS: Where does it come from? Who gets the disease? Why? What are your feelings and opinions about people with AIDS? Construct your response, keeping in mind the ethical principles of fidelity, autonomy, beneficence, and nonmaleficence. Because all of these principles collide in this example, it will be important to identify each and to recognize personal responses to the role that each plays in this narrative. Just as important is the role that nurses imagines they play for the client, especially as they differ from the nurse's own. For the sake of this discussion, it is illegal in your state for nurses to prescribe medicines. What are your possible courses of action?

4. You have been assigned the care of a 98-year-old woman who was recently admitted from home with a diagnosis of pneumonia. She has a history of cardiac disease and takes a number of medications. She had been fairly active until the past few days, when her cough worsened and a fever developed. You note that her pulse has become weak and thready and that her respirations are increasingly labored. The client is now too weak to respond to you. When you mention to the family that you may need to call the physician and even "call a code," the son and the daughter become distraught, saying that they do not want their mother to be kept alive on "machines." They report that they have discussed this situation with their mother. You find that documentation of these wishes is not in the chart. The family members have not discussed this situation with their doctor. What actions would you consider taking at this moment? Take into account the ethical principles of autonomy and beneficence. What are your personal values about interventions at the end of life?

Suggested Answers

1. For the cultural values exercise contained in Box 21-7, there are no wrong answers. The goal of the exercise would be the stimulation of discussion. Comparison of answers might reveal many common grounds, or it might reveal interesting differences. Either way, the students should gain insight into the valid differences that exist regarding values in our society.

2. This question continues to probe the issue of values. Students would probably gain most by answering this question privately and truly expressing personal thoughts about the ranking of this patient's needs in addition to opinions about addiction. Then sharing answers during a guided discussion with classmates might help to illustrate strategies for dealing with principles of autonomy, beneficence, maleficence, and advocacy.

3. As the question explains, the principles of fidelity, autonomy, beneficence, and nonmaleficence all collide in this narrative. Following the steps for processing an ethical dilemma, students should be able to practice values clarification while also coming to some conclusion about the ethical course of action in this situation. The use of ethics committees, pain management at the end of life, and personal concerns about AIDS should all become part of a group discussion about answers for this question.

4. In this not uncommon scenario, the nursing student should be able to practice use of the ethical process suggested in the text to come to a conclusion about realistic actions. This question is focused more on the use of one-to-one conversations and family care conferences than it is on an ethics committee as a solution, because the situation is fairly urgent. Discussion for this question would benefit from an examination of the difficult issue of death, dying, and personal expectations about dealing with this process as a nurse.

22

$\mathcal{L}$egal Implications in Nursing Practice

Classroom Discussion

1. Discuss the various sources of law that influence nurses and nursing practice.

2. Discuss standards of care and their application to nursing practice.

3. Review the Board of Nursing's role in regulating nursing practice, licensure, and disciplinary measures. Have students review the Nurse Practice Act and report on its content and focus.

4. Review licensed nurse versus student nurse liability. Ask students to identify possible situations in which the student nurse may be held liable.

5. Discuss intentional torts that may be committed by nurses.

6. Explain the criteria for professional negligence/malpractice. Ask students to respond to situations, giving their rationale as to whether the nurse may be held liable for malpractice.

7. Review the legal implications of nursing documentation.

8. Discuss nursing malpractice insurance and some of the conditions included in sample policies.

9. Review some of the case studies in the text (i.e., Darlene *v* Charleston Community Memorial Hospital), and ask students to provide their opinions on how each situation might have been avoided.

10. Invite a nurse who has appeared as an expert witness to speak to the class about court procedures and actual cases.

11. Review confidentiality and informed consent in respect to legal and ethical guidelines.

12. Discuss the responsibilities of the nurse in relation to informed and implied consent for the following or similar situations:
    a. An unconscious client
    b. Parents refusing treatment for a child
    c. A sedated client
    d. A 16-year-old parent
    e. An adult client involved in a research study
    f. An older client being prepared for surgery

13. Discuss the concept of shared liability of the nurse and physician, as well as the nurse's legal relationship with other members of the health care team. Ask students to provide examples of situations in which shared liability may occur.

14. Have students respond as to the action to be taken by the nurse during short staffing or when they are "floated" to another unit/client assignment.

15. Stimulate discussions as to the legal implications for nurses that may be associated with the following areas:
    a. Organ donation
    b. Abortion
    c. Acquired immunodeficiency syndrome (AIDS)/communicable disease
    d. Living wills/advance directives
    e. Assisted suicide

16. Discuss legal guidelines that may be specific to different health care agencies (i.e., Occupational Safety and Health Administration; OSHA regulations).

17. Invite a risk manager and/or nurse attorney to speak to the class about his or her role, educational preparation, and experience, and the concepts of nursing accountability, liability, and malpractice.

Interactive Exercises

1. Have the students role play examples of torts in client situations.

2. Provide students with examples of documentation, and have students critique and correct them according to legal guidelines.

3. Have students participate in role playing a courtroom experience in which a nurse must face malpractice charges. Assign students to the various roles, including judge, jury, prosecutor, defendant, etc. Provide the students with the background information from an actual or simulated experience. Have students develop the questions to be asked and the documents (possibly both good and bad examples) to be presented as evidence.

4. Assign students to attend a Board of Nursing meeting/hearing (if possible) or a legislative session to observe the procedures involved in establishing regulations, statutes, and legislation.

Resources for Student Activities

Worksheet on Torts
Chart on the Criteria for Professional Negligence/Malpractice

Worksheet on Torts

Tort	Definition	Nursing Example
Assault		
Battery		
Defamation		
Invasion of Privacy		
Professional Negligence/ Malpractice		

Criteria for Professional Negligence/Malpractice

Criteria	Explanation	Examples
1. The nurse (defendant) owed a duty to the client (plaintiff)		
2. The nurse did not carry out that duty		
3. The client was injured		
4. The cause of the client's injury was a result of the nurse's failure to carry out that duty		

Chapter 22: Legal Implications in Nursing Practice   111

Critical Thinking Exercises (from text page 420)

1. Nurse Smith and Nurse Jones are getting on an elevator to go down to the cafeteria. Several visitors are present in the elevator, as well as hospital personnel. Nurse Smith and Nurse Jones are talking about a client who is in the intensive care unit who has just tested positive for human immunodeficiency virus (HIV). They identify the client as the man in Room 14B. One of the visitors on the elevator who overhears this information is a woman who is engaged to the client in Room 14B.
   a. Have Nurse Smith and Nurse Jones breached a client's right to confidential health care?
   b. Will the client in Room 14B have any legal cause of action against the nurses?
   c. Even though the client's fiancée may have a right to know the HIV status of her future husband, does any duty exist on the part of the nurses to disclose confidential information to the fiancée?

2. While transporting a client down the hall on a stretcher, Nurse Black stops to chat with an orderly. The side rails on the stretcher are down, and while Nurse Black has her back to the stretcher, the client rolls over, falls off the stretcher, and fractures his hip. In a lawsuit by the client against Nurse Black, what must the client establish to prove negligence against the nurse?

3. Sally Green, a 16-year-old girl, is the mother of a newborn baby. While driving in her car, without having her newborn baby in an appropriate infant car seat, Sally Green has a car accident. Her newborn baby has a head injury. Physicians tell Sally Green that her baby has incurred severe brain damage and that she cannot be maintained without life support. They request her consent to have the baby's organs donated for transplant.
   a. Because Sally Green is a minor, is she able to give consent?
   b. Does the hospital have any duty to report Sally Green to the Division of Family Services for failure to have her child in a protective seat?
   c. If Baby Green should have a cardiac arrest, can the nurses and doctors perform cardiopulmonary resuscitation (CPR) on the baby without consent?

Suggested Answers

1. A. Yes, they have committed a breach of confidentiality.
   B. Yes, the same, plus invasion of privacy action
   C. No

2. The client must prove that Nurse Black had a duty to keep him safe from falling off the stretcher, that is, that the standard of care is to prevent falls.
   The client must prove that Nurse Black breached or failed in her duty.
   The client must prove that Nurse Black's breach of duty, her failing to prevent his fall, was the proximate cause, the most closely related cause of his injury, which is his fractured hip.
   The client must prove damages resulting from his injury.

3. A. Yes
   B. Yes
   C. Yes

23

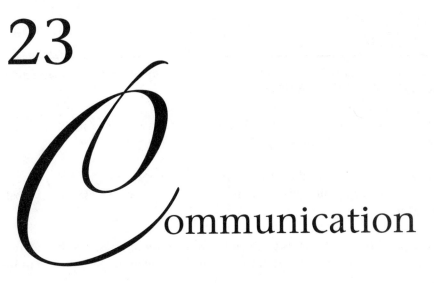

*C*ommunication

Instructor Media Resources

Instructor's Resource CD
evolve **Instructor's Resources**

Instructor's Manual
ExamView Test Bank
Image Collection
Power Point Slides
Weblinks

Student Media Resources

CD COMPANION

- Review Questions
- Glossary

evolve **WEBSITE**

- Review Questions
- Student Learning Activities
- Glossary

Classroom Discussion

1. Discuss the different levels of communication: intrapersonal, interpersonal, transpersonal, small group, and public. Provide examples of each level.

2. Explain the elements of the communication process: referent, sender, message, channels, receiver, feedback, interpersonal variables, and environment.

3. Discuss the aspects inherent in verbal, nonverbal, and symbolic communication, and meta-communication. Demonstrate situations in which the nurse may obtain assessment data from verbal and nonverbal communication.

4. Discuss the concept of perceptual bias as it relates to the process of communication. Ask students to share personal experiences in which they have been the sender or recipient of perceptual bias in an interaction.

5. Identify the factors that may influence communication. Ask students to identify how the use of space or distance between communicators (intimate, personal, social, or public) may be different depending on the type of nurse/client interaction.

6. Review the elements of professional communication and how the nurse communicates with other members of the health care team.

7. Discuss the techniques involved in therapeutic communication. Provide the students with examples of possible client statements/questions and ask the students to give appropriate responses.

8. Discuss the dimensions of a helping relationship, giving examples of the nurse's role in establishing an effective rapport.

9. Provide examples of how the communication process is integrated within the nursing process. Ask students to give examples of situations in which the opportunity for communication is available.

10. Invite a psychiatric nurse clinician and/or an interpreter to discuss specific elements of communication.

Interactive Exercises

1. Have students observe a live or videotaped role-playing situation to identify barriers to communication and methods that could have been used to facilitate communication.

2. Have students, working individually or in small groups, determine how communication is influenced by the following: language, sensory abilities, neurologic impairment, medication, mental status, and age/developmental level.

3. Assign students to investigate available resources within an affiliating agency for enhancement of communication (i.e., interpreters, speech therapy).

4. Ask students to identify how communication may be adapted for the following clients:
   a. 5-year-old child
   b. Hearing-impaired older adult
   c. Primarily Spanish-speaking adult
   d. Aphasic client (after a cerebrovascular accident [CVA])
   e. Extremely anxious adolescent

5. Have students follow through on a plan of care for a client with a nursing diagnosis related to ineffectual or impaired communication.

4. Videotape or audiotape students completing a basic health history with a peer. Review the tape individually or as a class, and ask students to critique the interaction and provide suggestions to enhance communication.

5. Have students demonstrate their response in dealing with a client who is:
   a. Angry
   b. Disoriented
   c. Unresponsive
   d. Silent/withdrawn
   e. Sexually inappropriate

Client Care Experiences

1. Assign students in the clinical setting to complete a basic health/admission history on clients of different ages and cultural backgrounds. Have the students self-evaluate the experience in relation to therapeutic verbal and nonverbal communication techniques.

2. Have students report on their client's status to their peers and other members of the health care team.

Resources for Student Activities

Facilitators of Communication
Barriers to Communication

Facilitators of Communication

Techniques	Examples/Nursing Behaviors
Active Listening	
Sharing Observations	
Sharing Empathy	
Sharing Hope	
Sharing Humor	
Sharing Feelings	
Using Touch	
Using Silence	
Asking Relevant Questions	
Providing Information	
Paraphrasing	
Clarifying	
Focusing	
Summarizing	
Self-disclosing	
Confronting	

Barriers to Communication

<u>Ineffective Techniques</u>	<u>Examples</u>
Asking Personal Questions	
Giving Personal Opinions	
Changing the Subject	
Automatic Responses	
Offering False Reassurance	
Sympathy	
Asking for Explanations	
Approval or Disapproval	
Defensive Responses	
Passive or Aggressive Responses	
Arguing	

Critical Thinking Exercises (from text page 445)

1. Mrs. Maria Ramirez, an American of Puerto Rican descent, is faced with the difficult decision of whether to continue chemotherapy in the face of a rapidly spreading malignancy. What communication techniques could the nurse use to help her at this point, and what traps must the nurse avoid in such a situation?

2. Jan, a nurse colleague, is having difficulty standing up to a physician who has an abrupt, intimidating communication style. She often ends up with a lot of unspoken anger, developing tension headaches, and easily becoming tearful. What could the nurse do to help?

3. Mr. Hess, a client with Parkinson's disease living at an extended care facility, has a stiff, expressionless face. He sits slumped in a recliner chair all day and seems lost in his own world, rarely looking at or interacting with anyone. When he does talk, he mumbles in a soft voice, and his words are difficult to understand. What kinds of things could the nurse do to establish a helping/healing relationship with Mr. Hess?

4. Jennifer Hughes, a new graduate, is very discouraged. In school, she had felt a great deal of anxiety about her own performance, and even now she finds it difficult to be positive about herself or her job. What knowledge about communication could she use to help improve her situation?

5. Mrs. Esther Larson, a client who has been recently admitted to a hospice program, confides in the nurse that she feels overwhelmed with the number of things she must attend to now that she's facing the possibility of death. She says, "My thoughts are all over the place. I don't know where to start." What communication techniques, based on the critical thinking model, could the nurse use to help her at this point?

Suggested Answers

1. The nurse could use several basic therapeutic communication techniques that will help Mrs. Ramirez feel safe and accepted and identify and understand her own values. These might include giving general openings ("Tell me about..."), paraphrasing and clarifying, acknowledging feelings with empathy statements, using caring touch, and using presence and silence. Helping her anticipate the consequences of her decision options would be useful. It is important for the nurse to avoid the trap of sympathy rather than empathy, so that he or she is not overwhelmed by Mrs. Ramirez's plight. The nurse should avoid trying to influence Mrs. Ramirez to make the decision that is close to the nurse's own values or beliefs and avoid giving personal opinions, approval, or disapproval. The nurse should stress that Mrs. Ramirez has the right to make her own decision but should be aware that in her culture, the husband is often a primary decision maker and needs to be included in discussions.

2. The nurse could help his or her colleague in several ways. First, provide a safe, private place away from client and family earshot for Jan to talk, reassure her of her confidentiality, listen empathetically, and encourage her to express her feelings. Offer to help her try out some assertive communication techniques through role play, and try to provide support by being present the next time the physician interacts with her. Adopt an optimistic stance and voice faith and hope that Jan will learn to cope well with future situations. Suggest some relaxation techniques to help her release muscle tension after such an encounter, and try a dose of humor.

3. The nurse can start building trust by getting to know Mr. Hess as an individual, including whether he is uncomfortable being called by his first name. Family members could be asked to provide information about his likes, dislikes, and personal history. The nurse could take opportunities to visit Mr. Hess for a few minutes just to say hello, comment on what is going on in his environment, and share social conversation. Touch could be used to communicate that he is accepted, and the nurse should realize that he or she cannot rely on Mr. Hess's facial expressions to make sure messages are understood. It is important to minimize environmental distractions, focus concentration when he talks, and patiently ask him to repeat words if they are not understood.

4. Jennifer could use intrapersonal communication techniques to build her self-confidence. She needs to identify her negative thoughts and replace them with positive assertions. She needs to find positive, caring colleagues who will support her through this period of role adjustment. She also could use transpersonal communication to find additional sources of strength and hope. Practicing positive intentionality and centering herself so that her worries about herself do not intrude also will help her feel more comfortable and competent.

5. **Specific Knowledge Base**, acquired through nursing education. Knowledge of therapeutic communication techniques. **Focusing** would help the client to identify key issues. For example: Nurse: "Do you have any unfinished business?"
    Client: "I must tell my daughter how very proud of her I am."
    Nurse: That sounds like a good idea. How do you want to go about telling her that?"
    Experience in nursing: nurse uses various therapeutic communication techniques to see what works best.
    Attitudes: nurse's response should convey attitudes of confidence, responsibility, curiosity, and integrity when communicating with client.
    Standards: nurse's response should display intellectual standards of being clear, precise, specific, logical, and precise when responding to client.

24

Client Education

Classroom Discussion

1. Discuss the standards and purposes established for client education. Review the distinction between teaching and learning.

2. Discuss teaching/learning with respect to the communication process.

3. Identify the aspects associated with the domains of learning. Provide and/or ask students to give examples of the type of information that may be conveyed with each domain.

4. Discuss the basic principles of learning, including the concepts of motivation, ability to learn, and learning environment.

5. Stimulate a discussion on how the learning environment may be adapted to facilitate the teaching/learning process.

6. Discuss the development of and demonstrate the format for learning objectives.

7. Review the basic principles and methods of teaching, and provide examples of their implementation in client situations.

8. Discuss available teaching tools.

9. By using the following example, or another simulated or actual situation, have students determine how they would approach and organize materials for a client with hypertension who needed information on medications, diet, activity, and recognition of complications.

10. Discuss the areas that are usually included in a teaching plan: topic(s), resources, recommendations for involving others, objectives, and strategies.

11. Ask students to consider which approaches they feel the most and least comfortable with in providing client education.

12. Discuss the use of reinforcement with individuals of varying ages.

13. Explain how teaching/learning principles and strategies are integrated into the nursing process. Ask students to identify nursing diagnoses associated with teaching/learning (i.e., *Knowledge deficit*), related objectives, and strategies. Have students give examples of where the opportunity for teaching may arise during daily client care activities.

14. Compare and contrast individual and group teaching/learning approaches.

15. Provide examples of agency documentation of client education.

16. Invite a nurse educator (i.e., diabetes educator, ostomy nurse) from an agency to speak to the class about client education.

17. In accordance with the teaching/learning approach used, explain how the methods of evaluation are determined by the nurse.

Interactive Exercises

1. Have students identify orally, or in writing, the factors that may influence the client's ability to learn.

2. Have students investigate and report on the resources available within an affiliating agency for client education (i.e., preoperative instruction, diabetes educator).

3. Provide examples of teaching plans and learning objectives for students to critique and correct according to the criteria.

4. Assign students a simple physical task that they will teach to another student or group of students. Have them identify the steps involved in demonstrating the procedure.

5. With the following, or other actual or simulated situations, have students develop a possible teaching plan that specifies the learning need/topic, available resources, objectives, and teaching strategies (see Resources for Student Activities):
   a. A new mother going home with her first child
   b. A group of teenagers who sunbathe frequently
   c. School-aged children who ride bicycles in a heavy traffic area
   d. Adult women and men in a community group who are unaware of breast and testicular self-examination techniques
   e. Older adults who inquired about diet and exercise
   f. An adolescent who is newly diagnosed with diabetes mellitus

Client Care Experience

1. Have students identify the learning needs of their assigned clients, and prepare and present a teaching plan based on the assessment of these needs.

Resources for Student Activities

Learning Domains and Teaching Strategies Worksheet
Teaching Plan Form

Learning Domains and Teaching Strategies Worksheet

Client Situation	Learning Domain	Teaching Strategies
Diagnostic Testing Tomorrow and Never Had the Test Before		
Self-injection of Medication Required		
Noncompliance with Treatment Regimen Demonstrated		
Need for Physical Hygiene Information Demonstrated		
Label Reading of Foods and/or Over-the-counter Medications Required		

Chapter 24: Client Education   123

Teaching Plan

Learning Need/Topic	Available Resources	Significant Others	Learning Objectives	Teaching Strategies

Critical Thinking Exercises (from text page 474)

1. Mrs. S. has a 10-year history of hypertension and a 5-year history of diabetes. Recently her hypertension has become uncontrolled, and she has been diagnosed with depression. Her medications, which have recently been changed, include captopril (Capoten), 25 mg 3 times a day; diltiazem (Cardizem CD), 240 mg every morning; metformin (Glucophage XR), 1500 mg before the evening meal; and sertraline (Zoloft), 100 mg by mouth at bedtime. The nurse identifies the priority nursing diagnosis as deficient knowledge related to change in medications. The nurse wants to develop a plan of care that uses the three domains of learning. What are the client's teaching priorities? Which learning needs would require a cognitive method? Which needs would be more appropriate to satisfy through affective or psychomotor methods?

2. The nurse is caring for a client who is being discharged after an appendectomy. He is taking medication for the treatment of attention deficit and hyperactivity disorder (ADHD). Which teaching strategies should the nurse use when providing discharge information to this client?

3. A 23-year-old man has recently sustained a spinal cord injury after being involved in a diving accident that has left him paralyzed from the waist down. He is verbally abusive to the staff and expresses anger toward his family and friends when they come to visit. He needs to begin learning transfer techniques. Which stage of grieving is this client experiencing? What approach should the nurse take in planning education for this client?

4. A 65-year-old woman is taking her 72-year-old husband home after a hip pinning. Which interventions should the nurse use in helping this couple make the transition to home smoothly?

Suggested Answers

1. The client's main teaching priorities include understanding the newly diagnosed medications and being able to take them accurately and correctly. Cognitive teaching interventions would include verbally teaching the client about her medications. Medication teaching sheets, if available, should be given. The nurse should provide some real-life experiences for the client to help improve decision making. For example, the nurse might ask the client what she would do if she forgot to take her morning medicine. Effective teaching interventions, such as discussion and role-play, should focus on allowing the client to verbalize her feelings about this change in her health status. If possible, she might benefit from a support group. Finally, the nurse should allow the client to prepare her own medications under supervision. This will give the client the ability to have feedback and will improve feelings of self-efficacy as she becomes more adept at setting up her medications. The client also should be included in deciding what times she should take her medications to enhance compliance with the medication regimen.

2. To ensure effective comprehension of discharge instructions, the nurse should present the information in a highly structured format. Goals and outcomes must be clearly stated, and brief, focused teaching sessions should be planned. Teaching should occur in an environment with minimal distractions. If the client has difficulty organizing information, providing a folder with only the essential reading material should be helpful. During teaching sessions, the nurse should assess the client's ability to pay attention and stay focused on the information presented. The nurse should have the client frequently verbalize understanding of what has been taught.

3. This client is in the stage of anger. At this moment, the nurse should not argue with the client. Allowing the client to verbalize feelings and anger and listening to the client's concerns are very important nursing interventions at this time. The client's family and friends need be assured that this is a normal stage experienced by people who are grieving. Helping the client work through the anger and introducing only information that the client must have at the moment may help the client begin to resolve these feelings.

4. Elderly clients learn best when they are rested, so it is important to plan teaching sessions around the clients' schedules. Both the husband and the wife should be active participants during teaching. A successful teaching plan would also ensure that the clients are involved in setting goals for education and would allow the clients to learn at their own pace. Building on existing knowledge and reducing environmental distractions also are helpful. Finally, written information that is given to the clients should be in large fonts and should be printed with contrasting colors.

25

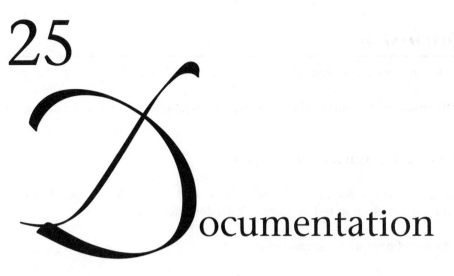

Documentation

Instructor's Resource CD
Instructor's Resources

Instructor's Manual
ExamView Test Bank
Image Collection
Power Point Slides
Weblinks

Student Media Resources

CD COMPANION

- Review Questions
- Glossary

evolve WEBSITE

- Review Questions
- Student Learning Activities
- Glossary

Classroom Discussion

1. Review and discuss different methods of communicating/reporting the client's status.

2. Ask students to identify what may be included in a client's record and how it varies, depending on the health care agency.

3. Discuss the purpose of documentation and record keeping.

4. Have students determine the role of accrediting agencies (i.e., Joint Commission on Accreditation of Healthcare Organizations; JCAHO) in setting standards for documentation.

5. Review general criteria/guidelines for documentation/recording.

6. Provide examples of nursing and multidisciplinary documentation.

7. Discuss the legal implications associated with client documentation, including federal regulations (Health Insurance Portability and Accountability Act; HIPAA) and confidentiality of records. Use video resources, if available, to highlight this concept.

8. Stimulate a debate on the concepts of "charting by exception" versus "care not documented is care not done."

9. Provide examples of client records/forms from a variety of different health care agencies for students to review.

10. Discuss the following methods of recording, including similarities and differences and advantages and disadvantages of each:
Problem-oriented medical records, source records, charting by exception, and focus charting.

11. Review the use of a multidisciplinary critical pathway in a case-management approach.

12. Ask students to identify the specific documentation needs in acute care, home care, and long-term care agencies.

13. Discuss the positive and negative aspects of the computer-based client care record and computerized nursing documentation. Compare and contrast the use of computerized documentation with that of traditional formats.

14. Review the information that should be included in the various types of nursing reports.

15. Ask students to identify what situations may warrant the completion of an incident report.

16. Discuss the nursing responsibilities associated with a verbal or telephone order.

17. Invite a Quality Assurance nurse and/or attorney to discuss the legal implications of nursing documentation.

Interactive Exercises

1. Have students critique and correct sample documentation entries according to the guidelines.

2. Assign students to observe or participate in the use of a computerized documentation system, or have students attend a workshop on available systems.

3. Provide an example of an incident report form, and have students practice completing the necessary documentation for a simulated occurrence.

4. Working individually or in small groups, have students write their responses to the following and/or similar situations that may be encountered in the documentation of client care:
   a. Another nurse asks you to chart for him or her.
   b. Mistakes are made when writing notes on the record.
   c. Coffee is spilled over a whole page of the record.
   d. Students from different schools are caring for the client.

5. By using the following simulation, have students document in problem-oriented medical record (POMR; SOAP/SOAPIE), PIE, and/or Focus (DAR) formats:
   A client, newly diagnosed with diabetes mellitus, was just admitted to the acute care agency. The client was anxious about learning the technique for self-injection of insulin. The nurse discussed with and demonstrated the procedure to the client and his wife. Self-injection technique improved after the first three attempts. A dietary referral was made for the client, as he expressed minimal knowledge about necessary restrictions.

Client Care Experiences

1. Assign students to observe and/or participate in an end-of-shift report or client conference at an affiliating agency.

2. In actual client care situations, have students maintain an index card with accurate times of nursing assessments and interventions. Use the cards to facilitate documentation and to stimulate postcare discussions of daily experiences.

3. Have students complete written or computerized documentation for their assigned clients according to expected guidelines. Critique their documentation before actual entry, and provide recommendations for improvement, as indicated.

Resources for Student Activities

Problem-oriented Documentation Form (SOAPIE)
Focus Documentation Form (DAR)

Problem-oriented Documentation Form

Subjective	
Objective	
Assessment (Nursing Diagnosis)	
Plan	
Interventions	
Evaluation	

Focus Charting Form

Data	

Actions	

Response	

C*ritical Thinking Exercises* (from text page 498)

1. Joseph Page is an 80-year-old man admitted with a diagnosis of possible pneumonia. He complains of general malaise and a frequent productive cough, worse at night. Vital signs are as follows: blood pressure, 150/90 mm Hg; pulse rate, 92 beats per minute; respirations, 22 breaths per minute; and temperature, 38.5° C (101.3° F). During your initial assessment, he coughs violently for 40 to 45 seconds without expectorating. His lungs have wheezes and rhonchi in both bases and are otherwise clear. He states, "It hurts in my chest when I cough." Differentiate between objective and subjective data in this case example.

2. The nurse positions Mr. Page in a semi-Fowler's position, encourages increased fluid intake, and gives acetaminophen (Tylenol), 650 mg PO as ordered for fever. One hour later, the client is resting in bed. Vital signs are as follows: blood pressure, 130/86 mm Hg; pulse rate, 86 beats per minute; respirations, 22 breaths per minute; and temperature, 37.7° C (99.8° F). He states that he has been unable to sleep. His fluid intake has been 200 ml of water. Use the given information to write a nurse's progress note in the PIE format.

3. At the end of your shift, you have identified *Deficient fluid volume* as a nursing diagnosis for Mr. Page. Since his admission, he has had fluid intake of about 600 ml, and his urine output was 300 ml of dark concentrated urine. His temperature is back up to 38.3° C (101° F), his mucous membranes are dry, and he states that he feels very weak. Record significant data. List what should be included in the change-of-shift report.

4. Several days later, after treatment with intravenous antibiotics, Mr. Page is feeling much better, and preparations are being made for discharge. He is to take cephalexin (Keflex), 500 mg every 6 hours for the next 10 days, continue to drink extra fluids, and get extra rest. He lives alone. Although he is generally cooperative, he does not like drinking water or taking pills. He is to make an appointment with his physician for 1 week from today and should call the physician if symptoms of recurrence develop. Write a discharge summary that is concise and instructive.

Suggested Answers

1. Subjective: complains of general malaise and frequent productive cough, worse at night. "It hurts in my chest when I cough."

   Objective: vital signs, coughs violently for 40 to 45 seconds with expectorating, wheezes and rhonchi both bases. BP, 140/90; pulse, 110; respirations, 32 per minute; temp, 101.6° (F) orally.

2. P: It hurts in my chest when I cough. Unable to sleep. Vital signs: BP, 150/90; pulse, 92; resp, 22; and temp, 38.5° C.
   I: Tylenol, 650 mg PO as ordered for fever. Positioned in semi-Fowler's position. Lying and resting in bed. Encouraged increased fluid intake.
   E: Vital signs: BP, 130/86; pulse, 86; respirations, 22; temperature, 37.7° C. Fluid intake, 200 ml in 1 hour.

3. Report should include: Nursing diagnosis of *Fluid volume deficit*. Fluid intake since admission was about 600 ml, and his urine output was 300 ml of dark concentrated urine. His temperature is back up to 38.4° C (101° F), his mucous membranes are dry, and he states that he feels very weak.

4. Discharge Summary: Mr. Page is to take cephalexin (Keflex), 500 mg every 6 hours for 10 days, drink five to six 8-oz glasses of fluid per day, and make a follow-up appointment for 1 week from today. He will need encouragement to drink, as he tends not to drink fluids easily. His compliance with medication therapy must be monitored because, although cooperative, he does not like to take pills and may tend to omit them because he is feeling better. He is aware of the need to call the physician if a painful cough, fever, difficulty breathing, or malaise develops.

26

*S*elf-concept

Instructor Media Resources

Instructor's Resource CD
Instructor's Resources

Instructor's Manual
ExamView Test Bank
Image Collection
Power Point Slides
Weblinks

Student Media Resources

CD COMPANION

- Review Questions
- Glossary

WEBSITE

- Review Questions
- Student Learning Activities
- Glossary

Classroom Discussion

1. Ask students what self-concept is, what it means to them, and how it may be associated with nursing care.

2. Discuss the development of self-concept within the life span.

3. Discuss the components of self-concept (identity, body image, self-esteem, and role performance) and how each may be positively or negatively influenced. By using a case study example, identify how the components of self-concept are manifested and how they may be affected.

4. Review the role of stressors in relation to self-concept and how the nurse may determine the presence of stressors. Bring multicultural considerations into the discussion.

5. Review how self-concept is developed and changed throughout the life span. Use a theorist (e.g., Erikson, Piaget, Freud) as a reference framework.

6. Discuss the assessment of a client's self-concept.

7. Ask students to provide specific examples of how the nurse may be a positive or negative influence on a client's self-concept and how a supportive environment may be established to promote self-exploration, self-awareness, and self-evaluation.

8. Guide students in the application of the nursing process for an actual or simulated client who is experiencing an altered self-concept.

Interactive Exercises

1. Assign students to investigate and report on resources that are available in the school, community, or affiliating agency to support/promote self-concept.
   Have students attend a meeting of a self-help group in the community and share with the class how the group supports individual self-concept.

2. Have students, working individually, or in small groups, identify nursing diagnoses, client goals and outcomes, nursing interventions, and evaluation criteria for the following client experiencing stress and an altered self-concept:
   Maria is 40 years old, has been married for 15 years, and is the mother of an 8-year-old boy. Maria provides the sole financial support for the family, as her husband has been unemployed for 2 years, with no immediate job prospects. She is currently concerned about the status of her company and the possibility of losing her income and medical coverage. Maria has returned to school to acquire additional knowledge and skills in the event that she loses her position. Although she enjoys the classes, the work is time consuming and tiring, especially with the long hours she puts in at work. Maria also feels guilty about not being as involved as she would like to be in her son's activities. She is currently experiencing severe headaches and gastric distress and has a tendency to cry easily.

Client Care Experiences

1. Have students assess their client's self-concept and report their findings in postclinical conference. Discuss possible interventions to promote or maintain their clients' self-concept.

2. Have students incorporate interventions to promote and support self-concept, as indicated, into the client's plan of care.

Resource for Student Activity

Stressors Affecting Self-concept

Self-concept Components	Examples of Stressors	Health Promotion Activities
Identity		
Body Image		
Self-esteem		
Role Performance		

Critical Thinking Exercises (from text page 520)

1. You are assigned to care for a 23-year-old Asian-American client who was in a motor vehicle accident and sustained multiple fractures to his face and a fractured femur (which was fixated through surgery on the evening of admission 4 days ago). He grew up in the United States; he and his mother came to the United States when he was a young child. He works as a janitor for a local university. He lives with his girlfriend and their 7-month-old daughter. You have been with him for most of the morning and found that he is in moderate pain, which has been treated with morphine. The morphine has decreased his pain rating from a 6 to a 3 on a scale of 0 to 10 but has left him somewhat drowsy. During the morning, he has shared with you some of his concerns about when he will be able to return to work. You are in the room when the surgeon tells him about his upcoming surgery. A temporary tracheotomy is planned because of the extensive surgery needed in the nasal and throat area. After the surgeon leaves, the client tells you that he does not want the tracheotomy. He indicates that he is unclear about what it actually entails, even though the surgeon explained it in fairly simple terms. He says to you, "I just want to get back to my normal self." How would you address his comment regarding "get back to normal" and his lack of understanding regarding the tracheotomy?

2. A 16-year-old girl is preparing for discharge from the hospital after giving birth 2 days earlier. She is unmarried, not involved with the baby's father, and has minimal familial support to care for the child. Before admission, she arranged to terminate rights and give the baby up for adoption. She reaffirms this as a good decision because she will be able to return to school immediately and graduate, as scheduled, in 2 years. The client confides in you that her biggest concerns right now are how she feels about herself and how she looks. Taking into account developmental needs of this adolescent, how will you collaborate with her to establish priority interventions to address her self-concept deficits?

3. As a part of your community health experience, you are assigned to visit a 75-year-old woman who has gone to her daughter's home after being hospitalized for agitation and aggression secondary to Alzheimer's disease. When you go to the home, you find the 55-year-old daughter tearful. She says, "I just don't know if I can do this. She doesn't like anything I cook. She calls me two or three times during the night to sit with her; sometimes she doesn't even recognize me. I've been missing a lot of work, and even when I'm there, I'm not as productive as I was before she came to stay with us." What additional assessment data would be important to gather? What provisional nursing diagnosis could be made for the daughter?

Suggested Answers

1. Assess client's specific concerns regarding tracheotomy; note verbal and nonverbal communication. Allow opportunities for client to discuss anxiety and fear; nurse may need to initiate conversation regarding overt changes in body image with opportunities to explore other alterations in self-concept (i.e., temporary loss of role as financial provider; concerns regarding the impact physical change in appearance may have on intimate relationship with girlfriend). Keep in mind that the client is experiencing a significant amount of pain, which may affect current perceptions; further be cognizant of impact of pain medication on ability to make decisions and to benefit from nursing interventions such as teaching. Specifically be astute to informed consent issues as the client prepares for another surgery. Statement regarding "getting back to normal" could reflect denial of the severity of the current condition. An empathic approach by the nurse will facilitate further opportunities to assess the

magnitude of the client's concerns; a need exists to present matter-of-fact data regarding current condition, including the need for a temporary tracheotomy, to both the client and his family.

2. The nurse needs to clarify her own values before interacting with this client and may benefit from reviewing developmental needs of a 16-year-old. Specifically, the nurse must be careful to not superimpose her perception of what is needed (i.e., dealing with the loss of this child), as the client has verbalized a different priority issue. The client is focused on other losses (loss of ideal body image and loss of normalcy regarding school). Further, because of her lack of support systems, she may be most focused only on basic needs consistent with the developmental tasks of adolescence. The client has verbalized her perceived need of addressing body-image concerns, which must be respected by the nurse to facilitate trust. The adolescent needs to be actively involved in establishing goals to address body-image concerns; follow-up care must be secured. Identifying community resources is essential.

3. A priority nursing diagnosis for the daughter is *Caregiver role strain*. In addition to the verbalizations of uncertainty regarding her effectiveness in the role as her mother's caregiver, she has expressed the negative impact it is having on her other roles, including her employment role. Further assessment regarding other roles (wife, mother, friend) is needed. Additional data are needed regarding the daughter's mood (including suicidality or homicidality) and her own self-care needs (including eating and sleeping patterns). An appraisal of her coping strategies and her support network is essential. The daughter's knowledge of community resources must be assessed, with appropriate referrals by the nurse. Further, ongoing assessment regarding everyone's safety is needed because of the mother's aggression and agitation; the nurse may have to guide the daughter in making decisions regarding alternative placement.

27

*S*exuality

Classroom Discussion

1. Discuss concepts of sexuality. Ask students to share their perceptions of sexuality and its relation to nursing care.

2. Discuss the dimensions of sexuality in relation to the past and current society.

3. With examples from today's media and societal culture, discuss the concept of sexual identity.

4. Discuss sexual development throughout the life span and strategies for health promotion that may be implemented with parents, children, and clients at each stage (see Resource for Student Activity).

5. Ask students to share their perceptions and/or those perceptions common in society about different sexual orientations. Provide examples of variations in client sexual orientation that the nurse may encounter.

6. Have students review, identify, and describe male and female sexual anatomy and physiology and sexual response.

7. Discuss issues related to sexuality, the role of the nurse, and the resources and referrals that are available to the nurse and client.

8. Have students identify how illness may affect sexuality and sexual functioning.
   Use the following or similar examples:
   a. A 56-year-old man after a myocardial infarction
   b. A 16-year-old female client receiving chemotherapy
   c. A 38-year-old woman after a mastectomy
   d. A 25-year-old paraplegic man
   e. An 85-year-old woman in a nursing home

9. Discuss how the nurse may recognize sexuality issues in the health care environment. Provide or ask students to give examples of possible situations that may occur with clients in the acute or long-term care environment. Ask how they should respond to each situation.

10. Guide students in the application of the nursing process for a simulated situation in which a client is experiencing an alteration in sexuality.

11. Provide specific examples of and interventions for male and female psychological and physiological sexual dysfunction.

12. Provide basic information on bacterial and viral sexually transmitted diseases (STDs), including methods of transmission and complications.

13. Review methods of contraception and the advantages and disadvantages of each.

14. Discuss how physical, relationship, lifestyle, and self-esteem factors may influence an individual's sexual behavior.

15. Invite a nurse therapist/counselor who deals with sexuality to speak to the class about the role of the nurse.

Interactive Exercises

1. In a small group, ask students to share their feelings about sexuality and the role of the nurse.

2. For discussion, have students bring examples from the media of sexual issues that may influence nursing and health care.

3. Organize a debate on a controversial issue relating to sexuality and the role of the nurse, such as a nurse's participation in versus refusal to participate in abortion procedures.

4. Assign students to visit available community agencies (i.e., Planned Parenthood, a fertility or woman's health clinic), and report to the class on the services offered to clients.

5. Organize a role-playing situation in which the student is the nurse who must complete a sexual health history and/or physical assessment.

6. Have students, working individually or in small groups, identify nursing diagnoses, client goals and outcomes, nursing interventions, and evaluation criteria for an actual and/or simulated client who is experiencing alterations in sexual health.

Client Care Experiences

1. Have students identify possible sexual health needs for assigned clients. Discuss interventions that may be incorporated into the plan of care to meet these needs.

2. Have students document identified sexual health needs in the client's record and/or student care plan.

Resource for Student Activity

Health Promotion for Sexuality Chart

Health Promotion for Sexuality Across the Life Span

Life Stage	Sexual Development	Health Promotion Strategies
Infant		
Toddler/Preschooler		
School-aged		
Adolescent		
Adult		
Older Adult		

Critical Thinking Exercises (from text page 541)

1. Your current clinical experience is in a community health care setting. You are conducting the initial interview with a 48-year-old man who started taking antihypertensives 2 weeks ago. You take his blood pressure and find it to be 136/74 mm Hg. You ask him how he has been doing since his last visit. He looks down at the floor and says, "Oh, OK, I guess. Seems like I'm just getting old now." What kind of follow-up would be indicated based on this information?

2. You are assigned to care for a 15-year-old girl who was admitted after a motor vehicle accident. Yesterday she had an internal fixation of a fractured ankle. In gathering her nursing history, you explore sexuality and learn that she has just recently become sexually active with her boyfriend of 3 months. When you ask about safe sex and the use of birth control, she tells you that she knows she does not have to worry about STDs with him because he is just not one of those kinds of boys. In regard to birth control, she says that her boyfriend has reassured her that because he is pulling out before ejaculation, there is no risk of her becoming pregnant. How would you proceed, given these assessment data?

3. You are working on a rehabilitation unit and caring for a 67-year-old man who had a stroke 3 weeks ago. He shares a room with another man who is recovering from a stroke. He has been progressing in his self-care skills and is now able to get around with a cane, feed himself, and do most of his bath. His wife is in fairly good health, and the plan is for him to return home within the next 1 to 2 weeks. As you work with him one morning, he says to you, "You know, one of the things that is hardest about being here is not being able to sleep in the same bed as Greta. I miss her so much. Even though she visits every day, it is just not the same." How would you explore his comment, and what planning would you consider?

Suggested Answers

1. The client's verbal response and nonverbal behavior (looking down at the floor) suggest that he may have concerns. You might want to make an opportunity for him to discuss any concerns. Possible openings could be "You sound kind of discouraged" or "Sometimes when people begin antihypertensive medications they notice various side effects. Have you noticed anything different since you began the medicine?"

2. Two issues are evident here. One issue is her assumption that she is not at risk for STDs, and the second is her misconception about pregnancy risk. Because she has shared this information with you, she likely trusts you enough to continue with some discussion regarding sexuality. No one way exists to approach this situation. Several approaches may be successful. One approach would be to inquire about her knowledge of STDs. When you have a sense of her background, you could either provide information to clarify or fill in missing information regarding her possible risk for STDs. Another valuable intervention would be to inquire about sexual history, safe sex, and/or contraception with her partner. Often adolescents are uncomfortable discussing sexually related issues with a partner. Providing her with an opportunity to role play how she might ask these questions could be very helpful to her. Finding the words to say it and the concern about how the conversation might flow are often the most difficult aspects of bringing up a sexually related topic with a partner. Once the topics are openly discussed, you can provide information and referral, as appropriate.

3. First, you would want to gather information to determine what aspects of sleeping with his wife he misses. You might say something like "What part of sleeping with her do you miss most?" or something that acknowledges more clearly a possible sexual concern such as "Many couples are sexually active after one partner has had a stroke. Is sexuality part of your concern?" The tactic that you use will likely depend on several factors: your own comfort with discussing sexuality; the amount of assessment data that you have gathered thus far; trust and comfort level; and observations that you have made about the couple's relationship (i.e., presence of touching and closeness). If privacy for physical intimacy (whether it is touching or more intimate sexuality) is part of what he misses, you will want to explore the possibilities for privacy within the facility. In a rehabilitation situation, privacy for sexual expression is likely an issue for clients. The facility may have made arrangements for private space. If a private space is unavailable, exploring how to make his room available while providing an acceptable space for the roommate may be a viable option.

28

*S*piritual Health

Classroom Discussion

1. Discuss the concepts of spirituality, faith, religion, and hope.

2. Ask students to share their own meaning of spirituality and how it may be incorporated into nursing practice and a holistic approach to health.

3. Ask students to determine how critical thinking may be used to meet the client's spiritual needs.

4. Review the development of spirituality across the life span in relation to overall health and well-being.

5. Ask students to identify situations that may result in spiritual distress, and the behaviors/responses that may be exhibited by the client.
   Use the following or similar examples to discuss possible client reactions and spiritual needs:
   a. A 40-year-old man who has had a heart attack
   b. A 20 year old who has been paralyzed after an automobile accident
   c. A 32-year-old mother of two children who has been diagnosed with breast cancer
   d. A 70 year old with severe, painful arthritis
   e. Parents of a child born with severe neurologic impairments

6. Discuss religious needs, problems, and conflicts that the nurse may encounter in working with clients.

7. Ask students to share examples of their own religious practices and how they may relate to or interfere with health care delivery.

8. Ask students to identify how recognition of spiritual needs may be viewed outside of specific religions.

9. Discuss specific examples of how the nurse intervenes to meet clients' spiritual needs in the following:
   a. Providing presence
   b. Establishing a healing relationship
   c. Determining support systems
   d. Promoting dietary needs
   e. Supporting rituals
   f. Providing for prayer and meditation
   g. Supporting grief work

10. Identify and/or ask students to identify how illness and hospitalization may interfere with an individual's spirituality and religious practices.

11. Review the association of cultural and religious beliefs and practices. Compare and contrast the differences and similarities in spiritual practices of different ethnic/cultural groups.

12. Guide students in the application of the nursing process for an actual client, or simulated case-study situation, in which evidence of spiritual distress is found.

Interactive Exercises

1. Assign students to report, orally or in writing, on the available support systems/resources that are available within an affiliating agency or community for clients experiencing spiritual needs.

2. Have students identify examples of specific nursing interventions that will enhance a client's spirituality. Ask students to determine how the routine of an acute or restorative care facility may be adapted to meet a client's spiritual needs.

3. Have students, working individually or in small groups, identify nursing diagnoses, long-/short-term goals and client outcomes, nursing interventions, and evaluation criteria/measures for the following, or similar, case-study situation:

   The client is a 28-year-old homosexual man who is terminally ill with acquired immunodeficiency syndrome (AIDS). He was raised in a Catholic home by parents who have maintained a strong belief in their religion and its practices. Although he has denied being a practicing Catholic, the client has made occasional statements that may indicate a conflict in his beliefs and a desire for spiritual assistance.

Client Care Experiences

1. Have students identify possible spiritual needs for their assigned clients in a variety of health care settings. Discuss how the clients' spiritual needs may be met by the nurse or spiritual counselor in pre- and/or postclinical conferences.

2. Have students incorporate the clients' identified spiritual needs into the plan of care/critical pathway.

Critical Thinking Exercises (from text page 564)

1. Mr. Jackson is a 40-year-old businessman who employs more than 100 employees. A 12-hour-a-day work week is not unusual for him. Last evening he was admitted to the cardiac care unit with severe chest pain resulting from a myocardial infarction (heart attack). He is now stabilized but is making frequent requests of his nurses and doctors, asking about his diagnostic tests and what he needs to do to be able to go home. He tells his nurse, "My doctor tells me I will need surgery once I am more stable. I hope he can do that soon. I just can't believe this is happening. I worry about what will happen to my business while I am gone."
   a. Applying the Framework of Systemic Organization, what behaviors is Mr. Jackson demonstrating?
   b. Identify three approaches you might use as his nurse to conduct a spiritual assessment with Mr. Jackson.

2. Celia is a new graduate nurse caring for Ms. Rosenbaum for the first time. Ms. Rosenbaum has been diagnosed with uterine cancer. Celia is helping Ms. Rosenbaum with her meal tray when she says, "I noticed that the information in your chart says you are Jewish. Would you like me to call a Rabbi to visit? Are there any diet considerations we should be making for you?" Are Celia's assessment and resultant interventions appropriate for this situation?

3. Critical thinking is an ongoing process. When you learn that you are assigned to Julio Gonsaga, you note that the Kardex information includes his religion, Catholic, and his place of birth, Cuba. A colleague tells you he can speak some English. The client is 80 years old and reportedly has a bit of a hearing deficit. What knowledge might you wish to reflect on critically before beginning a spiritual assessment of this client?

Suggested Answers

1. A. Mr. Jackson is attempting to practice control. He tries to control the threat of a serious heart condition by re-establishing pre-existing conditions. He seeks knowledge to minimize the uncertainty and fear of becoming disabled (system change). His desire to have surgery as soon as possible is a form of deliberate planning (system maintenance). His concern over the welfare of his business is a fear of loss of control.
   B. First begin by having an unhurried conversation, showing attentiveness and presence, and listen to what Mr. Jackson has to say. Determine what is important to him in his life. Ask Mr. Jackson what is his personal source of strength or faith. Also assess who Mr. Jackson relies on for support during difficult times.

2. In an acute care setting where client contact is often time limited, it is appropriate for Celia to focus on the client's religious affiliation and practices. Asking about dietary considerations during meal time shows good timing, although it would have been ideal to assess this need before the first meal. Determining whether a pastoral care referral is needed is quite appropriate. If Ms. Rosenbaum remains in the hospital, it will be important for Celia to extend her assessment to understanding the client's faith and belief system.

3. It will be important to know how to communicate appropriately with a client who has a hearing deficit. It would also be useful to know what health means to Hispanics. Finally, it would be very valuable to identify whether a family member or friend is available who can speak both Spanish and English fluently.

148   Chapter 28: Spiritual Health

29

The Experience of Loss, Death, and Grief

Classroom Discussion

1. Discuss the concept and categories of loss. Have students give examples for each of the categories, using personal experiences whenever possible.

2. Review the possible multicultural differences that may be seen in response to loss and grieving. Ask students to share their own or family experiences.

3. Discuss and provide examples of normal, anticipatory, complicated, and disenfranchised grief responses.

4. Compare and contrast the theories of grief and how the nurse may use each one to assess and respond to clients.

5. Review what is included in the assessment of a client's response to loss (see Resource for Student Activity).

6. Provide the students with the following or similar client situations, and ask them to identify how the individuals may progress through the grieving process. Encourage students to apply the theories of grieving.
   a. A 50-year-old man who has been laid off from his sales position of 20+ years; he is the sole income earner in the family
   b. An 86-year-old woman who has just lost her pet cat that she has owned since her husband died
   c. A 20-year-old woman who just had a miscarriage
   d. A 5-year-old child who has experienced the death of a parent or grandparent
   e. The middle-aged parents of a young adult man who was killed as an innocent bystander in a robbery

7. Discuss the specific approach and goals of hospice care.

8. Invite a nurse who is employed in a hospice to discuss his or her role, the challenges of the position, client and family reactions, and the needs of the nursing staff.

9. Guide students in the application of the nursing process for an actual or simulated client who is experiencing or having difficulty experiencing grief.

10. Discuss nursing measures to palliative care measures for the terminally ill client.

11. Describe postmortem care. Have students discuss their feelings about the procedure, and identify what adaptations may be made according to religious or cultural beliefs.

12. Use popular (e.g., films, TV) or educational media to stimulate a discussion on loss and grieving.

13. Discuss legal and ethical issues associated with death and dying [e.g., organ transplants, do not resuscitate (DNR) orders, advance directives].

Interactive Exercises

1. Assign students to investigate the resources available in the affiliating agency and community to assist clients, families, and nurses to deal with loss and the grieving process.

2. Ask students to specify nursing interventions that will assist clients and families to work through loss and the grieving process. Incorporate creative strategies for clients of different ages and sociocultural backgrounds.

3. Videotape students in a role-playing situation in which they are to apply therapeutic communication skills in an interaction with a client who is terminally ill. Have students critique the interaction and offer suggestions to their peers for improvement.

4. Have students, working individually or in small groups, identify nursing diagnoses, client goals and outcomes, nursing interventions, and evaluation criteria for an actual or simulated client who is experiencing loss, grieving, or dysfunctional grieving.

Clinical Skill/Technique

1. Demonstrate postmortem care in a simulated or actual client situation.

Client Care Experience

1. Assign students to participate in the care of clients who are experiencing loss and grief. In pre- or postconference, discuss the nursing care approach and the feelings of the students in working with the clients.

Resource for Student Activity

Response to Loss: Assessment Tool

Response to Loss: Assessment Tool

Criterion	Assessment Data	Health Promotion Activities
Personal Characteristics		
Nature of Relationships		
Social Support System		
Nature of Loss		
Cultural/Spiritual Beliefs		
Loss of Life Goals		
Hope		
Phase of Grieving		
Family's Grief		
Risk Factors in Survivors		
Nursing Role Perceptions		

*C*ritical Thinking Exercises (from text page 593)

1. Mr. Jamison visits the community health clinic and tells the nurse, "I do not know what is wrong with me. I lost my wife 6 months ago, and I still get angry that God let her die. I still miss her so much. I have been going out with friends, but I just do not enjoy it that much. There are times when I wake up at night and I think my wife is still here. What is wrong with me? I thought I would be feeling better by now." As the nurse, how would you respond to Mr. Jamison?

2. You are assigned to care for two different clients. Mrs. Rouse has rheumatoid arthritis and is experiencing severe joint pain in both hands. Mrs. Nester has bone cancer and has experienced ongoing deep pain in the back and hips, with some discomfort also in the lower extremities. Refer to Chapter 42 on content about pain. Then discuss in what way management of pain will differ between the two patients.

3. A nursing colleague is discussing her client with you. She says, "My client is a 48-year-old man with a degenerative neurologic disease. The disease is progressive. He is having trouble walking and taking care of his daily needs. The only thing I can do is assist him with bathing, feeding, and walking. He really is not a candidate yet for palliative care." What would be your response to your colleague?

Suggested Answers

1. Mr. Jamison is experiencing normal grief. No time frame exists for the resolution of his grief. He is experiencing normal anger, acceptance, and denial. It is normal for persons who have had loss to move back and forth between different stages of grief.

2. Mrs. Rouse's pain is the result of a well-defined diagnosis. Therapies will be directed specifically at the inflammation of her joints. Her care providers will be able to give clear expectations as to how the pain will respond to therapy. Mrs. Nester is likely to have symptom distress. Her pain from cancer is progressing. Care providers cannot tell Mrs. Nester how the pain will change and whether treatment will be effective. Mrs. Rouse will likely benefit from anti-inflammatory medications and appropriate analgesics. Mrs. Nester will likely benefit from opioid analgesics; however, her anxiety and uncertainty as to the course of her disease also must be managed with care.

3. Your colleague's client is an excellent candidate for palliative care. Palliative care is for any age, any diagnosis, at any time, and not just during the last few months of life. Caring for a client with a progressive disease, the nurse's goal is to prevent, relieve, reduce, or soothe symptoms without affecting a cure. In addition, the nurse focuses on providing physical, psychological, social, and spiritual aspects of the client's progressive illness. Palliative care allows clients to make informed choices and to work on issues of life closure.

30

S tress and Adaptation

Instructor Media Resources

Instructor's Resource CD
evolve **Instructor's Resources**

Instructor's Manual
ExamView Test Bank
Image Collection
Power Point Slides
Weblinks

Student Media Resources

CD COMPANION

- Review Questions
- Glossary

evolve **WEBSITE**

- Review Questions
- Student Learning Activities
- Glossary

Classroom Discussion

1. Discuss the concept of stress and provide examples of stressors.

2. Describe the physiological adaptation to stress and its limitations.

3. Discuss the different models, such as Neuman's and Pender's, that the nurse may use to understand and respond to stress. Guide students in the way these models may be applied to an actual and/or simulated personal or client situation.

4. Describe Selye's General Adaptation Syndrome (GAS), providing examples for each component (see Resources for Student Activities).

5. Discuss the psychological responses to stress. Ask students to provide examples and/or to share with the group their personal responses to stress.

6. Ask students to provide specific examples of how the following indicators may be assessed in an individual experiencing stress: physiological, psychological, developmental, emotional/behavioral, intellectual, sociocultural, family, lifestyle, and spiritual.

7. Guide students in the application of the nursing process for an actual or simulated client who is experiencing stress.

8. Invite a psychiatric nurse practitioner and/or psychologist from an employee-assistance program to speak with the class about stress and responses particular to nurses.

9. Describe stress-reduction techniques that the nurse may implement for himself or herself and clients. Have students participate in a stress reduction and/or relaxation exercise.

10. Discuss methods of avoiding or reducing stressful situations and responses. Ask students to provide examples or share personal experiences with improving responses to stress.

11. Review different coping mechanisms, and provide examples of each.

12. Invite a student who is close to graduation, or who has recently graduated, to speak to the class about strategies to reduce stress while enrolled in nursing school.

13. Discuss crisis and crisis-intervention strategies.

14. Stimulate a discussion on student perceptions of job-related stress for nurses: burnout.

15. Review the relation of stress to illness. Provide examples of specific illnesses that have been directly linked to stress.

Interactive Exercises

1. Assign students to report orally or in writing on available support systems/resources within the school or an affiliating agency for students, nurses, and clients.

2. Have students develop a questionnaire or use an available tool to assess stressors for themselves, their peers, or assigned clients.

3. Have students, working individually or in small groups, identify nursing diagnoses, client goals and outcomes, nursing interventions, and evaluation criteria for one of the following or similar client situation:
   a. A 48-year-old professional man who has been laid off from his job after 20 years with the company.
   b. A 14-year-old newly diagnosed diabetic who requires dietary adjustment and insulin injections.
   c. A 21-year-old first-time mother of a 4-month-old infant who has just moved to a community far from her family and friends.
   d. A 70-year-old woman who has experienced increasing difficulty with activities of daily living as a result of arthritic changes in her arms and legs.
   e. A 30-year-old student who is trying to balance school assignments, a full-time job, and family responsibilities with her husband and school-aged daughter.

Clinical Skill Technique

1. Demonstrate stress-reduction techniques that the nurse may implement for himself or herself and clients. Have students participate in a stress reduction and/or relaxation exercise.

Client Care Experiences

1. Have students assess assigned clients for indications of stress. Discuss how stress-reduction activities may be incorporated into the plan of care for the clients.

2. Assign students to prepare and present a teaching plan for a small group of clients on the recognition and reduction of stress.

Resources for Student Activities

Chart for GAS

General Adaptation Syndrome

GAS
General Characteristics
Alarm Reaction
Resistance Stage
Exhaustion Stage

Critical Thinking Exercises (from text page 614)

1. You are caring for a 30-year-old single mother who has recently received a diagnosis of metastatic breast cancer. She is the sole provider for three young children (all younger than 7 years). Discuss the various stressors that must be considered when writing an appropriate discharge plan.

2. A client comes to the emergency department with complaints of dizziness, not related to any physical finding on examination. During the health history, the client reports that her life is very stressful, and she is barely coping. She finalized her divorce 3 months ago, is working 32 hours per week, and is attending college. Her ex-husband recently lost his job and can no longer pay child support. Finally, she tearfully confesses that she thinks she might be pregnant but does not want her ex-husband to know. Develop nursing diagnoses related to this situation.

3. An older adult woman is admitted to the hospital with a fractured hip. Before her injury, she lived with her husband, who has advancing Alzheimer's disease. While she is hospitalized, he is staying with a niece who lives 100 miles away, but this cannot be a permanent situation because her niece also is in frail health. The client has no children who can help her when she returns home. She is concerned not only about who will care for her after she is discharged but also about her husband. What approach would be the best to take in establishing goals for treatment?

Suggested Answers

1. First determine the patient's perception of the stressors. They will not necessarily be the same stressors that the nurse would identify. Possible stressors she might identify are uncertainty about
   - who will care for the children when she is no longer able to provide their care and after her death,
   - how she will cope with pain,
   - how she will decide about treatment,
   - how to deal with the children's reactions to her illness, and
   - how to provide for the children's basic needs.

2. *Coping, ineffective, related to multiple life stressors*
   Fear related to increased demands on her limited resources
   Powerlessness related to loss of control over personal finances

3. Determine the woman's perception of the situation. Assess her support systems, including neighbors, friends, and church, and coping skills. Explore available community resources. Include the woman in the planning process.

31

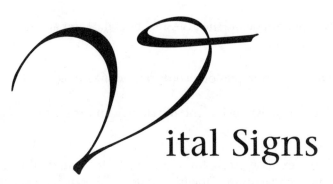

ital Signs

Instructor Media Resources

Instructor's Resource CD
evolve Instructor's Resources

Instructor's Manual
ExamView Test Bank
Image Collection
Power Point Slides
Weblinks
Skills Checklists

Student Media Resources

CD COMPANION

- Review Questions
- Glossary

evolve WEBSITE

- Review Questions
- Student Learning Activities
- Glossary

Classroom Discussion

1. Discuss general guidelines for taking vital signs, including frequency, parameters, etc.

2. Ask students to identify what information is important before the assessment of vital signs and how the findings are correlated with other assessment data.

3. Explain the documentation of vital signs, providing examples of records from different agencies.

4. With the aid of educational media (e.g., video, models), review the physiology and regulation of body temperature.

5. Discuss factors that affect body temperature: age, exercise, stress, hormone levels, circadian rhythm, and environment. Have students identify how each factor may increase or decrease body temperature.

6. Discuss potential changes in body temperature that the nurse may encounter, including their causative factors and the client's physiological responses.

7. Ask students to identify the following:
   a. How body temperature may differ from one site to another
   b. Advantages and disadvantages of different types of thermometers

8. Review the conversion of Fahrenheit to/from centigrade temperatures.

9. Discuss the assessment of and interventions that may be implemented for increases and decreases in body temperature.
   Have students identify specific examples of client responses and nursing interventions for situations involving significant increases and decreases in body temperature.

10. With the aid of educational media, review the physiology and regulation of the pulse.

11. Discuss factors that affect the pulse: fever, anxiety, blood loss, exercise, pain, and medications. Have students identify how each factor may influence the pulse.

12. Discuss the assessment of and nursing interventions that may be implemented for alterations in a client's pulse. Have students identify specific indications of pulse alterations and the resultant nursing responsibilities.

13. With the aid of educational media, review the physiology and regulation of respiration and the mechanics of breathing.

14. Discuss factors that may influence the rate, rhythm, and depth of respirations. Have students identify how each factor may alter respiration.

15. Discuss the assessment of and interventions that may be implemented for alterations in respiration. Have students identify specific indications of respiratory alterations and the resultant nursing responsibilities.

16. With the aid of educational media, review the physiology of blood pressure.

17. Discuss factors that affect blood pressure: age, stress, race/ethnicity, medical conditions, medications, diurnal variation, and gender. Have students identify how each factor may increase or decrease blood pressure.

18. Discuss potential changes in blood pressure (hypertension/hypotension) that the nurse may encounter, including their causative factors and the client's physiological response.

19. Ask students to identify how vital signs change in accordance with growth and development (see Resources for Student Activities).

20. Review the new parameters for assessment of blood pressure and subsequent referral when screening is conducted in a community setting/health fair.

21. Ask students to determine the following:
    a. How the environment may influence the measurement of vital signs or the assessment findings.
    b. How the environment may be manipulated to promote accurate findings and enhance client comfort.

22. Discuss how the measurement and evaluation of vital signs may be incorporated into a client's care plan/critical pathway.

23. Have students identify how the assessment of vital signs may be influenced and adapted in the following or similar situations. The client:
    a. Has just finished drinking coffee.
    b. Returned a few minutes ago from a rigorous physical therapy session.
    c. Has evidence of a dysrhythmia.
    d. States he or she feels lightheaded when getting out of bed.
    e. Is currently taking a medication for a cardiac or respiratory condition.
    f. Is 6 months old.
    g. Is experiencing rectal bleeding.
    h. Is an obese adult.
    i. Has a history of seizure activity.
    j. Was in an auto accident and has casts on both upper extremities.
    k. Is experiencing moderate to severe pain.
    l. Has had a right mastectomy.
    m. Has a dialysis shunt to the left arm.

Interactive Exercises

1. Provide practice fahrenheit (Fahrenheit not capitalized?)and centigrade temperatures for students to convert.

2. Provide a list of clients of various ages and their vital signs, and ask students to determine if the findings are within expectations.

3. Working individually or in small groups, have students design a teaching plan for a client's self-measurement of pulse and/or blood pressure.

Clinical Skills/Techniques

1. Assessment of body temperature:
   a. Explain and demonstrate, by using different body sites and equipment, the assessment of body temperature. (Use simulation mannequins/models and/or volunteers to demonstrate the assessment of the vital signs.)
   b. Have small groups of students practice, on mannequins and/or their peers, the assessment of body temperature by using:
      (1) Electronic, glass (optional), and/or disposable thermometers.
      (2) Oral, rectal, axillary, and tympanic sites.
   c. Evaluate the students' ability to accurately assess and record body temperature through return demonstration/skill testing before clinical experiences.

2. Assessment of the pulse:
   a. Explain and demonstrate, by using different sites, the assessment of the pulse, including the correct use of the stethoscope. Use audiotapes, if available, and a dual-earpiece stethoscope to facilitate the explanation and demonstration of apical pulse and blood pressure assessment.
   b. Have small groups of students practice, on simulation mannequins and/or their peers, the assessment of the pulse by using:
      (1) Temporal, carotid, brachial, radial, ulnar, femoral, popliteal, posterior tibial, and dorsalis pedis sites (see Resources for Student Activities).
      (2) A stethoscope for apical pulse determination.
   c. Evaluate the students' ability to assess and record the pulse accurately through return demonstration/skill testing before clinical experiences.

3. Assessment of respirations and oxygen saturation:
   a. Explain and demonstrate the assessment of respirations, identifying how the assessment is integrated into the procedure to avoid altering the findings.
   b. Explain and demonstrate the assessment of oxygen saturation through the use of the pulse oximeter.
   c. Have small groups of students practice the assessment of respirations and use of the pulse oximeter.
   d. Evaluate the students' ability to assess and record respirations accurately and use the pulse oximeter through return demonstration/skill testing before clinical experience.

4. Assessment of blood pressures:
   a. Explain and demonstrate, by using different sites and equipment, the assessment of blood pressure.
   b. Have small groups of students practice the assessment of blood pressure by using:
      (1) Aneroid, mercury, and electronic sphygmomanometers.
      (2) Ultrasound and palpation.
      (3) Upper and lower extremity sites.
   c. Evaluate the students' ability to assess and record blood pressure accurately through return demonstration/skill testing before clinical experiences.

Client Care Experiences

1. Assign students to assess, report, and record vital signs for clients of different ages in the clinical setting. Discuss expectations before and the students' findings and interventions after the experience. Ask students how the client's status was reflected in the vital signs assessed.

2. Have students participate in a community blood pressure screening.

3. Have students complete a care plan/pathway for an assigned client, incorporating the measurement and evaluation of vital signs.

4. Have students present a teaching plan on self-measurement of pulse and/or blood pressure to a client in an agency or community setting.

Resources for Student Activities

Pulse Measurement Form
Comparison Chart: Vital Signs across the Life Span
Vital Signs Assessment Form

Pulse Measurement Form

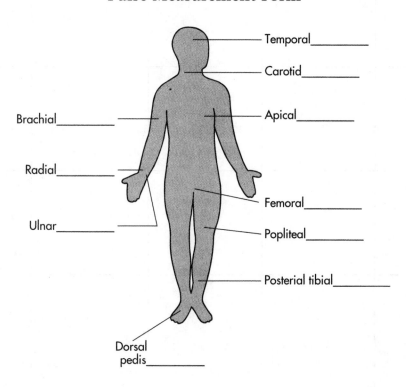

Temporal_____

Carotid_____

Apical_____

Brachial_____

Radial_____

Femoral_____

Ulnar_____

Popliteal_____

Posterial tibial_____

Dorsal pedis_____

Comparison Chart: Vital Signs Across The Life Span

	Temperature	Pulse	Respiration	Blood Pressure
Infant				
Toddle				
Preschool Child				
School-age Child				
Adolescent				
Adult				
Older Adult				

Vital Signs Assessment Form

Age: Height:

Sex: Weight:

Known Medical Conditions:

Vital Signs	Findings	Comparison with Norms
Temperature Site		
Pulse Site(s) Rate Rhythm Strength Equality		
Respiration Rate Depth Rhythm		
Blood Pressure Site Sitting/Standing/Supine		

Critical Thinking Exercises (from text page 699)

1. A 47-year-old African-American man is coming to the health clinic for a physical examination by the nurse practitioner for a routine employment physical. The nursing assistant obtains the following routine vital signs: tympanic temperature, 36.9°C (98.4° F); right radial pulse rate, 96 beats per minute and irregular; BP, sitting, right arm 162/82 mm Hg, left arm, 150/70 mm Hg; SpO$_2$, 95% on room air; respiratory rate, 22 breaths per minute.
   a. As the admitting nurse, what questions would you ask this client to evaluate his risk for hypertension?
   b. Based on these vital signs, what actions should you take?

2. A teenage mother brings her 3-year-old child to the walk-in health center. She notes that he has been fussy, has not had much of an appetite, and is not his active self. The boy is crying and struggling to get out of his mother's lap during your interview. You note that he is small for his age, but otherwise well developed.
   a. Describe the sequence you would use for obtaining vital signs.
   b. When selecting the appropriate equipment for obtaining the vital signs, what, if any, special considerations are needed?
   c. The nursing assistant reports she has obtained a temperature of 37.7°C (99.8°F). What additional information do you request from the assistant?

3. A 52-year-old woman is admitted to the medical unit for chronic dyspnea and discomfort in her left chest with deep breathing and coughing. She has been smoking for 35 years and has a 20-year history of emphysema. Over the past 4 months, she has lost 10 pounds and currently weighs 110 pounds.
   a. When delegating the vital signs to assistive personnel, what information and directions should you provide?
   b. The blood pressure and heart rate are within acceptable ranges. The temperature is 37.5°C (99.5°F), obtained with an oral electronic thermometer; the respiratory rate 32 breaths per minute and shallow; the SpO$_2$ is 89%. Based on these results, list your actions in priority.

4. An 82-year-old resident in your subacute extended care facility is being treated for pneumonia with antibiotics. She has been on bed rest for the past 2 days. She has a history of hypertension, treated with diuretics, but is otherwise healthy. She has been afebrile for the past 24 hours and is eager to walk to the activity room. She has activity orders "up ad lib."
   a. Should you delegate the ambulation assistance to a nursing assistant?
   b. What places this client at risk for fainting?
   c. Explain to this client the reason you are obtaining orthostatic measurements.

5. A 25-year-old Hispanic woman arrives at the prenatal clinic for her first visit. She is 8 months pregnant. The nursing assistant checks her vital signs and height and weight. The client weighs 230 pounds and is 5 feet 3 inches tall; BP in right arm is 210/92 mm Hg; HR, 104 beats per minute; respiratory rate, 24 breaths per minute; tympanic temperature, 98.8°F. You are concerned with the client's blood pressure and repeat the measurement. You obtain 148/86 mm Hg in the right arm and 144/84 mm Hg in the left arm.
   a. What blood pressure measurement should be recorded? Provide some possible explanations for the difference in the measurements by you and the nursing assistant.
   b. How might you explain the abnormal vital signs to the client?
   c. What will be included in your discharge teaching?

Suggested Answers

1. a. One hypertension risk factor for this client is his ethnic background. The nurse should assess the client for dietary habits (sodium and fat intake), smoking history, and participation in daily exercise. Questions related to the client's genetic risk factors, such as family history of hypertension and heart disease, would be appropriate.
   b. The admitting nurse should repeat the measurements in both arms. The nurse practitioner should be notified of the findings.

2. a. In children, vital signs are obtained with the least stimulating procedure occurring first to avoid influencing the measurement values. However, in this case, the respiratory rate and heart rate may be affected by crying and struggling. Obtain oxygen saturation, temperature, heart rate, respiratory rate, and then blood pressure.
   b. Special consideration is needed by using the appropriate temperature device. A tympanic thermometer or axillary thermometer is appropriate for this developmental age. The correct size blood pressure cuff is required. Heart rate should be obtained by auscultating the apical rate.
   c. It is necessary to know what type of device and what route was used to obtain the temperature.

3. a. Respiratory rate should be obtained by counting for a full minute, as should apical heart rate. Inform the unlicensed assistant to note the position of comfort of the client when obtaining vital signs. This client will not be comfortable lying supine for vital signs.
   b. The client is showing defining characteristics for the nursing diagnosis of *Ineffective breathing pattern and impaired gas exchange*. Compare these values with previous measurements. Check for a standing order for supplemental oxygen therapy by nasal cannula, and administer if indicated. Inform the nurse in charge. Assess lung sounds and limit the client's activity level. Place the client on continuous oxygen-saturation monitor until evaluated by nurse or physician in charge.

4. a. No. The client has not been out of bed for 2 days; with a history of hypertension and fever, she is at risk for orthostatic hypotension.
   b. Clients receiving hypertensive medical treatments have a reduced ability to adjust to position changes because of potential fluid volume deficits. The febrile episode also placed this client at risk for fluid volume deficit, which can lead to orthostatic hypotension.
   c. The nurse explains to the client that the nurse wishes to make sure the patient can safely ambulate without feeling dizzy because of a low blood pressure.

5. a. Record the BP measurements that you obtained. The client is obese. Most electronic BP machines have a standard-size cuff; it is likely that the cuff was too narrow for this client, causing a false high reading. Other reasons for a false high reading could have included arm below heart level, deflating cuff too slowly, cuff wrapped too loosely.
   b. The elevation in blood pressure may be caused by the weight gain of pregnancy, stress, or anxiety of the clinic visit. The heart rate is elevated perhaps because of the hemodynamic changes of pregnancy. The respiratory rate is elevated because of the reduced lung expansion.
   c. In addition to prenatal teaching, diet, and smoking cessation, the client should be urged to make and keep frequent clinic visits as requested.

32

$\mathcal{H}$ealth Assessment and Physical Examination

Instructor Media Resources

Instructor's Resource CD
Instructor's Resources

Instructor's Manual
ExamView Test Bank
Image Collection
Power Point Slides
Weblinks

Student Media Resources

CD COMPANION

- Review Questions
- Glossary

evolve WEBSITE

- Review Questions
- Student Learning Activities
- Glossary

Classroom Discussion

1. Discuss the purposes of a physical examination/health assessment.

2. Review the importance of determining baseline information to compare findings from the physical examination/assessment.

3. Ask students to identify how cultural awareness and sensitivity may be incorporated into the physical examination/assessment. Have students provide specific examples of how client preparation and the performance of the examination may be adapted by the nurse.

4. Review general concepts of growth and development in relation to the approach taken in the performance of the physical examination for different age groups. Have students provide specific examples of how client preparation and the performance of the examination may be adapted to meet the needs of clients of different age and developmental levels.

5. Stimulate a discussion on how physical assessment may be incorporated into nursing interactions with clients in the health care setting.
   Ask students what information may be obtained during the following or other similar nursing activities:
   a. Taking the health history.
   b. Providing hygienic care.
   c. Assisting the client to dress.
   d. Administering medications.

6. Identify infection-control measures that should be implemented in the performance of a physical assessment. (Refer to Chapter 33)

7. Discuss the arrangement of the environment in preparation for the physical assessment.

8. Stimulate a discussion on how the physical assessment may be made more comfortable for the client and for the nurse. Have students provide specific examples of nursing interventions that should promote overall comfort for clients of different ages and backgrounds.

9. Review the role and importance of communication with the client throughout the procedure. Ask students to specify possible points in the assessment at which an opportunity for client teaching may arise.

10. Discuss the general organization and sequence of the assessment. Have students identify situations in which the usual sequence may be altered (e.g., client in severe pain).

11. Describe the documentation of the findings from the physical assessment, focusing on the utilization of appropriate terminology. Provide examples of documentation from different agencies/resources.

12. Invite a nurse practitioner to speak to the class about the implementation of the physical examination/assessment and the application of findings into the care of the client.

13. Discuss the responsibilities of the nurse on completion of the physical examination/assessment.

14. Ask students to identify how the physical assessment may be adapted for the following clients:
    a. A 4-year-old child.
    b. A 16-year-old anxious girl.
    c. An adult man with abdominal pain.
    d. An older adult woman with arthritis.
    e. A client who does not speak/understand the nurse's language.
    f. A young adult regaining consciousness after an automobile accident.

15. Discuss how the physical assessment and resultant findings may be integrated into the client's care plan/critical pathway.

16. Review the recommended preventive screenings for adults.

Interactive Exercises

1. Organize a role-playing experience with the students simulating the client's physical and psychological preparation for the assessment.

2. Have students identify the expected norms and possible alterations that may be found during the physical assessment.

3. Have students, working individually or in small groups, design a teaching plan for adult clients on breast or testicular self-examination, or another preventive health measure.

4. Have students practice recording and reporting physical assessment findings.

5. Provide students with a list of physical assessment findings and have them identify the expected and unexpected findings (e.g., cloudy pupils, transparent conjunctiva, rebound tenderness).

Clinical Skills/Techniques

1. Explain and demonstrate (by using a simulation mannequin or volunteer) the skills of physical assessment: inspection, palpation, percussion, auscultation, and olfaction.
   Ask students to identify where and when each skill would be best used, and what information each skill elicits (see Resources for Student Activities).
   Use educational media, such as audiotapes/videotapes to reinforce the skills and the assessment findings that are expected.

2. Have students prepare a simulated setting for a client assessment.

3. Describe and demonstrate, by using simulation mannequins/models or volunteers, the client positions during the physical assessment.

4. Explain and demonstrate (by using simulation mannequins/models, volunteers, or videotapes/computer program) the systematic approach to the physical assessment as follows:

> General survey
> Skin, hair, nails
> Head and neck
> Thorax and lungs
> Heart
> Vascular system
> Breasts
> Abdomen
> Female genitalia (speculum examination, if appropriate for class)
> Male genitalia
> Rectum and anus
> Musculoskeletal system
> Neurological system

Review normal anatomy and physiology, as indicated.

5. Explain and demonstrate the use of specific equipment (as appropriate to the class) used in the physical assessment: ophthalmoscope/otoscope, speculum, reflex hammer, etc.

6. Have the students, working in pairs or small groups, practice selected areas and/or the entirety of the physical assessment, with supervision.

7. Evaluate students' ability to perform and document selected areas and/or an entire physical assessment through return demonstration/skill testing before clinical experience.

Client Care Experiences

1. Have students present a teaching plan on breast and/or testicular self-examination to a client group in an acute care or community setting.

2. Assign students to observe and/or perform a physical assessment (as appropriate to the class) for a client in a health care setting; provide supervision, as indicated. Have students record and report their findings. Discuss the expectations with the group before the experience and their findings and personal observations/feelings after the assessment.

3. Have students complete a care plan/pathway for an assigned client, incorporating the physical assessment and evaluation of findings.

Resources for Student Activities

Chart of Physical Assessment Skills
Comparison Form: Physical Assessment Findings

Physical Assessment Skills

Assessment Skill	Area(s) Assessed	Information Obtained
Inspection		
Palpation		
Percussion		
Auscultation		
Olfaction		

Comparison Form: Physical Assessment Findings

Assessment Area	Expected Findings	Unexpected Findings
General Appearance/Behavior		
Vital Signs Height/Weight		
Skin, Hair, Nails		
Head, Neck		
Thorax, Lungs		
Heart		
Vascular System		
Breasts		
Abdomen		
Female/Male Genitalia		
Rectum, Anus		
Musculoskeletal		
Neurological		

Critical Thinking Exercises (from text page 769)

1. A 32-year-old client entering a neighborhood clinic has the following symptoms: frequent productive cough, fatigue, decreased appetite, and persistent fever. What focused assessment should the nurse conduct?

2. The nurse is performing an abdominal assessment and observes a pulsating midline abdominal mass. What is the nurse's next line of action?

3. A 75-year-old black man is being visited 1 week after surgery by the home care nurse to assess his peripheral vascular status after a femoral-popliteal bypass graft for arterial insufficiency. What assessment data should be obtained by the nurse?

4. Develop a teaching plan for a female client (age 40 years) with a family history of breast cancer who acknowledges that she does not perform a monthly breast self-examination (BSE).

5. What physical examination techniques does the nurse use during assessment of the following clients:
   a. A client suspected of having a head injury
   b. A client with a cast on the lower leg
   c. A client reporting abdominal pain

6. A 55-year-old client is to be evaluated for osteoporosis. Which specific questions would the nurse ask to ascertain the client's risk? What physical examination techniques would the nurse use?

Suggested Answers

1. The nurse should perform a detailed history, identifying that this client is at risk for lung disease (i.e., tuberculosis, HIV pulmonary disease, pneumonia). All techniques of respiratory assessment should be completed (i.e., inspections, palpation [excursion, tactile fremitus, percussion, auscultation]); as well as P, BP, temperature.

2. The nurse must not palpate abdominal mass; the physician should be notified.

3. Assessment criteria: color, temperature, pulse, edema, and skin changes. Systems assessed: skin and neurovascular. Client's history: especially pain, helps to identify occlusion (3 Ps: pain, pallor, pulselessness). Pallor in the dark-skinned client: normal brown skin appears yellow brown, and normal black skin, an ashen gray.

4. Teaching plan should include:
   Review for and educate client about why BSE is important.
   Provide literature from the American Cancer Society regarding breast cancer
   Discuss risk factors for breast cancer.
   Discuss ACS's recommendations for early detection of breast cancer.
   Demonstrate how to perform BSE.
   Have client return-demonstrate BSE.
   Schedule appointment with client's primary care giver for examination.

4. Physical examination measures used for:

Head injury: client's history, complete neurological examination (most important, Glasgow Coma Scale and cranial nerves II, III, IV, VI).

Cast on lower leg: inspection and palpation of skin, neurovascular assessment as well.

Abdominal pain: client's history and palpation of affected area.

5. Health history questions:

Family history?

Presence of osteoporosis risk factors? (See Table 32-3).

Level of exercise?

Alcohol/caffeine intake/smoking?

History of fractures/presence of pain/history of falls?

Calcium intake?

Women: Onset of menopause? Use of estrogen replacement therapy (ERT)?

Physical examination:

Musculoskeletal system examination checking for kyphosis, gait impairments, muscle weakness.

33

$\mathcal{J}$nfection Control

Classroom Discussion

1. Discuss the chain of infection, including factors that contribute to the development of an infection.

2. For each step of the chain of infection, ask students to provide specific examples of different possible infectious agents, reservoirs, portals of exit, modes of transmission, portals of entry, and susceptible hosts.

3. Review what is entailed in the infectious process. Have students identify positive and negative nursing interventions in response to the infectious process.

4. Review normal body defenses against infection.

5. Describe the inflammatory process and immune response and resultant physiological manifestations.
   Have students specify client signs and symptoms that indicate that body defenses have been mobilized against an infection.

6. Review the types of immunity and the role of vaccines/immunizations.

7. Discuss nosocomial infections: iatrogenic, endogenous/exogenous. Ask students to determine what may contribute to or reduce the development of these infections in the health care setting.

8. Explain the concept of asepsis in the health care environment, including the differences between medical and surgical aseptic practices.
   Ask students to identify the type of asepsis that is used for the following:
   a. Catheterization
   b. Dressing removal
   c. Wound care
   d. Bathing
   e. Injections
   f. Tracheostomy care

   Have students provide additional situations in which each type of asepsis should be applied.

9. Discuss factors that may put the client at a greater risk for infection: age, altered nutrition, stress, heredity, disease processes, medications, and medical treatments.
   Have students specify assessment findings that would indicate that the client may be at greater risk for developing an infection (e.g., infancy, diabetes, urinary catheterization).

10. Describe local and systemic signs/symptoms of infection (see Resource for Student Activity).

11. Discuss the laboratory tests used and the results that are indicative of an infectious process. Provide students with a list of laboratory results, and have them identify whether they are within normal limits and, if not, what the possible etiology is for each alteration.

12. Guide students in the application of the critical thinking model and the nursing process for a client who is experiencing an infectious process.

13. Discuss nursing interventions that may be implemented to reduce or eliminate the infectious process. Ask students to specify additional strategies to break the chain of infection.

14. Have students discuss what they believe is meant by an "infection control conscience." Demonstrate breaks in aseptic technique, and have students identify them.

15. Identify and/or have students identify supportive measures that may be used to promote the client's defenses against infection.

16. Describe the specific measures that are incorporated in medical asepsis and the nurse's role in the implementation of this type of asepsis.
    Have students identify what principles/procedures of medical asepsis should be applied in the following, or similar examples:
    a. Disposing of an exudate-filled dressing.
    b. Removal of contaminated body fluids.
    c. Changing of bed linens.
    d. Discarding used equipment: syringes, needles, tubing.

17. Explain the different types of isolation measures/barrier precautions, per Centers for Disease Control (CDC) guidelines.

18. Discuss the application of and measures included in Standard Precautions, including the two-tier approach.

19. Ask students to identify how clients, before the CDC guidelines, may have been over- or underisolated.

20. Stimulate a discussion on how the frequent use of nonsterile gloves may have a negative impact on the client or how health care providers may "misuse" them.

21. Identify the basic principles of isolation, commonly used equipment (gloves, gowns, masks, protective eyewear) and specific guidelines for selected disease processes (e.g., tuberculosis [TB]).

22. Ask students how the psychological effect of isolation may be minimized for the client.

23. Invite a nurse who is a Risk Manager or Infection Control nurse to speak to the class about his or her role in infection control and promotion of client defenses.

24. Describe the principles and measures that are specific to surgical asepsis, including when objects are considered contaminated. Ask students to provide examples of breaks in sterile technique.

25. Discuss the difference between routine hand hygiene and a surgical scrub.

26. Have students whether the following nursing interventions require clean or sterile gloves:
    a. Changing a surgical dressing.
    b. Taking an oral temperature.
    c. Obtaining a venous blood sample.
    d. Providing hygienic care.
    e. Inserting a urinary catheter.
    f. Preparing an intramuscular injection.

27. Ask students how aseptic practices may be amended, without being abandoned, in the client's home environment.

Interactive Exercises

1. Have students, working individually or in small groups, design a teaching plan on measures to implement to control the spread of infection for a client in the acute or home care environment.

2. Provide students with the following or another similar list of client situations, and ask students to identify what precautions should be implemented in the acute care setting (including transfers within the institution) or home environment:
    a. A child with gastroenteritis.
    b. Purulent drainage seeping from a client's surgical wound.
    c. Clients with hepatitis A, B, or C.
    d. A middle adult client with TB.
    e. An adolescent with leukemia.

3. Assign students to participate in an affiliating agency's in-service programs on infection control and health care worker responsibilities (as available).

4. Have students investigate and report on resources pertinent to infection control that are available for nurses within an affiliating agency.

5. Organize a role-playing experience with one group of students demonstrating both good and bad aseptic technique, and the other students identifying the positive and negative examples.

Clinical Skills/Techniques

1. Have students simulate the preparation of an acute care room for a client who requires second-tier precautions.

2. Explain and demonstrate the procedure for opening a sterile package, and have students practice the technique.

3. Explain and demonstrate (by using appropriate supplies and equipment, and educational media, as available) the following skills associated with medical or surgical asepsis:
   a. Hand hygiene
   b. Isolation precautions
   c. Applying a surgical mask
   d. Preparing a sterile field
   e. Performing a surgical scrub
   f. Applying a sterile gown and performing closed gloving
   g. Performing open gloving

4. Have small groups of students practice the skills of medical and surgical asepsis, by using the appropriate equipment and supplies.

5. Evaluate the students' ability to implement the skills of medical and surgical asepsis through return-demonstration/skill testing before clinical experience.

Client Care Experiences

1. Have students present a teaching plan on measures to control the spread of infection to a client/family experiencing an infectious process.

2. Assign students to observe and participate in the nursing care of clients experiencing, or at risk for developing, an infectious process within an acute, extended, rehabilitation, and/or home care setting.
   Discuss expectations with the group before the experience, and have students report on their interactions, specific to infection control, after the assignment.

3. Have students complete a care plan/pathway for an assigned client who has an infection present or is at risk of developing an infection.

Resource for Student Activity

Comparison of Local and Systemic Infection: Client Responses

Comparison of Local and Systemic Infection

Type of Infection	Client Responses
Local	
Systemic	

Critical Thinking Exercises (from text page 819)

1. Mrs. Jaycock had an indwelling urethral catheter for 1 week. The catheter has now been out for 2 hours. She complains of frequency and pain on urination. Mrs. Jaycock suggests reinsertion of the catheter because of the need to get up frequently. Of what can frequency or pain on urination be an indication? Should the catheter be reinserted? Why or why not? Describe at least one appropriate assessment measure and independent nursing action for Mrs. Jaycock.

2. You are caring for Mr. Huang, who has a large, open, and draining abdominal wound. You notice another health care worker changing Mr. Huang's dressing without wearing gloves or using sterile supplies or sterile technique. When you question the health care worker regarding his or her practice, this person says, "Don't worry, the wound is already infected, and the antibiotics and draining will take care of any contaminants." How would you respond to this comment? What would your next steps be in following up on this incident?

3. Mrs. Niles is 83 years old and lives alone. She has difficulty walking and relies on a church volunteer group to deliver lunches during the week. Her fixed income limits her ability to buy food. Last week Mrs. Niles's 79-year-old sister died. The two sisters had been very close. As a home care nurse, explain the factors that might increase Mrs. Niles's risk for infection.

4. Mr. Vargas is admitted to the facility with a history of recent weight loss, a cough that has persisted for 2 months, and hemoptysis. His chest radiograph film shows a cavity in one lung, and his physician suspects TB. What type of isolation precautions would you use for Mr. Vargas? What protection would you use to provide care? What education would you provide for the client and his family?

Suggested Answers

1. A urinary tract infection. No, this may aggravate the infection and promote spread to the bloodstream. Increase fluid intake if not clinically contraindicated, and check her urinalysis.

2. It is important not only to protect Mr. Huang from additional contamination, but also to protect ourselves from becoming contaminated. Report the incident to your supervisor.

3. Her age, potential for poor nutrition, potential for depression.

4. Airborne precautions, wear an N95 mask and keep the door closed, educate the client and family on transmission of TB and reasons for isolation.

34

*M*edication Administration

Classroom Discussion

1. Discuss terminology related to drugs: names, classifications, and forms.

2. Identify legislation and standards associated with the administration and use of drugs.

   Ask students to identify how legal guidelines influence the nurse's role in the control (e.g., double-lock) and administration of medications.

3. Describe the different drug actions, including the pharmacokinetics: absorption, distribution, metabolism, and excretion of drugs.

   Have students provide specific examples of how drug actions are influenced by the following factors: type and dosage of drug administered, route of administration, and individual client status (age, weight, medical condition, etc.).

4. Discuss how the following effects of a medication may be differentiated, and the nursing responsibilities associated with each:
   a. Therapeutic effect
   b. Side effect
   c. Toxic effect
   d. Idiosyncratic reaction
   e. Allergic reaction
   f. Drug interaction
   g. Dose responses

5. Review factors that influence the actions of drugs: genetics, physiological/psychological variables, environment, and diet.

   Ask students to provide examples of how the influence may be therapeutically increased or decreased.

6. Identify the different routes by which medications may be administered and the factors involved in the selection of different routes.

   Ask students to identify the advantages and disadvantages that are associated with each route.

7. Review the metric, apothecary, and household measurement systems and the conversion/calculation of drug dosages.

   Review the specific calculation for pediatric dosages.

8. Discuss the roles of the physician, pharmacist, and nurse/nurse practitioner in the preparation and administration of medications.

9. Invite a nurse practitioner to speak to the class about his or her preparation for and the responsibilities entailed in the prescription of medications.

10. Guide students in the application of the critical thinking model and the nursing process for clients requiring medications

11. Ask students what client-assessment information is crucial to obtain to administer medications safely.

12. Describe the documentation required after the administration of client medications.
    Review the legal and safety implications of accurate and timely documentation.

13. Discuss what is incorporated in the nurse's evaluation of the client responses to medications and the resultant responsibilities based on the evaluation.

14. Discuss the "six rights" of medication administration. Have students identify how each "right" is determined.
    Ask students what should be done in the following situations:
    a. Two clients on the unit have the same name.
    b. Client has no identification (ID) band.
    c. Client questions the medication being given.
    d. Nurse cannot read the smeared label of the medication bottle.
    e. Tablets must be scored or crushed.
    f. Child requires an extremely small liquid dose.
    g. Client is not able to tolerate swallowing pills.
    h. An intramuscular (IM) site appears hard.
    i. An as-needed (PRN) pain medication is ordered.
    j. A medication to be given is more effective when given on an empty stomach.

15. Have students suggest possible reasons for medication errors, and how they might be prevented, and identify the responsibilities of the nurse if an error does occur.

16. Discuss special considerations associated with the administration of medications to infants, children, and older adults.
    Have students identify particular examples of how the nurse may adapt his or her approach in administering medications for clients in these age groups.

17. Ask students to identify the nurse's responsibility for each of the following client situations:
    a. One of the end-of shift narcotic counts is incorrect.
    b. A needle stick occurs after the injection is given.
    c. The client refuses to take the medication that is ordered.
    d. Blood is aspirated back into the syringe during an IM injection.
    e. The client's vital signs, pulse, respiration, and/or blood pressure have decreased significantly.
    f. A rash is noted on the client's upper chest and arms.
    g. The client cannot hold the medication cup to swallow the tablets.
    h. Another nurse requests that you give his or her already prepared medications.
    i. The dosage of the medication ordered is double the usual amount for the drug.
    j. The client is at physical therapy when the medications are ready to be given.
    k. An extremely thin or obese client requires IM injections.
    l. A medication to be given IM is extremely irritating to the tissues.
    m. A newborn requires an IM injection.
    n. A 1-year-old child has an intravenous (IV) infusion to be maintained.

Interactive Exercises

1. Provide students with a variety of drug calculations for practice and/or determination of competence in preparation to administer drugs. Use the following and/or similar examples:

   a. Ordered: Demerol, 75 mg IM   Available: Demerol, 100 mg/ml
   b. Ordered: Digoxin, 0.25 mg PO   Available: Digoxin, 0.125-mg tablets
   c. Ordered: Atropine, 0.4 mg IM   Available: Atropine, gr 1/150/0.5 ml
   d. Ordered: Tylenol, 40 mg PO   Available: Tylenol, 80 mg/0.5 tsp

2. Organize a debate on the topic of whether the nurse or another ancillary health care worker (e.g., pharmacy technician) should be responsible for the administration of medications.

3. Arrange for students to visit the pharmacy in an acute care facility to observe the preparation and dispensing of medications. Ask the pharmacist to discuss his or her role in drug preparation and distribution, and coordination with the nursing staff.

4. Have students, working individually or in small groups, design a teaching plan for clients related to self-administration of medications (e.g., home IV therapy, insulin injections).

5. Assign students to investigate the resources available to clients in the affiliating agency or community that will facilitate self or family administration of medications in the home.

   Students may report, orally or in writing, on available referral sources (i.e., Home Care, Visiting Nursing Services) that have been determined and the criteria for client referrals.

6. Provide examples of forms from different agencies for students to review and practice documentation.

7. Have students develop creative strategies to enhance medication compliance that may be implemented for an older adult client who lives alone and has diminished vision and occasional lapses of memory.

Clinical Skills/Techniques

1. Explain and demonstrate (by using simulation mannequins/models, appropriate equipment, and educational media), the preparation and administration of medications as follows:
   a. Oral administration
   b. Parenteral administration

Injections:	Preparation from an ampule or vial
	Mixing of medications
	Subcutaneous, intramuscular, and intradermal routes/sites
	Z-track and air-lock techniques
	Safe handling and disposal of equipment
IV infusions:	Large volume
	Bolus (if appropriate for class)
	Volume controlled
	Piggyback
	Intermittent access

    c. Topical applications: Skin applications
                                   Eye, ear, nasal instillations
                                   Vaginal instillations
                                   Rectal suppositories

    d. Metered-dose inhalers and/or dry-powder inhalers

    e. Irrigations

2. Have small groups of students practice, with supervision, the preparation and administration of medications via the specified routes by using simulation mannequins/models, grapefruit (or similar "practice" fruits), and/or injection pads. Focus on the selection of the appropriate equipment (e.g., needle length and gauge, syringe, IV setup) for the specific administration route and the accurate calculation of dosage to be administered.

3. Describe the preparation and administration of medications through enteral tubes (NG, J-tube, G-tube, feeding tube). Demonstrate the procedure by using available educational media, appropriate equipment, and simulation mannequin/model.

4. Have students practice the preparation and administration of medications through enteral tubes (as available).

5. Evaluate, through return-demonstration/skill testing, the students' ability to prepare and administer medications accurately and safely, and document the procedure appropriately before clinical experience.

$\mathcal{C}$lient Care Experiences

1. Have students present a teaching plan on self-medication administration to an adult client/parent.

2. Assign students to observe and participate, with supervision, in the preparation and administration of medications to clients in a health care setting.

3. Discuss expectations with the group before the experience, having students follow through on the "six rights." Have students identify the therapeutic use of the medications for their clients. Review general observations of their medication administration with the group. Have students report back on their experience.

4. Ask students to identify situations that may have been noted in the clinical area that could contribute to medication errors, and have them suggest strategies that may eliminate the problems.

5. Have students complete a care plan/pathway for an assigned client in which the administration of medications is integrated into the approach.

$\mathcal{R}$esources for Student Activities

Effects of Medications Chart
Comparison Chart of Subcutaneous, Intramuscular, and Intradermal Injections
Routes of Medication Administration: Nursing Responsibilities

Effects of Medications

Effects	Nursing Assessment
Therapeutic Action	
Side Effect	
Toxic Effect	
Idiosyncratic Reaction	
Allergic Reaction	
Drug Interaction	
Drug Dose Response	

Subcutaneous, Intramuscular, and Intradermal Injections

	Subcutaneous	Intramuscular	Intradermal
Needle Gauge/Length			
Sites Used			
Angle of Injection			
Maximum Amount of medication			
Specific Medications Given by Route			

Routes of Medication Administration: Nursing Responsibilities

Routes	Nursing Responsibilities
Oral	
Parenteral	
Topical	
Inhalation	
Intraocular	

Critical Thinking Exercises (from text page 907)

1. Mrs. O'Toole, a 69-year-old woman, recently experienced a stroke. She is experiencing right-sided weakness. The neurological clinical nurse specialist wrote orders to start oral medications today. What steps should the nurse take to ensure that it is safe for this client to receive her oral medications? What should the nurse do if the client is unable to swallow?

2. Marissa is a 25-year-old who just delivered a healthy infant. She is to receive RhoGAM, 300 μg IM, today. What size needle and which injection site and technique should the nurse use when administering this medication?

3. Jack, a 70-year-old retired farmer, has been experiencing new respiratory difficulties. His physician has ordered him to start using an albuterol inhaler with a spacer. What steps will the nurse take to ensure that he can self-administer his metered-dose inhaler (MDI)?

4. The nurse receives an order to give furosemide (Lasix), 40 mg IV push. The nurse has never given this medication while working on this unit. What steps should the nurse take before administering the furosemide?

Suggested Answers

1. One common physiological complication in clients who have experienced a stroke is difficulty in swallowing, or dysphagia. Clients who have dysphagia are at risk for aspirating fluids or foods taken by mouth. Before beginning oral medications for a client at risk for aspiration, the nurse should assess the client's cough and gag reflexes. If these are intact, the nurse should begin by placing the client in a sitting position. Because the client has weakness on the right side, the medication should be placed in the left side of her mouth. Fluids may be thickened, or the nurse may offer fruit nectars to help prevent aspiration. Medications should be administered one at a time, and the client should not be rushed to take her medications. If the nurse suspects the client cannot swallow safely, the medications should be held, and the clinical nurse specialist should be notified of the client's difficulty in swallowing. The nurse should suggest a referral to a speech therapist for a complete swallow workup before giving medications orally. If the client really needs the medications, alternate routes or medications must be explored.

2. First, the nurse must determine that the IM order is appropriate and that the medication cannot be given in any other route. After verifying that it is appropriate for Marissa to receive RhoGAM IM, the nurse uses knowledge about the various IM sites to determine the most appropriate site and needle to use in giving the injection. The nurse chooses the ventrogluteal site because it is situated away from major nerves and blood vessels and is the preferred site for medications that are irritating and viscous. For healthy, well-developed adults, the appropriate needle size is 1.5 inches in length. The nurse administers the injection by using the Z-track method to ensure the medication stays in the muscle and does not seep into the subcutaneous tissue.

3. Because of Jack's age, the nurse first must ensure that he has enough strength and dexterity to manipulate the MDI and spacer to administer the medication safely. The best way to teach Jack is to use a "practice" inhaler that does not contain the medication so that he can practice several times before actually using his inhaler. He should complete the following steps in administering the inhaler:

   • Remove mouthpiece from MDI and spacer, and inspect spacer for foreign objects.
   • Insert MDI into spacer and shake vigorously 5 to 6 times.
   • Because the inhaler is new, he should push a "test spray" into the air to be sure the inhaler is assembled and works properly.
   • Jack should then completely exhale and then close his mouth around the spacer, avoiding covering the small exhalation slots with the lips.
   • Jack should then depress the medication canister, spraying one puff into the spacer.
   • He should inhale deeply and slowly through the mouth for 3 to 5 seconds and then hold his breath for 10 seconds.
   • Finally, he should remove the spacer before exhaling.

   Jack also will need instruction in how to clean his inhaler and spacer and how to determine when he needs to have his inhaler refilled.

4. Different patient units in a medical center or hospital have different guidelines for administering IV push medications. One of the most common complications clients experience from receiving IV push medications results from not having the appropriate monitoring completed after the medication is given. Therefore the nurse should locate the policy and procedure manual for the unit the client is on and verify that the medication can be safely given on this unit. If the medication requires special monitoring that is not available on the unit, the nurse must contact the prescriber and determine if a different dosage or medication can be substituted for this medication. If this is not possible, the client may need to transfer to a different unit for the medication to be safely given. If the medication can be administered on the unit safely, the nurse will need to look in a drug reference guide or consult with a pharmacist to determine if the medication should be diluted, if any special filters or other considerations are necessary, and how fast to push the drug.

35

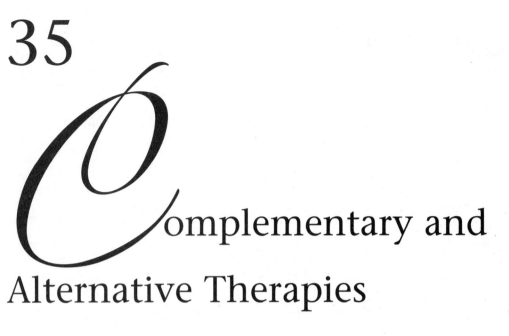

*C*omplementary and Alternative Therapies

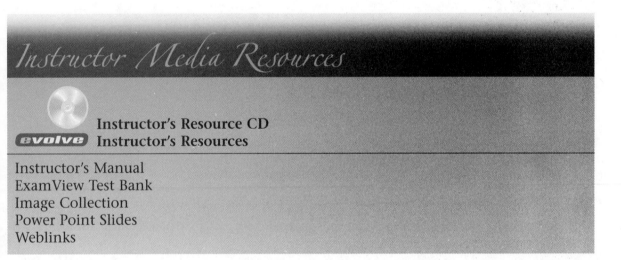

Instructor Media Resources

Instructor's Resource CD
evolve Instructor's Resources

Instructor's Manual
ExamView Test Bank
Image Collection
Power Point Slides
Weblinks

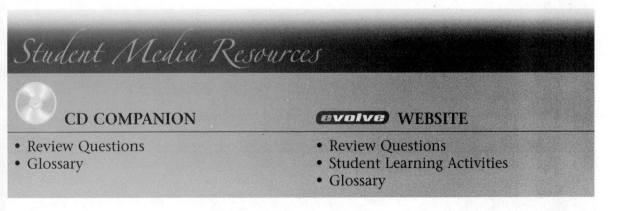

Student Media Resources

CD COMPANION

- Review Questions
- Glossary

evolve WEBSITE

- Review Questions
- Student Learning Activities
- Glossary

Classroom Discussion

1. Define and explain complementary and alternative therapies and their relation to conventional Western medicine. (Refer to the text for examples.)

2. Describe the following nurse-accessible therapies, including their advantages and limitations:
   a. Relaxation therapy, progressive and passive
   b. Meditation and breathing
   c. Imagery

3. Ask students how the biobehavioral therapies may be used for clients experiencing:
   a. Dysfunctional grieving
   b. Sleep disorders
   c. Hypertension
   d. Cardiac dysrhythmias
   e. Cerebrovascular or neurological injury
   d. End-stage cancer

4. Describe the following training-specific therapies, including their advantages and limitations:
   a. Biofeedback
   b. Therapeutic touch
   c. Chiropractic therapy
   d. Traditional Chinese medicine
   e. Acupuncture
   d. Herbal therapies

5. Ask students to identify how training-specific therapies may be applied to clinical situations.

6. Discuss the role of the nurse in relation to complementary and alternative therapies, including the assessment of clients who may benefit from their use and the support of clients who select these therapies.

7. Stimulate a discussion on different complementary and alternative therapies to elicit students' attitudes or perceptions about their use in client care.

8. Ask students to share personal or family experiences with the use of complementary and alternative therapies.

9. Compare and contrast the different complementary and alternative therapies.

10. Guide students in the application of the nursing process for clients selecting complementary or alternative therapies.

Interactive Exercises

1. Organize a debate on the benefits versus the dangers of alternative therapies.

2. Assign students to investigate available community resources for complementary and/or alternative therapies.

Clinical Skill/Technique

1. Demonstrate and have students practice appropriate nurse-accessible therapies.

Client Care Experiences

1. Have students assess their clients to determine, if they are not already in use, whether complementary or alternative therapies may be beneficial. Discuss how the client and the primary health care provider may be approached to suggest the use of selected therapies.

2. Assign students to incorporate the use of complementary and/or alternative therapies into the care plan/critical pathway for their assigned clients, as indicated.

Resource for Student Activity

Comparison Chart of Nurse-accessible Therapies

Biobehavioral Therapies

	Description/ Effects	Clinical Applications	Limitations
Relaxation			
Meditation			
Breathing			
Imagery			

Critical Thinking Exercises (from text page 926)

Client Profile: Margaret is a 76-year-old Catholic woman who has been diagnosed with a slow-growing renal tumor. She has been scheduled for surgery in 2 weeks. She is afraid of both the surgical procedure and the outcome. Is it cancer? Will the surgery result in a disability? After surgery, she becomes depressed.

1. What specific nursing-accessible CAM interventions can the nurse offer Margaret to prepare for the surgery and reduce her anxiety?

2. What CAM therapi.es may be appropriate to help her deal with her depression?

Suggested Answers

1. Nursing-accessible interventions: To help reduce the anxiety of the situation, the nurse can teach Margaret relaxation breathing and meditation exercises to do several times a day; help her create visualizations of the surgery as a healing experience; help her ask her church congregation to pray for her, especially during the surgery; help her find relaxing music to listen to before and after the surgery by using a portable CD or tape player and headphones; make sure that supportive members of Margaret's family are with her before and after the surgery to provide comfort and support, etc. Teach the use of guided imagery, relaxation breathing, or meditation to reduce postoperative pain

2. CAM therapies to help depression: Music therapy using songs that Margaret enjoyed when she was younger can stimulate pleasant memories to elevate her mood. Suggest using St. John's wort as an herbal remedy for depression.

36

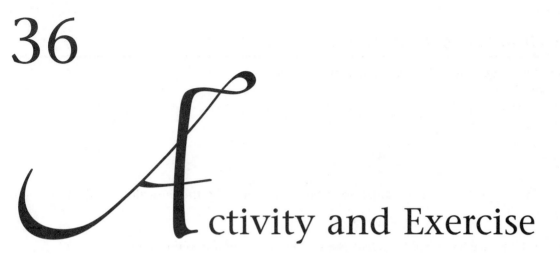

$\mathcal{A}$ctivity and Exercise

Instructor Media Resources

Instructor's Resource CD
evolve **Instructor's Resources**

Instructor's Manual
ExamView Test Bank
Image Collection
Power Point Slides
Weblinks

Student Media Resources

CD COMPANION

- Review Questions
- Glossary

evolve **WEBSITE**

- Review Questions
- Student Learning Activities
- Glossary

Classroom Discussion

1. Discuss body mechanics, exercise, and activity, including:
   a. Body alignment
   b. Body balance
   c. Coordinated body movement
   d. Friction
   e. Exercise and activity

2. Review the regulation and coordination of body movement by the musculoskeletal and nervous systems.

3. Discuss the principles of body mechanics and their integration into nursing care.

4. Describe pathological influences on body alignment and mobility, including pathological influences; congenital abnormalities, disorders of the bone, joints, and muscles; central nervous system (CNS) damage; and musculoskeletal trauma.
   Ask students to identify specific pathological problems that may be experienced by clients.

5. Review growth and development across the life span in respect to musculoskeletal and neurological function and mobility. Ask students to identify specific changes that may influence mobility status and place the individual at risk.

6. Discuss the following in relation to an individual's activity and exercise:
   a. Behavioral aspects and lifestyle
   b. Environmental issues: work, school, community
   c. Cultural and ethnic influences
   d. Family and social support

7. Describe the assessment of client mobility in the following areas:
   a. Posture/positioning
   b. Mobility/gait
   c. Activity tolerance

   Ask students what constitutes expected or abnormal findings in the assessment of mobility.

8. Describe the general effects of exercise on the body systems, as well as the specific benefits of specific types of exercise (e.g., isometric).

9. Guide students in the application of the nursing process for clients who need to maintain or regain their activity and exercise abilities.

10. Discuss joint mobility and range of motion (ROM). Explain the use of the continuous passive range-of-motion machine (CPROM). Have students identify how ROM exercises may be integrated into other nursing care activities.

11. Ask students to identify possible situations in which additional assistance may be needed to position or ambulate a client.

12. Invite a physical therapist to speak to the class about measures to promote exercise and activity for clients in the community and acute and restorative care agencies.

13. Review the importance of safety and comfort measures when assisting clients with activity and exercise.

14. Ask students to share their own activity and exercise regimens.

$\mathcal{I}$nteractive Exercises

1. Have students develop a teaching plan that incorporates basic exercise for an older adult or correct use of an assistive device.

2. Have students identify the activity and exercise needs and the nursing approaches for the following or similar client situations:
   a. An 8-year-old child with acute asthma
   b. An 86-year-old who has had a cerebrovascular accident (CVA) with resultant left-sided hemiplegia
   c. A 45-year-old overweight client
   d. A 16-year-old with a casted fracture of the right tibia and limited weight bearing (crutches required)
   e. A 65-year-old with peripheral neuropathy
   f. A 48-year-old with hypertension
   g. A 56-year-old who has had a myocardial infarction (MI)

$\mathcal{C}$linical Skills/Techniques

1. Explain and demonstrate (by using simulation mannequin/model or volunteer, appropriate equipment, and educational media, as available) specific nursing interventions that may be implemented to promote proper body alignment and mobility, including:
   a. Lifting (by the nurse)
   b. Use of assistive devices for ambulation: walking belt, walker, cane, crutches

2. Have small groups of students practice the skills to promote body alignment and mobility, by using the appropriate equipment and supplies, and document the procedure and status of the client accordingly. Supervise activities such as lifting and crutch walking.

3. Evaluate the students' ability to implement and document selected skills through return-demonstration/skill testing before clinical experience.

$\mathcal{C}$lient Care Experiences

1. Assign students to observe and participate in the nursing care of clients in acute, restorative, or home care settings, with focus placed on the promotion of body alignment and mobility.

   Discuss expectations of students before the experience, specifically emphasizing client safety and requesting assistance in moving clients.

   Review the students' assessments, strategies used, and evaluation of clients' mobility status after the experience.

2. Have students complete care plans/pathways for their assigned clients, incorporating interventions designed to promote activity and exercise.

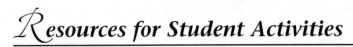

Resources for Student Activities

Musculoskeletal Development across the Life Span
Benefits of Exercise

Musculoskeletal Development Across the Life Span

Age Group	Musculoskeletal Changes
Infants	
Toddlers	
Preschool to Adolescents	
Young to Middle Adults	
Older Adult	

Benefits of Exercise

Target	Benefits of Exercise
Client with Coronary Heart Disease	
Client with Hypertension	
Client with Chronic Pulmonary Disease	
Client with Diabetes Mellitus	
Older Adult Client	
Immobile Client	
Client with Multiple Sclerosis	

Critical Thinking Exercises (from text page 956)

1. Ms. Moushey is an 52-year-old woman. She sustained a fracture of the left femur and must use crutches for 1 week until her follow-up visit at the orthopedic clinic. Her physician has ordered no weight bearing on the left leg. You are conducting the first home visit after her discharge from the hospital. What is the appropriate crutch gait for Ms. Moushey? List several teaching strategies that focus on crutch safety.

2. Mr. Neel has just undergone extensive abdominal surgery. What assessment parameters should be considered before ambulation of this client? What precautions should you take before helping him to ambulate for the first time?

3. The family of Mrs. Parks made the decision to care for her at home. She is a quadriplegic, weighs 72 kg, and is in total care. You are her nurse and responsible for instructing her family on several aspects of her care. Develop a list of basic principles describing body mechanics to protect Mrs. Parks's family members from injury.

Suggested Answers

1. The appropriate crutch gait for Ms. Moushey is the three-point alternating, or three-point gait that requires the client to bear all of the weight on one foot. Several teaching strategies can be used for Ms. Moushey. It is important that these be individualized to meet the learning needs of the client. Some examples of teaching strategies are:
   - Teach client with axillary crutches about the dangers of pressure on the axillae, which occurs when leaning on the crutches to support body weight.
   - Explain why client must use crutches that were measured for him or her.
   - Show client how to inspect crutch tips routinely. Rubber tips should be securely attached to the crutches. When tips are worn, they should be replaced. Rubber crutch tips increase surface friction and help prevent slipping.
   - Explain that the crutch tips should remain dry. Water decreases surface friction and increases the risk of slipping.
   - Show client how to dry the crutch tips if they become wet; client may use paper or cloth towels.

2. Assessment parameters for Mr. Neel should include physiological parameters such as vital signs, muscle strength, weakness, endurance, pain, fatigue, and level of consciousness. Precautions before helping Mr. Neel to ambulate should focus on securing drains and tubes, assessing for dizziness, applying a gait belt, using the help of another staff member, and applying nonskid shoes to prevent slipping and provide support.

3. Each of the following principles of body mechanics should be demonstrated to the family members. Allow each family member to provide a return demonstration to evaluate understanding and correct body mechanics. The following principles of body mechanics are:

The wider the base of support, the greater the stability of the nurse.

The lower the center of gravity, the greater the stability of the nurse.

The equilibrium of an object is maintained as long as the line of gravity passes through its base of support.

Facing the direction of movement prevents abnormal twisting of the spine.

Dividing balanced activity between arms and legs reduces the risk of back injury.

Leverage, rolling, turning, or pivoting requires less work than lifting.

When friction is reduced between the object to be moved and the surface on which it is moved, less force is required to move it.

Reducing the force of work reduces the risk of injury.

Maintaining good body mechanics reduces fatigue of the muscle groups.

Alternating periods of rest and activity helps to reduce fatigue.

37

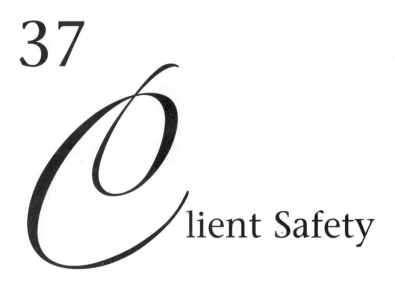

Client Safety

Instructor Media Resources

Instructor's Resource CD
evolve **Instructor's Resources**

Instructor's Manual
ExamView Test Bank
Image Collection
Power Point Slides
Skills Checklists

Student Media Resources

CD COMPANION

- Review Questions
- Glossary

evolve **WEBSITE**

- Review Questions
- Student Learning Activities
- Glossary

Classroom Discussion

1. Discuss the concept of a "safe environment" in respect to health care and community settings.

2. Review the basic needs that should be met in a safe environment: oxygen, nutrition, temperature, and humidity. Ask students to provide specific examples of how those needs may be met by the client and/or nurse in diverse health care settings.

3. Discuss the major causes of accidents/accidental deaths in the home and health care environment. Ask students to contribute the possible underlying causes of these accidents.

4. Identify physical hazards and how they may be reduced in the home and health care setting. Have students indicate specific measures that may be implemented to reduce hazards. Ask students to share personal experiences of safety hazards that have been identified and/or eliminated in their home or occupational setting.

5. Review concepts of growth and development that have an impact on safety throughout the life span. Review specific safety concerns of different age groups from infancy to older adulthood. Ask students identify target areas for prevention of age-related injuries (e.g., helmets for bicycle riding).

6. Review how the reducing the transmission of pathogens contributes to overall client safety and well-being. Have students specify nursing interventions and client instruction that may be implemented to reduce pathogens in the home and health care setting.

7. Given the following, or similar situations, have students determine possible safety hazards and preventive measures:
   a. New parents going home with their first child.
   b. An older adult living alone in a third-floor apartment that has wooden floors, throw rugs, cluttered areas, and dark hallways and stairwells.
   c. A single-parent family living in an inner city area where crime and drug abuse are prevalent.
   d. New homes built on and around an old chemical plant site.
   e. A client with tuberculosis (TB) going home to live with his large family.
   f. An individual whose sexual partner is a known drug user.

8. Discuss the types of pollution present today and their affects on people and the environment. Ask students what the role of the nurse should be in reducing or eliminating environmental pollution.

9. Guide students in the application of the nursing process for clients who are at risk of injury.

10. Describe the components of a home safety assessment.

11. Discuss bioterrorism, possible biological agents that may be used, and how it may be recognized and responded to by health care workers. Review the components of an emergency management plan.

12. Identify and/or ask students to identify risk factors that contribute to safety hazards, including lifestyle behaviors, mobility, sensory impairment, and overall awareness.

13. Discuss safety risks (falls, accidents) that are specific to the health care setting, including client-inherent, procedure-related, and equipment-related situations. Ask students to identify potential risks and preventive measures in acute, extended, rehabilitative, and home care settings. Stimulate a discussion on similarities and differences in these different settings with respect to safety hazards and prevention of accidents.

14. Explain the nursing responsibilities associated with the following interventions:
    a. Seizure precautions
    b. Use of restraints
    c. Intervening in poisoning
    d. Fire, electrical, and radiation safety
    e. Disaster readiness/emergency management in response to bioterrorism or natural catastrophes

    Ask students to provide examples of situations in which these interventions may be implemented, and the decision making that is required of the nurse.

15. Ask students to identify hazard-prevention resources that are readily available to consumers, such as carbon monoxide and fire/smoke detectors, bicycle helmets, child proof locks, etc

16. Review overall measures to promote and maintain client safety in the home, community, and health care setting.

17. Invite a nurse risk manager to speak to the class about his or her role in reducing or eliminating safety hazards in the health care environment.

18. Invite a representative from a local fire department to speak to the class about home and health care agency fire-safety measures, and the nurse's responsibility for fire control and evacuation.

19. By using the following, or similar, situations, have students identify the health and safety risks for clients and families, and specify possible measures to alleviate or prevent them:
    a. A living environment with flaking paint, crowding, poor lighting and ventilation
    b. An adolescent having unprotected sex
    c. An older adult with diminished eyesight and peripheral sensation

*I*nteractive Exercises

1. Have students investigate the types of pollution that may be evident in their own neighborhood and/or work environment.

2. Assign students to complete the Home Hazard Assessment and report, orally and/or in writing, on their findings.

3. Assign students to investigate and report on media examples, such as public service announcements, that focus on safety issues.

4. Have students investigate where hazard-prevention resources (e.g., smoke detectors) may be obtained if the client/family does not have sufficient finances.

5. Arrange for students to attend, if possible, a mandatory employee-safety program in an acute care facility.

6. Assign students to investigate and report on safety statistics (e.g., client falls) within an affiliating health care agency, and the agency's plans to reduce the overall incidence of accidents/injuries.

7. Have students contact the local poison-control center and ask about common poisoning situations and treatments.

8. Assign students to obtain information on a health care institution's emergency-management or disaster-readiness plan. If possible, have students attend a workshop on this topic.

Clinical Skills/Techniques

1. Explain and demonstrate the following skills (by using simulation mannequin/model, appropriate equipment, and available educational media):
   a. Applying restraints
   b. Seizure precautions

2. Have small groups of students practice the skills by using the appropriate equipment and supplies and document the procedure.

3. Evaluate the students' ability to implement and document the hazard-prevention skills through return-demonstration/skill testing before clinical experience.

Client Care Experiences

1. Have students identify and implement a hazard-prevention plan for a specific target group/community, such as home childproofing, sport injury prevention, adolescent suicide, or fire and burn safety for older individuals.

2. Assign students to observe and participate in the nursing care of clients within an acute, restorative, community, and/or home care environment, focusing on the promotion of safety and reduction of hazards.
   Discuss expectations with the group before the experience, identifying the parameters for assessment of client risk, and the implementation and evaluation of preventive strategies.

3. Have students report back on their clients' teaching/learning needs, interactions, and other identified risks for injury.

4. Have students complete a care plan/pathway for an assigned client who is at risk for injury.

Resources for Student Activities

Safety Concerns across the Life Span Chart

Safety Concerns Across The Life Span

Age Group	Specific Safety Concern	Preventive Measures/Teaching
Infant		
Toddler/Preschool Child		
School-age Child		
Adolescent		
Adult		
Older Adult		

Critical Thinking Exercises (from text page 998)

1. Mrs. Santiago, who is 88 years old, was recently admitted to the hospital. Although she was independent at home, the admission assessment reveals she is at risk for falling because of urinary frequency, an unsteady gait, and recent mental status changes. Design specific interventions to ensure the client's safety in the hospital.

2. Mrs. Carr, a 76-year-old nursing home resident with Alzheimer's disease, has been refusing food and fluids for the past month. The family has agreed to placement of a nasogastric (NG) tube to improve her fluid and nutritional status. Shortly after the first tube feeding was started, Mrs. Carr became more restless, and she has been picking at the tube.
   a. What might be precipitating Mrs. Carr's behavior of picking at the tube?
   b. What approaches can be used to eliminate interference with the treatment?
   c. If a restraint is necessary to avoid disruption of therapy, what interventions are necessary to ensure the client's safety while in restraints?

3. A family member reports that a lit cigarette dropped on the client's mattress, but they were able to put out the small fire. What actions are needed to ensure the safety of clients?

Suggested Answers

1. Interventions should focus on elimination of environmental risks and prevention of injury during ambulation. Make sure the bed is in the low position with wheels locked. Orient the client on how to use the call light at the bedside and in the bathroom. Instruct her to call for help before getting up. Place all needed items within reach, such as eyeglasses, dentures, and hearing aid. Provide frequent checks and scheduled toileting. Make sure the client wears well-fitting shoes or slippers with nonskid soles when ambulating. Provide a clear pathway to the bathroom and adequate room lighting. Evaluate the need for a bedside commode during the night hours. Put the top bed rails in the up position and instruct client on how to use them to assist in turning or to sit up. If available, place an electronic monitoring device on the client that triggers an audio alarm when the client attempts to ambulate unassisted. Evaluate the need for a physical therapy (PT) referral or an assistive device to increase stability during ambulation. In addition, investigate what might be the cause of her recent mental status changes, such as multiple medications, an electrolyte imbalance, or an emotional response to a recent loss of a loved one.

2. a. Mrs. Carr's behavior might be precipitated by the discomfort associated with the NG tube, such as dry mouth, irritation of the nares due to friction or crusting of nasal secretions, or perhaps the adhesive tape holding the tube in place is causing irritation. Mrs. Carr also may lack the understanding of why the tube was inserted and may be frightened by the pump alarms.
   b. Based on your assessment of the reason for Mrs. Carr's behavior, multiple approaches should be attempted to prevent interference with the prescribed treatment. Orient Mrs. Carr to the device and its purpose. Explain why the tube is in place and how it is connected to a feeding pump. Show Mrs. Carr the pump and explain how and why the alarm sounds. To address the discomfort associated with the tube, provide nasal and oral care at least every shift or more often as needed. If possible, continue oral intake and periodically reassess the continued need for the treatment. If physical causes have been ruled out, intensify supervision of the client by having a family member, sitter, or assistive personnel stay with the client. As a last resort, and only if alternative measures are unsuccessful at preventing interruption of therapy, consult with the physician and family for consideration of a mitten or wrist restraint.

c. To ensure Mrs. Carr's safety while in a restraint, it is essential that the device be correctly applied. The nurse should review the manufacturer's instructions before application and any agency-specific restraint policies. Pad the client's skin if needed to protect the skin from irritation. Secure the device to the bed frame, not the side rails, by using a quick-release tie. Secure the call light within reach of the client. Provide frequent monitoring of the client in restraints. Check Mrs. Carr at least every hour, assessing for proper placement, presence of pulses, temperature, color, and sensation of the restrained extremity. Remove the restraints at least every 2 hours to provide range of motion, skin care, toileting, food/fluid, exercise, and opportunities for socialization. Monitor the client's response to application of the device and frequently reassess for continued need. Discontinue the restraint at the earliest possible time.

3. After receiving this report from the family, immediately go to the client's room and assess the situation. Although the fire on the surface of the mattress may appear to be out, smoldering can occur inside the mattress. Assess the client for the presence of any injury. Call for assistance in evacuating those clients that are in immediate danger. Get help if needed when moving the client from the bed. Activate the fire alarm after all clients and visitors are out of danger. Take measures to contain or put out the fire by closing the door to the room, turning off any oxygen or electrical equipment, and locating the nearest fire extinguisher. After fire department personnel are on the scene and the situation is under control, perform a more thorough assessment of the client and notify the physician. Finally, thank the family for reporting the event. Review with the patient and family why smoking in the room is unsafe (e.g., oxygen is in use and is combustible, placing other clients at risk for injury), and if necessary, identify alternative means to allow the client to smoke safely.

38

$\mathcal{H}$ygiene

Classroom Discussion

1. Discuss the measures that constitute personal hygiene and the usual hygienic care that is provided in the acute and extended care health setting.

2. Discuss factors that may influence hygienic care practices. Have students identify how these factors may alter the nurse's approach to the client.

3. Review the anatomy and physiology of the integumentary system.

4. Review the physical assessment of the skin, hair, nails, mouth, teeth, and feet (refer to text, Chapter 32). Use photos, illustrations, models, and videos, as available.
   Ask students to identify how the physical assessment may be integrated into hygienic care and to specify expected and unexpected findings of the assessment.

5. Review developmental changes that occur in the skin, hair, nails, and teeth throughout the life span.

6. Ask students to identify the information about the client's self-care abilities and personal hygienic practices that determines the type of hygienic care and amount of assistance provided by the nurse.

7. Review possible risks for skin impairment. Have students provide additional situations in which preventive measures may be indicated for the client.

8. Explain the multiple purposes of hygienic care, including cleanliness, exercise, relaxation, improved self-image, and stimulation of circulation and respiration.
   Ask students how the hygienic care routine may provide an opportunity for communication with the client.

9. Review the guidelines for bathing a client: privacy, safety, warmth, and independence.
   Have students provide specific examples of how the nurse achieves these guidelines.

10. Discuss the principles of perineal care for male and female clients.

11. Ask students how the bath of a newborn/infant and young child differs from that of an adult.

12. Discuss general foot care and appropriate footwear.
    Describe and demonstrate special foot care that is provided for clients with reduced peripheral circulation (e.g., clients with diabetes).

13. Identify and/or ask students to identify risk factors that may contribute to oral hygiene problems. Describe common oral problems that the nurse may encounter (use photos/illustrations).

14. Discuss general guidelines for oral hygiene. Ask students to identify the special considerations that would be indicated for clients who are unconscious, prone to stomatitis, diabetic, or experiencing an oral infection.

15. Identify common hair and scalp problems.

16. Describe general measures that may be implemented to assist the client with hair care, including brushing, combing, shampooing, and shaving. Ask students to identify specific precautions that should be taken to avoid client injury.

17. Review the physical assessment of the eyes, ears, and nose (refer to text, Chapter 32).
    Discuss the expected and unexpected findings that may be assessed by the nurse.

18. Describe general measures that are incorporated into the hygienic care of the eyes, ears, and nose, and the maintenance of sensory aids (e.g., glasses, contact lenses, artificial eyes, and hearing aids).

19. Ask students how the client's environment, in the home or health care setting, may be modified to increase comfort, cleanliness, and a feeling of security.

20. Discuss general principles of bed making, including the situations that warrant making unoccupied or occupied beds.

21. Have students discuss how sociocultural practices may influence a client's hygienic care.

22. For the following situations, have students identify how hygienic care measures may be adapted by the nurse to meet the client's needs:
    a. A client with right-sided weakness after a cerebrovascular accident (CVA)
    b. An obese client with shortness of breath, residing at home, who has access to only a bathtub
    c. An older client with some difficulty in balance
    d. A newborn, a 2-year-old, or an 8-year-old
    e. A client with casts on both arms and/or legs
    f. An unconscious client
    g. A severely depressed client
    h. An adolescent client with acne
    i. A middle-aged adult client with diabetes mellitus

Interactive Exercises

1. Assign students to design a teaching plan for the following, or similar client situations, with respect to hygienic care practices:
   a. New parents with a 3-day-old newborn
   b. A client with diabetes
   c. An older client with dry skin
   d. A client taking anticoagulant medication

2. Ask students to determine what resources may be available and what adaptations may be indicated for implementation of hygienic care in the client's home environment (e.g., availability of hot water).

Clinical Skills/Techniques

1. Have students modify a simulated acute/restorative care client environment to increase client comfort and privacy by manipulating available equipment and furniture.

2. Explain and demonstrate (by using simulation mannequin/model or volunteer, appropriate equipment/supplies, and educational media, as available) the following selected nursing interventions for promotion of client hygiene:
   a. Bathing/perineal care/back rub/"bag bath"
   b. Nail and foot care
   c. Mouth care/denture cleansing
   d. Hair/scalp care
   e. Care of sensory aids: contact lenses and hearing aids
   f. Unoccupied and occupied bed making

3. Have small groups or pairs of students practice the performance and documentation of the skills by using the appropriate equipment and supplies.

4. Evaluate the students' ability to implement and document the selected hygienic care interventions through return-demonstration/skill testing before clinical experience.

Client Care Experiences

1. Assign students to participate in the nursing care of clients in a variety of health care settings, specifically focusing on the implementation of hygienic care measures.

   Discuss with the group, before the experience, the decision making involved in determining the client's hygienic care needs.

2. Have students complete a care plan/pathway for an assigned client in whom a self-care limitation exists that influences the achievement of hygienic care.

Resource for Student Activity

Comparison Chart of Hygienic Care Measures from Infant to Adult

Specific Hygienic Care Measures Across the Life Span

Age Group	Specific Hygienic Care
Newborn	
Infant	
Toddler/Preschooler	
School-age Child	
Adolescent	
Adult	
Older Adult	

Critical Thinking Exercises (from text page 1064)

1. Mrs. Truman is a 62-year-old woman being seen in the internal medicine clinic during her follow-up appointment for management of her diabetes mellitus. During the nurse's conversation with Mrs. Truman, the client says, "You know, last week I found a sore on my left foot; I didn't even know it was there." What type of assessment should the nurse conduct for Mrs. Truman, and what recommendations are needed for Mrs. Truman's foot care regimen?

2. Mr. Golf had abdominal trauma in a motorcycle accident. Abdominal surgery resulted in an ileostomy, which is leaking liquid fecal material on his skin. In addition, he has a postoperative infection, is diaphoretic and has a high fever, and has a nasogastric tube in place. What factors must you consider when providing hygiene care? Include rationales for assessments and interventions.

3. Peter Nixon is an 18-year-old admitted to the neurosurgical intensive care unit after a head injury. Peter is currently unconscious, responsive only to painful stimulus. What assessment is critical for the nurse to perform before providing oral hygiene?

Suggested Answers

1. The nurse should assess Mrs. Truman's feet for sensory perception, circulation, and observe for any red areas or indications of pressure. The nurse should review Mrs. Truman's daily foot care practices and use of cotton socks, appropriate footwear, frequency of going barefoot, etc. A referral to a foot care clinic or podiatrist is important to determine baseline information and observe for and treat any foot problems.

2. a. Assessments:
   i. Skin around surgical wound and around areas of fecal contamination: observe for impaired skin integrity.
   ii. Pressure areas due to decreased mobility, increased body temperature, and secretions increase risk for impaired skin integrity.
   iii. Oral mucosa fever: increases risk of dry mouth and impaired integrity of oral tissue.
   iv. Nasal mucosa, as client probably has a nasogastric tube
   b. Interventions
   i. Increased frequency of total and targeted skin care. Maintain skin dry and intact
   ii. Increased monitoring of skin integrity status to pressure areas, nares, and skin surrounding incision and ileostomy
   iii. Increased frequency of position change
   iv. Increase linen changes
   v. Increased frequency and specialization of oral hygiene

3. Clients who have had serious neurological injury involving the brain must be assessed for the presence of a gag reflex. Absence of a gag reflex will make the client more prone to aspiration during cleansing of the oral cavity.

39

$\mathcal{O}$xygenation

Classroom Discussion

1. Review normal anatomy and physiology and common pathophysiological changes in the cardiac and respiratory systems.

2. Discuss factors that affect oxygenation, including physiological, developmental, lifestyle, and environmental. Ask students to identify specific examples of how and why these factors affect oxygenation.

3. Describe the following alterations in cardiac function that influence oxygenation and the signs and symptoms associated with each: conduction disturbances, altered cardiac output, impaired valvular function, and myocardial ischemia.

4. Describe the following alterations in respiratory function and the signs and symptoms associated with each: hyperventilation, hypoventilation, and hypoxia.

5. Describe the assessment of the client's oxygenation status (refer to text, Chapter 32), including the history, physical examination, and diagnostic/laboratory tests.

6. Identify components of the nursing history relevant to the client's oxygenation status, such as fatigue, dyspnea, coughing, wheezing, pain, possible exposure, infections, risk factors, and medication administration.

7. Review the physical assessment techniques and components that are specific to determining a client's oxygenation status

8. Identify and describe diagnostic/laboratory tests that are used to determine the client's cardiopulmonary function and oxygenation status (see Resources for Student Activities).
   Have students identify the client preparation and education that is necessary before these diagnostic/laboratory tests.

9. Identify and/or have students identify nursing interventions that may be implemented for the promotion and maintenance of a client's oxygenation. Incorporate how the interventions may be adapted according to the client's developmental status.

10. Discuss the use of influenza and pneumococcal vaccines, including their indications and contraindications for use.

11. Discuss what clients are at a greater risk for reduced oxygenation because of occupational or geographical exposure.

12. Describe secondary and tertiary care for clients with alterations in oxygenation:
    a. Dyspnea management
    b. Maintenance of patent airway
    c. Mobilization of pulmonary secretions
    d. Suctioning

13. Ask students to identify the rationale for nursing interventions that promote oxygenation.

14. Describe the placement and suctioning of artificial airways by using photos/illustrations, and/or videos, as available.

15. Discuss oxygen therapy and the nurse's responsibilities associated with its use in the health care and home environments. Have students identify the specific safety measures that must be implemented in the presence of oxygen therapy.

16. Invite a respiratory therapist to speak to the class about client oxygenation needs. Ask the therapist to demonstrate different types of equipment, their uses, and monitoring requirements.

17. Discuss the purpose, insertion, maintenance, and removal of chest tubes.

18. Discuss the maintenance and promotion of oxygenation in the restorative and home care environments and the role of the nurse in client education and monitoring.

19. Guide students in the application of the critical thinking model and the nursing process for clients experiencing alterations in oxygenation.

Interactive Exercises

1. Have students investigate and report on environmental pollutants that are present in their community, what their influence may be on the health status of that community, and what measures may be taken to eliminate or reduce the level of pollutants.

2. Provide photos/illustrations of different types of oxygen equipment and have students identify the use, flow rate, and client considerations for each one.

Clinical Skills/Techniques

1. Demonstrate select cardiovascular and pulmonary assessment techniques to reinforce the information.

2. Demonstrate coughing, deep breathing, use of the incentive spirometer, positioning, chest physiotherapy, and postural drainage to the class. Have students practice the techniques individually and/or with a partner.

3. Explain and demonstrate (by using simulation mannequin/model, appropriate equipment/supplies, and educational media) the following nursing interventions for the promotion/evaluation of client oxygenation:
   a. Suctioning
   b. Care of an artificial airway
   c. Care of chest tubes
   d. Application of a nasal cannula and oxygen mask
   e. Use of home liquid oxygen equipment (as available)
   f. Pulse oximetry (refer to text, Chapter 31 for review)

4. Have pairs or small groups of students practice the implementation and documentation of the specified nursing interventions for promotion of oxygenation.

5. Evaluate the students' ability to implement and document the interventions to promote client oxygenation through return-demonstration/skill testing before clinical experience.

6. Discuss and demonstrate or show a video of cardiopulmonary resuscitation (CPR).

7. Assign students to complete a CPR class (preferably health care–provider level) through an approved provider and verify with possession of certification card.

Client Care Experiences

1. Assign students to observe and participate in the nursing care of clients with actual or potential alterations in oxygenation in a variety of health care settings.
   Focus on the assessment of the client's oxygenation status and the implementation of measures to support and/or improve cardiopulmonary function (e.g., positioning, coughing, deep breathing).

2. Supervise the administration of appropriate medications and oxygen therapy.

3. Evaluate the students' ability to implement and document nursing interventions for the promotion of oxygenation.

4. Have students design and implement a teaching plan for an assigned client with an oxygenation deficit, who requires oxygen therapy in the home.

5. Have students complete a plan of care/pathway for a client experiencing alterations in oxygenation and requiring strategies for the promotion of cardiopulmonary function.

Resources for Student Activities

Select Factors Affecting Oxygenation Chart
Diagnostic Tests for Oxygenation Status: Client Preparation and Data Obtained

Select Factors and their Affect on Oxygenation

Factors	Effect on Oxygenation Status
Hypovolemia	
Pregnancy	
Obesity	
Kyphosis	
Exercise	
Smoking	
Substance Abuse	
Anxiety	
Premature Birth	

Diagnostic Tests for Oxygenation Status

Focus	Diagnostic Tests	Client Preparation	Data Obtained
Cardiac Conduction			
Cardiac Contraction/ Blood Flow			
Ventilation/ Oxygenation			
Blood Studies			
Visualization of Structures			
Determination of Infection			

Critical Thinking Exercises (from text page 1132)

1. Ms. Wanda Johnson is a 56-year-old postmenopausal woman with a history of hypertension. She appears in her primary care office with complaints of nausea, indigestion, increased fatigue, and shortness of breath with increased activity for the past 16 hours. What questions would you ask Ms. Johnson in the history?

2. Mr. Jose Martinez has recently immigrated to the United States from his homeland of Cuba to join his family. He comes to the clinic because he has been increasingly fatigued, has a persistent cough, has been losing weight, and awakens at night with sweats. What questions would be important to ask when completing the health history?

3. Mrs. Amanda Miller, age 45 years, has been admitted to the hospital with community-acquired pneumonia. She has a productive cough, fever, chills, crackles, and wheezes on auscultation of her chest and a heart rate of 104 beats per minute. What nursing diagnosis would you consider for this client? What nursing interventions would be appropriate for Mrs. Miller? What health promotion interventions should be initiated before discharge from the hospital?

4. Mr. Chen Lee, age 72 years, has been having chest pain, shortness of breath, and pain down his left arm for about 2 hours. He comes to the emergency department because the pain has been getting worse over the past hour. What nursing interventions would you initiate?

Suggested Answers

1. Because women often have atypical symptoms for heart disease, the nurse must have a high suspicion and include questions that would differentiate chest pain from abdominal pain. Questions to include are (1) When did the pain start? (2) What made the pain better? (3) On a scale of 0 to 10, how would you rate the pain? 4) What have you eaten in the past 24 hours? (4) have you ever had anything like this before? (5) is there any history of heart disease in the family? Additional questions would include what medications she was currently taking.

2. Most likely he has tuberculosis (TB). Be sure to question him about the length of time he has had symptoms, if anyone else in his family has been told they have TB, if he has ever received any medication for TB, and who are his close personal contacts.

3. Nursing diagnoses could include *Airway clearance, ineffective*; *Breathing pattern, ineffective*; *Fatigue*; and *Fluid volume, deficient*. Nursing interventions to consider include hydration, coughing and deep breathing, administration of ordered medications, and monitoring of lung sounds and vital signs. It will be important that the client get a pneumococcal vaccine after the acute pneumonia has completely resolved. If flu season is near, an influenza vaccination also is indicated.

4. Nursing interventions would include elevation of the head of the bed, obtaining vital signs, obtaining orders for oxygen therapy, administration of aspirin, 325 mg, as ordered, sublingual nitroglycerine as ordered, monitoring of cardiac rhythm, and initiation of an IV, as ordered. The nurse would also provide emotional support to the client and family as the initial evaluation and therapies are initiated.

40

*F*luid, Electrolyte, and Acid-Base Balances

Classroom Discussion

1. By using educational media (e.g., illustrations, overhead transparencies), review the composition, distribution, movement, and regulation of body fluids, including:
   a. Extracellular fluid (ECF) and intracellular fluid (ICF) compartments
   b. Examples of body fluid movement
   c. Fluid intake
   d. Hormonal regulation
   e. Fluid output

   Provide examples of different types of intravenous (IV) solutions, and ask students how they will influence fluid movement within the body.

2. Review the major cations and anions, their functions, regulatory mechanisms, sources, and normal blood values. Ask students to provide examples of food sources for each electrolyte.

3. Discuss acid/base balance, and the chemical, biological, and physiological mechanisms of regulation within the body.

4. Discuss disturbances in fluid, electrolyte, and acid/base balance, including possible etiology, signs and symptoms, and clients with a greater risk of developing the imbalances.
   Ask students to give the rationale for the physiological manifestations and why particular clients are at risk to develop these imbalances.

5. Identify variables that affect fluid, electrolyte, and acid/base balance, including age, illness, environment, diet, lifestyle, and medication. Have students provide specific examples of the effects of these variables on different clients (e.g., why an infant is more susceptible to fluid imbalances).

6. Guide students in the application of the critical thinking model and nursing process for clients experiencing an alteration in fluid, electrolyte, and/or acid/base balance.

7. Describe the nursing assessment and physical examination of clients to determine actual or potential fluid, electrolyte, or acid/base disturbances.

8. Discuss common health problems and client situations in which a greater risk occurs for imbalances, including surgery, burns, cardiovascular disorders, respiratory disorders, renal disorders, cancer, head injuries, and gastrointestinal disturbances. Ask students to identify which imbalances may be present in these situations, and how they may be assessed by the nurse.

9. Explain the role of daily weights and intake (I) and output (O) measurement in the determination of fluid balance. Discuss what is included in fluid I & O, and have students practice the calculation and documentation of sample/actual client intake and output for a prescribed period.

10. Identify laboratory tests that may be used to determine fluid, electrolyte, and acid/base disturbances.

11. Discuss the following measures that may be implemented to correct fluid, electrolyte, and/or acid/base disturbances and the associated nursing responsibilities for each:
    a. Enteral replacement
    b. Fluid restriction
    c. Parenteral replacement

12. Discuss the initiation, monitoring/maintenance, and discontinuation of IV therapy. Review aseptic technique!

13. Describe potential complications associated with IV therapy, including phlebitis, infiltration, fluid overload, bleeding, and infection.

14. Discuss blood replacement and administration, nursing responsibilities, and precautions. Have students identify what nursing interventions are peculiar to the IV administration of blood products.

15. Discuss medical interventions and associated nursing strategies that may be implemented to correct problems underlying acid/base disturbances.

16. Discuss the assessment of fluid, electrolyte, and acid/base imbalances and how nursing strategies may be altered to monitor and assist clients in extended and community health care settings.

*I*nteractive Exercises

1. Provide students with sample client weights and have them calculate fluid volume changes (by using 5 lbs = 2.5 L).

2. Have students, by using the following and/or a similar sample situation, determine the client's I&O in milliliters:

1/2 cup ice cream	urine, 480 ml
1 cup coffee	wound drainage, 120 ml
1/5 cup cream	
2 cups corn flakes	
1/2 cup milk	
2 cups water	
IV began with 950 ml; currently 290 ml left in bag	

3. Provide students with sample test results and have them analyze the values and decide what imbalance the client may be experiencing (see Resources for Student Activities).

4. Provide examples and/or show students photos or illustrations of different IV complications, and ask them to identify each problem.

5. By utilizing the following or similar situations, ask students to identify what fluid, electrolyte, and/or acid/base disturbance the client may be experiencing and what nursing interventions may be implemented:
    a. A client in labor who is hyperventilating
    b. An individual working outside in extremely hot weather
    c. A 4 year old with a high fever
    d. An 80 year old living alone, with diminished appetite and thirst

e. An individual who has cut himself on a lawn-mower blade

f. An infant with gastroenteritis and severe diarrhea

g. An adult experiencing prolonged episodes of vomiting

h. A client with bone cancer

i. A client with known coronary insufficiency

j. A client who has smoked consistently for years and has emphysema

k. A child who ingests a large amount of aspirin

l. An adult with second- and third-degree burns over 30% of her body

m. A client in whom tachycardia, dyspnea, and chills develop in the first 5 minutes of a blood transfusion

n. A client who is experiencing renal failure

o. An individual who is diagnosed with syndrome of inadequate antidiuretic hormone (SIADH).

p. A client with a history of heart disease who is taking a cardiotonic medication and furosemide (Lasix).

q. An adult client with a history of alcohol abuse

r. An individual with diabetes mellitus who has had difficulty controlling blood glucose levels

s. A woman in her ninth month of pregnancy and is preeclamptic

Clinical Skills/Techniques

1. Explain and demonstrate (by using simulation mannequin/model, appropriate equipment, and educational media, as available) the following nursing interventions associated with intravenous (IV) therapy:

   a. Initiating a peripheral IV infusion

   b. Regulation of IV flow rate

   c. Changing a peripheral IV solution, tubing, and dressing

2. Have small groups of students practice, with supervision, the performance and documentation of the specified nursing interventions, by using appropriate equipment/supplies.

3. Evaluate the students' ability to implement and document the interventions for IV therapy through return-demonstration/skill testing before clinical experience.

4. Explain and demonstrate the procedure for an arterial puncture for blood gas analysis. Have students observe a nurse/skilled technician perform the procedure in an acute care setting.

Client Care Experiences

1. Assign students to observe and participate in the nursing care of clients in acute health care settings, focusing on the assessment of fluid, electrolyte, and acid/base disturbances. Discuss physical assessment and analysis of laboratory values with the group.

2. Supervise the initiation (if appropriate) and maintenance of IV therapy.

3. Have students design and implement teaching plans to meet client needs related to fluid, electrolyte, and acid/base imbalances. Review client discharge planning/referral with the students.

4. Have students complete a care plan/pathway for an assigned client who is experiencing an alteration in fluid, electrolyte, and/or acid/base balance.

Resources for Student Activities

Analysis of Blood Chemistry Values
Comparison Chart of Acid/Base Imbalances

Analysis of Blood Chemistry Values

Client Values	Normal Levels	Analysis
Sodium, 155 mEq/L		
Chloride, 95 mEq/L		
Calcium, 3.5 mEq/L		
Potassium, 3.0 mEq/L		
Magnesium, 3.2 mEq/L		
Phosphate, 5.2 mEq/L		
Urine Specific Gravity, 1.1		

Arterial Blood Gases
  pH 7.3
  $PaCO_2$, 50 mm Hg
  PaO_2, 82 mm Hg
  Bicarbonate, 19 mEq/L		

Comparison Chart: Acid/Base Imbalances

Body State	Etiology	Signs/Symptoms	Treatment
Metabolic Acidosis			
Metabolic Alkalosis			
Respiratory Acidosis			
Respiratory Alkalosis			

Critical Thinking Exercises (from text page 1196)

1. Mrs. Emanuele is an 81-year-old admitted to the hospital with a 3-day history of vomiting and diarrhea. She has had only ice chips since the first episode of vomiting and is now complaining of malaise, cramping muscles, and a temperature of 101°F. Which laboratory findings would you expect to be abnormal, based on her complaints? What interventions would you expect the physician to order?

2. Caroline has just received a new client on her unit who is to receive 1 unit of red blood cells (RBCs) within the next hour. What nursing actions are necessary before administering blood? What are the signs and symptoms of a transfusion reaction? Can Caroline delegate the administration of blood to a licensed practical nurse or a nursing assistant on her team?

3. Bob is caring for a 52-year-old man who has been seen in the emergency department after being involved in a motor vehicle accident. He is complaining of difficulty breathing and a respiratory rate of 40 breaths per minute. Bob's client is transferred to the intensive care unit, intubated, and placed on a ventilator. After the client leaves, a nursing student asks Bob to interpret his client's last arterial blood gas (ABG) results: pH, 7.30; PaO_2, 70; $PaCO_2$, 50; HCO3, 24. What interpretation will Bob give to the student nurse? What is the relation between the ABG results and the client's being intubated and ventilated?

4. Jane is the nurse caring for Betty, a 59-year-old who has just had a total knee replacement. The physician has ordered cefazolin (Ancef), 1 g in 50 ml, to run over 30 minutes IV piggyback tid. Betty has a continuous infusion of Ringer's lactate at 75 ml/hr in the left forearm. What type of tubing will Jane use to administer the IV piggyback medication? Calculate the drops per minute of the piggyback by using both microtubing (60 drops/ml) and macrotubing (15 drops/ml).

5. John Patrick, a 24-year-old tennis professional, was admitted to the clinic with a temperature of 105°F. He has a history of playing in a 5-hour tennis match in 100°F heat. His coach brought him to the clinic because he was weak and lethargic. What assessment findings would the nurse expect to find? What interventions would be necessary? Describe a teaching plan for John on discharge.

Suggested Answers

1. Any of the following laboratory values may be low, normal, or below normal, related to the diarrhea and vomiting episodes. Serum potassium low or below normal, <3.5 mEqL; urine specific gravity, >1.025; increased hematocrit, >50%; and an increased blood urea nitrogen (BUN) level, >25 mg/100 ml (hemoconcentration), all related to fluid volume deficit. The nurse can anticipate that the physician will order IV therapy and blood work. The physician will begin to investigate the etiology of the vomiting and diarrhea, and, based on the assessment, the physician may begin to treat the symptoms and underlying cause.

2. Administering a blood transfusion is a professional nurse's responsibility, and Caroline would not be able to delegate this activity. Transfusing blood requires an assessment of the IV site, vital signs, client status, and potential and actual signs and symptoms related to a transfusion reaction, before, during, and after the infusion. Additionally, because a transfusion reaction can be fatal, it is imperative that the unit of blood be checked properly. (Review the explanation of blood transfusion.)

3. The client's increased respiratory rate is a compensatory method to increase oxygenation that has been ineffective. A client who is laboring to breathe runs the risk of extensive systemic and cerebral hypoxia that may lead to irreversible deficits. The blood gases demonstrate the inability of the client's system to compensate, and ventilatory assistance is required.

4. Jane can use either microtubing or macrotubing. Some hospitals have a policy regarding the appropriate tubing for 50 ml/hr or less IV rates. If Jane used microtubing, 60 gtts/ml, she will calculate the IV rate at 100 gtts/min. If she uses macrotubing, 15 gtts/ml, she will calculate the IV rate at 25 gtts/min.

5. John Patrick is experiencing deficient fluid volume related to heat exhaustion. The nurse should expect the following physical assessment findings. Dry mucous membranes, flat neck veins, weak pulse, decreased capillary filling, decreased blood pressure, oliguria with increased urine specific gravity, and skin cool and clammy to touch. Interventions are directed at correcting the deficient fluid volume. Monitor vital signs, and ensure temperature is decreasing. Replace fluid and electrolyte loss with intravenous solutions. Monitor serum and urinary electrolytes. Weigh and measure I&O to monitor fluid balance. Assess skin turgor and mucous membranes. Watch for ominous changes toward deterioration. A discharge teaching plan for John Patrick would include the need for oral hydration before, during, and after strenuous exercise and heat exposure. Monitor urinary output for amount and color. Weigh himself before and after match to determine fluid loss. Understand signs and symptoms of heat exhaustion, and implement strategies to correct them in a timely manner.

41

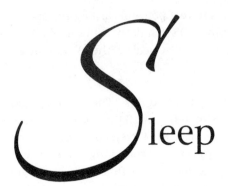

*S*leep

Instructor Media Resources

Instructor's Resource CD
evolve **Instructor's Resources**

Instructor's Manual
ExamView Test Bank
Image Collection
Power Point Slides
Weblinks

Student Media Resources

CD COMPANION

- Review Questions
- Glossary

evolve WEBSITE

- Review Questions
- Student Learning Activities
- Glossary

Classroom Discussion

1. Review the physiology of sleep, including the sleep/wake cycle, circadian rhythm, regulation of sleep, and stages of sleep. Discuss how the physiological mechanisms are determined through the use of selected instruments (e.g., EEG [electroecencephalogram], EMG [electromyogram], EOG [electrooculogram]).

2. Stimulate a discussion on how the physiology of sleep may be disrupted in the home and health care environment.

3. Describe the difference between rest and sleep, and discuss how the nurse may promote rest. Have students share what makes them feel "rested."

4. Describe the functions of sleep in restoration and healing, and the importance of rapid-eye-motion (REM) sleep and dreams.

5. Identify the average sleep requirements and specific concerns for individuals across the life span. Ask students to provide examples of how sleep patterns change with growth and development.

6. Identify factors that may affect sleep patterns, including:
   a. Physical and psychological illness
   b. Drugs/substances
   c. Lifestyle
   d. Usual sleep patterns and excessive sleepiness
   e. Emotional stress
   f. Environment
   g. Exercise and fatigue
   h. Food and caloric intake

   Ask students to provide specific examples of how and why each factor may affect normal sleep patterns.

7. Have students discuss how the acute care environment specifically may interfere with sleep patterns and how the nurse may eliminate or reduce this interference.

8. Describe common sleep disorders, including insomnia, sleep apnea, narcolepsy, sleep deprivation, and parasomnias.

9. Discuss the assessment of sleep patterns/habits, the possible sources of data that the nurse may use to elicit information (e.g., parents, spouse, sleep partner), and questions that may be asked to determine the client's routines.

10. Review the components of a sleep history.

11. Discuss how the sleep history may be correlated with the client's medical history, life events, emotional and mental status, and/or alteration in bedtime routine or environment.

12. Identify behaviors that may be associated with sleep deprivation.

13. By using the following or similar situations, have students identify how the individual's sleep patterns may be disturbed, and what interventions the nurse may implement to promote adequate sleep and rest:
    a. An employee who has been rotated to the night shift (12 AM to 8 AM) every 3 weeks
    b. A 3-year-old child admitted to the acute care environment with a respiratory condition
    c. A middle adult who is fearful of losing his or her job.
    d. An older adult with chronic arthritic pain
    e. A young adult preparing for her upcoming wedding
    f. A student who is working, caring for a family, and preparing for college examinations
    g. An individual with a bed partner who is restless and snores
    h. Parents who have just brought their newborn home
    i. A client in the intensive care unit for several days

14. Guide students in the application of the critical thinking model and the nursing process for clients with a sleep-pattern disturbance.

15. Identify interventions that may be implemented to promote a client's sleep and rest.
    Ask students to specify measures to achieve the following for clients:
    a. A restful and safe environment
    b. Promotion of bedtime routine (as close as possible).
    c. "Sleep friendly" scheduling of treatments, etc.
    d. Stress reduction
    e. Physical comfort
    f. Pharmacological management

16. Invite a counselor/therapist who specializes in sleep-pattern disturbances to speak to the class about measures to promote relaxation and rest and the recognition of sleep-deprivation behaviors.

Interactive Exercises

1. Have students complete a sleep questionnaire with a peer, family member, or client.

2. Have students determine what resources are available in the health care setting and community for clients who are experiencing sleep-pattern alterations.

Client Care Experiences

1. Assign students to observe and participate in the nursing care of clients in a variety of health care settings, focusing on the following:
    a. Assessment of actual/potential sleep-pattern disturbances
    b. Promotion of physical and emotional comfort and relaxation
    c. Administration, with supervision, of prescribed medications for promotion of comfort and rest
    d. Evaluation/documentation of client responses to sleep/rest promotion interventions

2. Have students determine client teaching/learning needs and design a teaching plan specific to the attainment of rest and sleep.

3. Have students complete a care plan/pathway specific to, or incorporating the client's needs for rest and sleep.

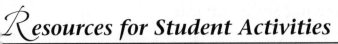

Resources for Student Activities

Comparison Chart for Sleep Patterns Across the Life Span
Factors Affecting Sleep Patterns

Sleep Patterns Across the Life Span

Age Group	Sleep Pattern/Needs
Neonate/Infant	
Toddler	
Preschooler	
School-age Child	
Adolescent	
Young Adult	
Middle Adult	
Older Adult	

Factors Affecting Sleep Patterns

Factors	Sleep-pattern Alterations
Physical Illness	
Drugs/Substances	
Lifestyle	
Usual Sleep Patterns	
Emotional Stress	
Environment	
Exercise & Fatigue	
Food/Caloric Intake	

236   Chapter 41: Sleep

Critical Thinking Exercises (from text page 1225)

1. Mr. Collins, age 45 years, comes to the doctor for a checkup. He tells you that he feels as if he is not getting enough sleep and that his wife says he snores loudly. What assessment data should you gather from Mr. Collins?

2. You are doing a presentation to a preschool parents group on the topic of sleep and rest. What information should you provide to parents to help promote sleep in preschool and school-age children?

3. Mrs. Augustine is a 75-year-old who recently moved into a nursing home. She says she has not been sleeping well since moving. Develop a plan of care to promote sleep for Mrs. Augustine.

Suggested Answers

1. Mr. Collins statement that he feels as if he is not getting enough sleep is an indication of a sleep problem. The report from Mrs. Collins about snoring can be an indication of an obstructive sleep apnea problem. A more in-depth assessment on Mr. Collins' sleep problem, sleep pattern, history, and sleep hygiene habits is needed. A 1- to 2-week sleep log or diary with entries by both Mr. and Mrs. Collins can provide additional assessment data related to the problem. Assessment data related to the problem should be collected from both Mr. Collins and his wife.

2. One of the most important topics for early in the presentation is that the establishment of a regular bedtime routine is very important in preschool and school-age children. This regular bedtime routine should be consistently reinforced nightly. Other information that will help promote good sleep habits could include:
   • Eliminate or reduce noise so bedroom is as quiet as possible.
   • Play soft music to help relax the child.
   • Do quiet activities before bed such as reading a story, listening to music, praying, or coloring.
   • Avoid exercise and stimulating activities 2 to 3 hours before bedtime.
   • Dress child in soft cotton nightclothes that are warm and comfortable.
   • Place a nightlight in the child's room to help decrease fears of the dark.
   • Have child go to the bathroom before bedtime.
   • Provide a light snack before bedtime.

3. Moving into the nursing home has disrupted Mrs. Augustine's regular sleeping pattern and habits. The change in environment and a different bed also are contributing to the problem. Ask Mrs. Augustine about her usual bedtime routines, and attempt to reestablish these routines with her. Additional points to consider for the plan of care include:
   • Administer any needed pain medication to promote comfort.
   • Provide personal hygiene measures such as a warm washcloth to wash face and hands, tooth brushing, brushing of hair.
   • Close door of room to cut down on environmental noise.
   • Provide Mrs. Augustine with a back rub.
   • Position Mrs. Augustine with pillows in a position of comfort.
   • Adjust temperature in room so that it is not too hot or cold.
   • Turn on TV or radio to soft music per Mrs. Augustine's preference.
   • Assist Mrs. Augustine to the bathroom before sleep.

42

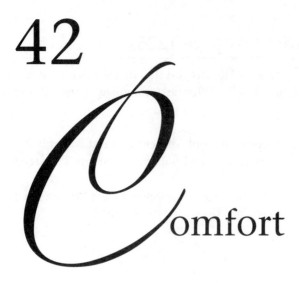

*C*omfort

Instructor Media Resources

Instructor's Resource CD
evolve **Instructor's Resources**

Instructor's Manual
ExamView Test Bank
Image Collection
Power Point Slides
Weblinks

Student Media Resources

CD COMPANION

- Review Questions
- Glossary

evolve **WEBSITE**

- Review Questions
- Student Learning Activities
- Glossary

Classroom Discussion

1. Explain the neurophysiology of pain. Ask students how alterations in the central nervous system may influence the physiological pain mechanism.

2. Discuss the concept of comfort and the holistic approach that the nurse may use in assisting clients to achieve comfort.

3. Discuss the nature of pain, including the objective and subjective aspects of the experience, sources of pain, and its protective mechanism.

4. Ask students to contribute their ideas about the prejudices and misconceptions that may be associated with the pain experience and how nursing care may be influenced/altered.

5. Identify physiological and behavioral responses to pain. Ask students to share personal or clinical experiences in which responses to pain have been manifested.

6. Explain the different classifications of pain: acute, chronic, and cancer related. Ask students how the client's activities of daily living may be influenced by each type of pain.

7. Discuss factors that influence the pain experience:
   a. Physiological
   b. Social
   c. Spiritual
   d. Cultural
   e. Psychological

   Ask students to provide specific examples of how and why each factor may influence an individual's pain experience.

8. Describe the assessment guidelines for clients experiencing pain, including:
   a. Expression of pain
   b. Classification of pain
   c. Characteristics of pain

9. Have students indicate how the client may express pain verbally and nonverbally, and therapeutic measures that may be used to promote nurse/client communication.

10. Discuss the importance of pretreatment or procedure explanation in reducing a client's discomfort (anticipatory pain).

11. Identify and describe specific pain-relief measures that the nurse may implement. Ask students to provide additional examples of possible interventions for different health care settings. Review non-pharmacological pain-relief measures, including indications for their use, precautions/contraindications, and nursing responsibilities associated with their implementation.

12. Discuss pharmacological pain therapy, including indications, precautions/contraindications, and nursing responsibilities associated with the following:
    a. Analgesics
    b. Patient-controlled analgesia
    c. Local/Regional anesthetics
    d. Topical analgesics/anesthetics
    e. Surgic3al interventions

13. Stimulate a discussion on the advantages of nonpharmacological and pharmacological pain-relief measures and situations in which they may be used most effectively.

14. Explain the treatment protocol for clients with intractable pain, including the goal of therapy, types of administration routes, and most effective pharmacological agents.

15. Review the evaluation and documentation of the client's responses to pain-relief measures.

16. Invite a nurse working in a hospice, or on an oncology unit, to speak to the class about client assessment, pain-relief measures, and nursing accountability.

17. Guide students in the application of the critical thinking model and nursing process for clients experiencing pain.

Interactive Exercises

1. Provide examples of different client situations, and ask students to identify whether the client may experience acute or chronic pain (e.g., a client with a ruptured appendix). Have students identify the possible signs and symptoms that the client may exhibit or express.

2. Have students investigate and report on different cultural responses to the pain experience.

3. Have students complete an assessment with another student or family member who is currently or has previously experienced pain.

4. Organize a role-playing situation with students explaining a procedure or treatment and the sensations that the client may expect (e.g., lumbar puncture).

5. Have students design a teaching plan for a client by using a PCA (patient-controlled analgesia) pump in the home.

6. Have students investigate and report on available resources in the health care setting or community for reduction or relief of pain (e.g., headache clinic).

7. Assign students to attend a nursing staff conference, if available, on pain-relief strategies.

3. Have students, working in small groups, plan how they may approach pain relief for the following clients:
   a. An older adult with arthritis
   b. A middle adult who has just had abdominal surgery
   c. A young adult with severe pain from advanced bone cancer
   d. A school-age child after a fracture or severe burn
   e. A toddler who is to have a lumbar puncture
   f. An adolescent with migraine headaches
   g. A client experiencing childbirth
   h. An adult client who is having a myocardial infarction
   i. An adolescent who has appendicitis and will have an appendectomy

Clinical Skills/Technique

1. Demonstrate selected nonpharmacological pain relief measures to the class, such as relaxation, guided imagery, biofeedback, distraction, and cutaneous stimulation (application of hot/cold, warm bath, transcutaneous electrical nerve stimulation [TENS], acupressure, and/or massage).

Client Care Experiences

1. Assign students to observe and/or participate in the nursing care of clients experiencing pain in one or more of the following or similar health care settings:
   a. Labor and delivery
   b. Oncology unit
   c. Postoperative/postanesthesia care unit
   d. Hospice care center/home care agency

2. Have students assess the presence and characteristics of a client's pain and the client's responses to the experience. Supervise the students' implementation and documentation of appropriate pain-relief measures in the clinical setting.

3. Have students complete a care plan/pathway for clients experiencing pain, and then identify how they individualized interventions to meet the specific clients' needs.

Resources for Student Activities

Factors Influencing the Pain Experience

Factors Influencing the Experience of Pain

Factors	Influence on/Response of Individual in Pain
Age	
Fatigue	
Genes	
Neurological Function	
Attention	
Previous Pain Experience	
Family/Social Support	
Spiritual	
Anxiety	
Coping Style	
Culture	
Meaning of Pain	
Ethnicity	

242   Chapter 42: Comfort

Critical Thinking Exercises (from text page 1268)

1. John is a 32-year-old construction worker who sustained an injury to the lumbar region of his back during a fall approximately 8 months ago. John is 6 feet tall and weighs 280 pounds. He continues to report pain intensity as a 5 (on a scale of 0 to 10), increasing with activity; he has limited flexibility and is unable to return to work. He has recently been admitted for treatment at a comprehensive pain clinic. What interventions might the health care team use?

2. Alexis is a 3-year-old admitted to the pediatric unit for a third-degree burn to her right lower extremity. What tools might be useful when assessing this child's pain?

3. You are caring for an unconscious client who was involved in an automobile accident and sustained multiple injuries. The client has several lacerations, wounds, and surgical incisions, as well as multiple lines and tubes. What measures might you take to promote the client's comfort?

4. Mary Beth Jones, a 55-year-old woman with metastatic breast cancer to the bone, has been receiving IV morphine sulfate (MSO_4) for a week for severe back and leg pain. Her frequently increased infusion of MSO_4 is not reducing her pain to an acceptable level, and she is becoming increasingly sedated. What other pharmacological interventions might be considered?

5. Ms. Wilkins, 65 years old, returns from surgery after a small bowel resection. The physician orders a 25-mg fentanyl patch applied to help manage the postoperative pain. Ms. Wilkins received one dose of morphine, 4 mg IV push, in the recovery room 1 hour ago, which relieved her pain. What actions would be appropriate for you to take at this time?

Suggested Answers

1. After conducting an extensive pain history and assessment, the team may recommend a variety of interventions. Pharmacological interventions may need to be implemented, but additional interventions would be helpful when dealing with chronic pain. The team may consider physical therapy, including activity and exercise, diet control, if necessary, and nonpharmacological interventions such as heat and cold application, biofeedback, distraction, and relaxation. A social worker might assist with any ramifications that his chronic pain has had on his financial status (e.g., unemployment).

2. The Oucher face scale is a very useful tool when assessing pain in toddlers. It also is important to involve the parent in the pain assessment.

3. Because of the extent of the client's injuries and altered level of consciousness, it will be necessary to assess for nonverbal cues of pain (e.g., grimacing). Pharmacological interventions would most likely be used. It would be the responsibility of the RN to assess the client routinely and consider around-the-clock dosing. Nonpharmacological interventions such as massage, range of motion, and positioning might be beneficial.

4. It might be helpful to start the client on a nonsteroidal antiinflammatory drug (NSAID) around the clock as an adjuvant to the morphine sulfate. If this is not effective, the client may benefit from an epidural analgesic with or without a local anesthetic. A test dose may be given to determine effectiveness, and an implantable catheter might be considered.

5. This is an inappropriate order. Fentanyl is not recommended for acute pain. It takes about 17 hours for it to become effective. Once applied, it also takes about 17 hours for the effect to diminish below therapeutic levels. In addition, it could increase the risk of respiratory depression after surgery (additive effect with anesthesia). It also is inappropriate for opioid-naïve clients. The nurse should call the physician and request an immediate-release opioid formulation and/or PCA.

43

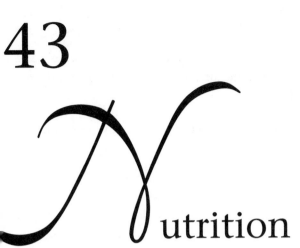

$\mathcal{N}$utrition

Classroom Discussion

1. Review the principles of nutrition, including basal metabolic rate, resting energy expenditure, nutrients, and nutrient density.

2. Identify the six categories of nutrients, the role and storage of each in the body, and current recommendations for daily intake:
   a. Carbohydrates
   b. Proteins
   c. Lipids
   d. Water
   e. Vitamins: fat soluble and water soluble
   f. Minerals

   Have students identify food sources for each nutrient.

3. Discuss the role of carbohydrates, lipids, and proteins in energy provision.

4. Review the processes of digestion, absorption, and elimination. Review body metabolism, anabolism, and catabolism, and present situations in which individuals may be in one of these states.

5. Discuss the current dietary guidelines. By using transparencies, photos, illustrations, and/or models, explain the food guide pyramid.

6. Discuss how the promotion of nutrition follows the *Healthy People 2010* objectives with guidelines for reducing saturated fat and sodium intake and increasing the intake of fruits and vegetables, etc.

7. Review developmental variables and nutritional needs across the life span. Have students provide specific examples of how growth and development alters nutritional needs (see Resources for Student Activities).

8. Explain the potential for nutrient/drug interactions. Ask students for additional examples of possible interactions.

9. Discuss alternative food patterns (e.g., vegetarianism) and the advantages and disadvantages in nutrient intake. Ask students to share personal or clinical experiences with alternative food pattern intake.

10. Identify and explain the aspects of a nutritional assessment and the information that is elicited through the following:
    a. Physical measurements: height, weight, anthropometric measurements, body mass index, ideal body weight
    b. Laboratory tests
    c. Dietary and health history, food records
    d. Clinical observation

11. Identify clients who may be at risk for nutritional problems. Use the following or similar situations, and ask students to provide the rationale for why nutritional problems may develop, and how the nurse could determine the presence of the problem(s).
   a. A postoperative client
   b. An immobilized client
   c. An older adult living alone
   d. A preschool child living in a poor socioeconomic setting

12. Guide students in the application of the critical thinking model and the nursing process for clients with an altered nutritional status.

13. Identify measures that may be implemented to promote nutrition for clients in a variety of health care settings. Have students provide additional specific nursing interventions for stimulating a client's appetite, meeting nutritional guidelines for disease-related treatment, and client/family counseling and teaching.

14. Stimulate a discussion on client situations in which referrals for nutritional needs may be indicated (e.g., Meals-on-Wheels, food stamps).

15. Discuss nutritional concerns for clients of diverse cultural and spiritual backgrounds (e.g., Kosher and Hindu requirements).

16. Invite a nutritionist/dietitian to speak to the class about dietary health promotion for clients in the acute, restorative, and/or home care setting.

17. Discuss enteral nutrition, including its purpose, uses, complications, and associated nursing responsibilities. Have students identify client situations in which enteral nutrition/tube feedings may be used to promote nutrition.

18. Discuss parenteral nutrition, including its purpose, use, specific solutions, contraindications, complications, and associated nursing responsibilities of assisting with central venous or peripherally inserted central catheter (PICC) line insertion and maintaining the infusion.
   Have students identify situations in which parenteral nutrition may be indicated for a client.

Interactive Exercises

1. Have students complete a food-intake record for themselves, a peer, or a family member (24 hours up to 3 days) and analyze the total nutrient intake for adequacy. Use a commercial computer program, if available.

2. Have students identify what is available to the consumer regarding nutritional information and guidelines (e.g., food labels, media presentations). Assign students to bring in examples of readily found nutritional information.

3. Provide students with client situations and have them, orally and/or in writing, identify potential nutritional problems/needs and appropriate nursing interventions. Use examples for clients experiencing one or more of the following: diabetes mellitus, gastrointestinal (GI) or cardiovascular disease, human immunodeficiency virus (HIV), or cancer (see Resources for Student Activities).

4. Have students design and present a teaching plan on dietary needs for one of the following simulated situations:
    a. Parents with an 8-month-old infant and/or a 2-year-old child
    b. An older adult with coronary disease
    c. A family member responsible for a client's gastrostomy tube care.

Clinical Skills/Techniques

1. Explain and demonstrate (by using simulation mannequin/model, appropriate equipment, and available educational media) the following nursing interventions for promotion of client nutrition:
    a. Insertion of a small-bore nasoenteric tube.
    b. Administration of enteral tube feedings via nasoenteric tubes.
    c. Administration of enteral feedings via gastrostomy or jejunostomy tube.
    d. Verification of tube placement

2. Have small groups of students practice the performance and documentation of these interventions, by using appropriate equipment (as available).

3. Evaluate the students' ability to implement and document the interventions to promote client nutrition through return-demonstration/skill testing before clinical experience.

Client Care Experiences

1. Assign students to observe and participate in the nursing care of clients, in a variety of health care settings, focusing on the assessment and promotion of nutritional intake. Have students prepare the environment and assist with oral care to stimulate the client's appetite.

2. Supervise the students' implementation of oral, enteral, or parenteral feedings, as indicated. Review and evaluate their assessment of the client's nutritional status, and discuss possible strategies for improvement, if needed. Have students work with clients in food selection, meal planning, and food preparation according to prescribed diet therapy.

3. Have students complete a care plan/pathway for an assigned client who is experiencing an alteration in nutritional status.

Resources for Student Activities

Chart on Nutritional Needs across the Life Span
Disease-related Dietary Management Chart

Nutritional Needs Across the Life Span

Age Group	Nutritional Needs
Infant	
Toddler/Preschooler	
School-age Child	
Adolescent	
Young & Middle Adult	
Pregnancy/Lactation	
Older Adult	

Disease-related Dietary Management

Pathophysiology	General Dietary Needs
Gastrointestinal	
Cardiovascular	
Diabetes Mellitus	
HIV/AIDS	
Cancer	

C *ritical Thinking Exercises* (from text page 1319)

1. Jean, age 35 years, has just had surgery for a bowel obstruction. Her medical history includes Crohn's disease. Before this exacerbation, 3 months ago, Jean's weight was 123 pounds (55.8 kg). Admission weight was 115 pounds (52.2 kg); 3 days after surgery, she now weighs 108 pounds (49.0 kg). Her height is 5 feet, 5 inches (165 cm). Reported laboratory values are white blood cell count, 8.3; lymphocytes, 13%; albumin, 2.3 g/dl. What is Jean's body mass index (BMI)? What is her percentage weight loss? What is her total lymphocyte count? Jean remains nil by mouth (NPO) with nasogastric suction; what intervention(s) would you discuss with her physician?

2. Darrin Thomas, 86, was admitted for a viral infection. He had a recent weight loss of 6 pounds in the week before admission. He lost an additional 4 pounds during the week of hospitalization. His appetite is poor; he has frequent nausea and vomiting. His abdomen is soft, nontender, and cancer free, and bowel sounds are present. Enteral feedings will be initiated.
   a. What type of tube should be selected?
   b. How will the tube placement be verified?
   c. Describe the type of feeding and initiation of feedings.
   d. What complications should be assessed?

3. Roberta is being treated for breast cancer with chemotherapy as adjunct to a lumpectomy. She has maintained a positive attitude as well as possible but is concerned about the side effects of the medication. Roberta has bleeding gums, stomatitis, nausea, and diarrhea. As a result she has no desire to eat. She is 85% of her usual body weight at present. How could you assist Roberta in improving her nutritional status?

Suggested Answers

1. a. Jean's body mass index is calculated by using the formula kg ÷ meters (ht) squared. Thus Jean presently weighs 49.1 kg and is 1.64 meters in height, which squared equals 2.69, and BMI is 18.25. A BMI of 18.25 places Jean within a high-risk category, in need of nutritional intervention.
   b. Jean's percentage weight loss is calculated with the formula: usual body weight (UBW) – current body weight (CBW) ÷ UBW × 100; thus 123 lb – 108 lb equals 15 lb, divided by 123, equals 0.122, times 100 equals 12.2%. 12.2% weight loss within a 3-month period is significant. A loss greater than 7.5% over 3 months and 10% over 6 months places client at high risk.
   c. Jean's total lymphocyte count (TLC) is calculated by % lymph × WBC count ÷ 100, thus a WBC of 8.3×10^9/L is equivalent to 8300/mm³; therefore 13 × 8300 equals 107,900 divided by 100 equals 1079. A TLC of less than 1500 cells/mm³ is associated with greater morbidity and mortality.
   d. Jean is a good candidate for parenteral nutrition (PN). When nasogastric suctioning is discontinued, and Jean has bowel sounds in all four quadrants, she should be transitioned to oral intake with calorie counts. PN is decreased as oral intake increases to full dietary requirements.

2. PEG or PEJ:
   a. Rationale, probably long-term EN or supplemental EN. Reduced risk of pulmonary aspiration, reduced risk of tube dislodgement. If accidental tube extubation occurs, tube is easily replaced.
   b. Verification: Initially via radiograph, and then pH strip verification. Abdominal assessment and evaluation of gastric residuals to determine presence of bowel sounds or delayed gastric emptying
   c. Probably whole-nutrient polymeric formula. May be given full strength if tolerated, rate of 10 to 20 ml/hr and advanced 10 to 20 ml/hr until target rate is achieved. If client resumes oral intake, EN may be used as supplemental (e.g., nocturnally) to improve and maintain nutritional status.
   d. Complications: diarrhea, fluid and electrolyte imbalance, increasing gastric residuals, and nausea and vomiting are common.

3. Perform a complete physical assessment. Focus on medications, food preferences, cues that induce nausea and what she does to cope, and frequency and amount of diarrhea. Establish Roberta's energy requirements, and estimate her usual intake. What is her illness/activity factor? Encourage exercise as tolerated.

Bleeding gums: Have Roberta use an extra-soft bristle, child-size toothbrush.

Stomatitis: Eat cool or room-temperature foods, increase fluids, avoid coarse-textured, highly seasoned or acidic foods, tobacco, alcohol, or commercial mouthwashes. Consult with physician about use of an analgesic mouth rinse. Supplement foods with protein powder or polycose (a carbohydrate liquid supplement).

Nausea: Suggest frequent, small, nutrient-dense meals. Include high-protein/kcal supplements, avoid excess fat, eat slowly, limit fluid intake with meals, rest after meals with head elevated, and consult with physician regarding antiemetic medication use.

Diarrhea: Suggest frequent, small meals. Avoid excess fat, drink fluids between meals, and consult with physician about antidiarrheal medication use. Avoid gas-forming foods.

44

$\mathcal{U}$rinary Elimination

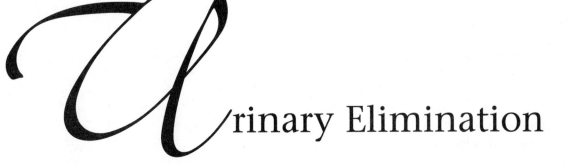

Instructor Media Resources

Instructor's Resource CD
evolve Instructor's Resources

Instructor's Manual
ExamView Test Bank
Image Collection
Power Point Slides
Weblinks
Skills Checklists

Student Media Resources

CD COMPANION

- Review Questions
- Glossary

evolve WEBSITE

- Review Questions
- Student Learning Activities
- Glossary

Classroom Discussion

1. Review the anatomy and physiology of the urinary tract (kidneys, ureters, bladder, urethra, and process of urination).

2. Discuss factors that influence urinary elimination:
   a. Pathophysiology
   b. Growth and development
   c. Sociocultural
   d. Psychological
   e. Muscle tone
   f. Fluid balance
   g. Surgical procedures
   h. Medications
   i. Diagnostic examination

   Have students identify specific examples of how each factor may influence an individual's urinary elimination (see Resource for Student Activity).

3. Identify and describe the following alterations in urinary elimination, including possible etiology, client signs and symptoms, and treatment:
   a. Urinary retention
   b. Lower urinary tract infections
   c. Urinary incontinence

4. Discuss the indications for, surgical treatment of, and resultant client alterations in elimination that are associated with urinary diversions.

5. Discuss the components of the nursing history that will elicit information on a client's urinary function, including patterns of urination, symptoms, and other related factors. Have students determine which initial and follow-up questions may elicit the most accurate information from the client.

6. Discuss the importance of hygiene and asepsis in the control of urinary infections. Ask students how the age, developmental level, and sociocultural practices of the client may have an impact on urinary hygiene.

7. Review the physical assessment of the client with respect to urinary elimination. Ask students to identify expected and unexpected findings from the assessment (e.g., distended bladder, inflamed mucosa).

8. Describe the nursing assessment of urinary output, including analysis of intake and output, and characteristics of urine.

9. Identify and describe common laboratory and diagnostic tests used to evaluate urinary function. Discuss client preparation for, and nursing responsibilities associated with the testing. Review normal results and the meaning of abnormal findings from urinary diagnostic testing.

10. Discuss the psychological and emotional factors involved in urinary elimination. Ask students to identify how the nurse may promote client dignity and alleviate anxiety in the health care setting.

11. Ask the students, by utilizing the following or similar situations, to specify how urinary elimination may be affected:
    a. A paraplegic client
    b. An older adult with rheumatoid arthritis
    c. A hospitalized 3-year-old child
    d. An adult female with recurrent urinary tract infections
    e. A client diagnosed with bladder cancer
    f. A woman who has had multiple pregnancies

12. Identify nursing interventions that may be implemented to promote urinary function, including client education, stimulation of function, bladder emptying, and prevention of infection. Have students provide additional specific examples of nursing interventions and the rationales for their implementation.

13. Discuss how nursing approaches/procedures to promote urinary elimination may be altered from the acute care setting to the restorative setting to the home care setting.

14. Discuss the types, purposes, complications, nursing responsibilities, and documentation associated with urinary catheterization. Have students identify measures that may be implemented to reduce the incidence of infection associated with catheterization.

15. Describe restorative nursing care measures for promotion of urinary elimination, such as teaching the client Kegel exercises or self-catheterization, maintaining skin integrity and comfort, and bladder retraining. Stimulate a discussion on how the nurse may be creative in implementing these measures with the client, especially in the home environment.

16. Invite a nurse who specializes in dialysis/renal care to speak to the class about specific client needs, assessment, and nursing responsibility for promoting and evaluating urinary function.

17. Guide students in the application of the critical thinking model and the nursing process for clients experiencing alterations in urinary elimination.

Interactive Exercises

1. Assign students to investigate and report on the resources available in an affiliating health care setting or community for clients requiring dialysis, urinary-diversion support groups, and/or special ostomy equipment (type available and cost).

2. Provide students with the results of this or a similar sample urinalysis and have them determine the normal and abnormal findings.
    a. pH 7.0
    b. Protein, 2 mg/100 ml
    c. Glucose, present
    d. Four red blood cells (RBCs)
    e. Specific gravity, 1.020
    f. Casts, present
    g. White blood cells (WBCs), two per low-power field

3. Provide small groups of students with the name of a urinary diagnostic test and have them design a teaching plan for and/or role-play the preparation of a client for that procedure.

4. Have students design and implement a teaching plan for an adolescent or adult female client in the community on the prevention of urinary tract infections.

Clinical Skills/Techniques

1. Explain and demonstrate the procedure for collection of a midstream (clean-voided) specimen. Ask students how the procedure may be altered for clients of different ages and self-care abilities.

2. Demonstrate measures to stimulate urinary elimination by having students place their hands in warm water or hear the sound of running water (if a rest room is available nearby).

3. Explain and demonstrate (by using simulation mannequin/model, appropriate equipment/supplies, and available educational media) the following nursing interventions to promote urinary elimination:
   a. Collection of a midstream (clean-voided) urine specimen
   b. Insertion of a straight or indwelling catheter
   c. Provision of indwelling catheter care
   d. Closed and open catheter irrigation
   e. Application of a condom catheter

4. Have small groups of students practice, with supervision, the performance and documentation of the specified interventions, by using appropriate equipment.

5. Evaluate the students' ability to implement and document the interventions to promote urinary elimination through return-demonstration/skill testing before clinical experience.

Client Care Experiences

1. Assign students to accompany clients (as possible) and observe urinary diagnostic procedures (e.g., cystoscopy). Have students share their observations after the experience.

2. Assign students to observe and participate in the nursing care of clients in diverse health care settings who may be experiencing alterations in urinary elimination. Discuss the assessment of urinary function with the group. Review laboratory/diagnostic test results and client manifestations that may indicate altered urinary function.

3. Discuss measures to be implemented to promote urinary elimination, focusing on the maintenance of client dignity, privacy, and control (as possible).

4. Identify actual and potential client educational needs regarding urinary elimination.

5. Have students complete a care plan/pathway for an assigned client who is experiencing an alteration in urinary elimination.

Factors Influencing Urinary Elimination

Factors	Influence on Urinary Elimination
Disease Conditions	
Growth and Development	
Sociocultural	
Psychological	
Muscle Tone	
Fluid Balance	
Surgical Procedures	
Medications	
Diagnostic Examinations	

Critical Thinking Exercises (from text page 1371)

1. Mrs. Rodriquez is a 77-year-old woman who has had problems with urgency for the past 2 years. The episodes are becoming increasingly frequent. She has been attempting to deal with the problem by using an absorbent pad in her underwear, but she feels as though everyone knows her problem. The embarrassment of having an odor often keeps her at home. She has given up attending daily mass at church.
   a. How can the nurse help her regain control of her urinary elimination?
   b. What are the actual nursing diagnoses that apply to Mrs. Rodriquez?
   c. For one diagnosis, give one goal/outcome and two nursing interventions.

2. Mrs. Brownell is a 37-year-old woman who has been admitted with back pain radiating down into her groin. She also has noticed blood in her urine for a week, but she was hoping it would go away. She is to undergo an intravenous pyelogram (IVP) in 4 hours.
   a. What is the purpose of the IVP?
   b. What nursing care is needed before she goes to the x-ray department?
   c. Give at least two nursing responsibilities for care of the client after undergoing an IVP.

3. Mrs. Fenton is a 70-year-old woman with physical limitations related to rheumatoid arthritis. Her daughter, with whom she lives, has brought her to her family practitioner's office. You are the family nurse practitioner in the practice. As you assess Mrs. Fenton, you ask her how she is coping. Mrs. Fenton begins to answer but then starts to cry. "I know when I have to go to the bathroom, but I often don't make it in time." The daughter asks you for suggestions on how to manage, as she noticed that her mother's perineal skin is reddened and sore. What assessments does the nurse need to complete before planning interventions for Mrs. Fenton's care?

Suggested Answers

1. a. Mrs. Rodriquez is suffering from a condition that is a source of embarrassment and shame for her. The nurse in assessing the situation knows that in order to make a difference the urine loss must be controlled. With increased muscle control, Mrs. Rodriquez can enhance the ability of the external urinary sphincter to control the urine loss. For long-term control, a regimen of pelvic floor exercise will accomplish that goal. For the immediate problem, the nurse needs to help her choose an appropriate absorbent pad product that will contain the urine, prevent odor, and be undetectable under her clothes. Medication may be needed to decrease the bladder irritability and the urgency episodes.
   b. Some possible nursing diagnoses for Mrs. Rodriquez are:
      Altered pattern of urinary elimination related to irritative voiding symptoms as evidenced by urgency and frequency.
      Situational low self-esteem related to reduced self-care ability as evidenced by shame and embarrassment.
      Social isolation related to perceived urinary odor as evidenced by self-imposed limited social interaction.
   c. Situational low self-esteem related to reduced self-care ability as evidenced by shame and embarrassment.

Goal/Outcome	Client will be able to relate effect of life events (incontinence) on feelings about self
Interventions	Actively listen to and demonstrate acceptance of client

2. a. Mrs. Brownell has been admitted with back pain radiating down into the groin and hematuia. The purpose of the IVP is to determine, if possible, a renal or urinary source of the pain and bleeding. The type pain described is often the result of trauma from the calculus or may be an early sign of either renal or bladder cancer. Early detection of either problem will greatly improve the success of medical treatment.

b. Before sending Mrs. Brownell to the x-ray department, it is important to assess her level of anxiety concerning both the procedure and the outcome of the study. In addition, it is important that any allergy to iodine or seafood be determined to prevent severe allergic reactions. A bowel prep will need to be completed to cleanse the bowel prior to the study.

c. When Mrs. Brownell returns to her room it is important for the nurse to:
   1) encourage fluids by mouth and monitor urine output
   2) monitor for delayed allergic reaction

3. In planning care for Mrs. Fenton, it is important and necessary to include assessment of her caregiver and her environment in order to have a complete picture of the situation.

a. Client assessment
   What is her ambulatory status? How well can she rise from the chair?
   What is the pattern of incontinence?
   What is the current condition of her perineal skin?

b. Caregiver assessment
   Is the daughter working outside the home? From home? Primary responsibilities in the home?
   Other constraints on daughter's time and energy? (Children at home, etc.)

c. Environmental assessment
   How long has Mrs. Fenton been in her current living situation?
   Does she need environmental changes in the home?
   Would a commode help to decrease distance from chair or bed to toilet facilities?
   Are there any physical barriers such as, only bathroom on the second floor or loose rugs?

45

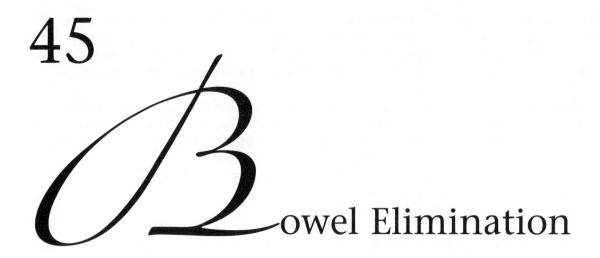

owel Elimination

Classroom Discussion

1. Review the anatomy and physiology of the gastrointestinal tract and the process of defecation.

2. Identify factors that affect bowel elimination. Have students provide specific examples of how bowel elimination may be affected by each factor.

3. Describe common bowel elimination problems, including their etiology, potential complications, and client signs and symptoms:
   a. Constipation
   b. Fecal impaction
   c. Diarrhea
   d. Incontinence
   e. Flatulence
   f. Hemorrhoids

4. Discuss psychological and emotional factors associated with bowel elimination. Ask students how the nurse may recognize and minimize disturbances in bowel elimination that may be related to the health care environment (e.g., lack of privacy, positioning).

5. Discuss the indications for, surgical treatment of, and resultant client alterations in elimination that are associated with bowel diversions: ileostomies and colostomies. By using educational media (photos/illustrations, videos, models), demonstrate how the incontinent and continent ostomies differ in location, drainage, and nursing/client care management.

6. Stimulate a discussion on the potential effect on a client's self-concept and body image after the creation of an ostomy.

7. Invite an enterostomal therapy nurse to speak to the class about specific physical and psychological needs of the client with an ostomy and measures that the nurse may implement to support the client.

8. Describe the aspects of the nursing history that will elicit information about the client's bowel elimination status.

9. Review the physical assessment of the client in relation to digestion and bowel elimination. Ask students to identify unexpected findings from the physical assessment that may indicate a problem with digestion and/or bowel elimination.

10. Discuss the nurse's analysis of fecal characteristics for determination of abnormalities.

11. Identify and describe laboratory and diagnostic tests that may be used to determine problems with digestion and bowel elimination. Discuss client preparation for and the nursing responsibilities associated with the testing. Review normal results and the meaning of abnormal findings from digestive and bowel elimination testing.

12. Explain the procedure for collection of a fecal sample for the measurement of occult blood. Ask students what information is necessary to provide to clients who will use the test at home.

13. Identify specific nursing measures that may be implemented to promote bowel elimination and support the client's self-concept, including bowel training, fluid and dietary intake, exercise, privacy, and proper positioning. Have students specify additional measures that may be used by the nurse, particularly in the acute and extended care setting, to establish client comfort and routine.

14. Discuss the use of medications (laxatives, cathartics, stool softeners, antidiarrheals) to promote or restore normal bowel elimination. Ask students how these medications may also create bowel elimination problems.

15. Discuss the types, purposes, and administration of enemas.

16. Review the indications and the procedure for the digital removal of stool.

17. Discuss the nursing care and client/family educational needs associated with ileostomies and colostomies. Ask students to provide specific concerns related to skin care, diet therapy, and body image.

18. Have students identify how bowel elimination may be affected and the nursing measures that may be implemented for the following client situations:
    a. A client with a cardiac condition
    b. A client with a new ileostomy or colostomy
    c. A truck driver who is on the road for long periods
    d. An immobilized client with a head trauma
    e. An adult client with multiple sclerosis
    f. A 3-year-old hospitalized for a minor surgical procedure
    g. A client after abdominal surgery
    h. An individual taking narcotic analgesics
    i. An older adult with osteoarthritis
    j. A salesperson who is under a great deal of occupational stress
    k. A client diagnosed with Crohn's disease or ulcerative colitis

19. Guide students in the application of the critical thinking model and the nursing process for clients experiencing alterations in bowel elimination.

Interactive Exercises

1. Assign students to investigate resources that are available within the affiliating agency and community for clients with an ileostomy or colostomy. Have students identify the types and costs of equipment that the client may need to purchase, and whether medical insurance will cover the expenses.

2. Have students practice completing the bowel elimination component of the health history with a peer, to better experience the embarrassment that may be felt by the client in response to these assessment questions.

3. Have students design and present a teaching plan based on one of the following:
    a. Client/family member care of an ileostomy or sigmoid colostomy
    b. Maintenance of regular bowel elimination patterns during pregnancy
    c. Bowel retraining
    d. Hazards of overuse of laxatives, cathartics, enemas
    e. Client scheduled to have an upper or lower gastrointestinal (GI) series

Clinical Skills/Techniques

1. Discuss and demonstrate the procedure for collection of a fecal sample for the measurement of occult blood.

2. Explain and demonstrate (by using simulation mannequin/model, appropriate equipment/supplies, and available educational media) the following nursing interventions to promote bowel elimination:
   a. Administration of a cleansing enema
   b. Pouching of an ostomy
   c. Insertion and maintenance of a nasogastric tube

3. Have small groups of students practice the performance and documentation of the specified interventions by using appropriate equipment/supplies.

4. Evaluate the students' ability to implement and document the interventions for promotion of bowel elimination through return-demonstration/skill testing before clinical experience.

Client Care Experiences

1. Assign students to accompany clients (as possible) and observe diagnostic testing for digestive or bowel elimination disorders. Have students share their observations after the experience.

2. Assign students to observe and participate in the nursing care of clients in a variety of health care settings with the focus on the assessment and promotion of bowel elimination.
   Discuss client manifestations and laboratory/diagnostic test results that may indicate a problem with bowel elimination.

3. Have the students collaborate with the nursing staff and clients to promote food and fluid intake, provide exercise and comfort, maintain skin integrity, and support client self-concept.

4. Evaluate the students' implementation of nursing measures, being alert to the maintenance of client dignity, privacy, and safety.

5. Have students complete a care plan/pathway for an assigned client who is experiencing an alteration in bowel elimination.

Resources for Student Activities

Factors Influencing Bowel Elimination Chart
Nursing Measures to Promote Bowel Elimination

Factors Influencing Bowel Elimination

Factors	Description of Influence on Elimination
Age	
Infection	
Diet	
Fluid Intake	
Physical Activity	
Psychological Factors	
Personal Habits	
Positioning	
Pain	
Pregnancy	
Surgery/Anesthesia	
Medications	
Diagnostic Tests	

Nursing Measures to Promote Bowel Elimination

Regular Bowel Pattern	
Fluid and Food Intake	
Exercise	
Comfort	
Skin Integrity	
Self-concept	
Positioning	
Ostomies	

Critical Thinking Exercises (from text page 1418)

1. A 19-year-old man with a history of good health and regular exercise is seen by the college health service nurse practitioner. He complains of increasing diarrhea and abdominal cramping; he has no weight loss. He states that on rare occasions, he has noticed blood on the toilet paper he has used. What additional pieces of assessment data do you need?

2. The nursing long-term care center has invited you to do a presentation concerning prevention of bowel incontinence in their residents. What points of information would you want to include in your presentation?

3. A 22-year-old man is to undergo surgery for Crohn's disease. He will have a new pouching ileostomy. He and his mother need teaching about what this means for his future elimination needs. What would you tell them?

Suggested Answers

1.
- Complete medical history, especially family information on colorectal and other cancer
- Depending on setting, complete physical examination including digital rectal examination; obtain fecal specimen for fecal occult blood
- Determine what colorectal screening practices client has used
- Determine medication use: prescribed, over-the-counter (OTC) and herbal and dietary supplements
- Do a dietary assessment over a 3-day period to determine balanced intake and adequate fiber
- Do not assume hemorrhoids
- Three-day screening for fecal occult blood
- Colonoscopy baseline

2. Information in your presentation should include the need for an adequate fluid intake (intake and output is a must). Many nonpharmaceutical methods exist for treating or avoiding constipation, including fruits, fiber, and activity; the use of bowel charts is very helpful in identifying problems early. Many clients think that they are drinking enough, when really they are not; be especially attentive to those with dementia or Alzheimer's disease who are unable to recognize the thirst mechanism. Other information to include is:
- Impact of fiber on continence
- Differentiating diarrhea incontinence from diarrhea due to impaction
- Bowel training programs
- Avoid excessive use of laxatives, cathartics, and enemas
- Impact of exercise on continence
- Addressing client's defecation needs promptly

3. Teaching for this family should include the following:
   - The anatomical changes associated with this bowel surgery
   - The amount of fecal material that the pouch will hold and how often it will need emptying
   - The method of evacuating stool from the pouch
   - The fact that he will be able to live as he did before; that he can swim, run, participate in any activity that he chooses
   - Dietary needs will be important; constipating foods, such as corn, chips, and popcorn, may cause a constipation-like action in the bowel contents

46

*M*obility and Immobility

Instructor Media Resources

Instructor's Resource CD
Instructor's Resources

Instructor's Manual
ExamView Test Bank
Image Collection
Power Point Slides
Weblinks
Skills Checklists

Student Media Resources

CD COMPANION

- Review Questions
- Glossary

WEBSITE

- Review Questions
- Student Learning Activities
- Glossary

Classroom Discussion

1. Review body mechanics and the maintenance of body alignment, balance, coordinated movement, exercise and activity, gravity, and friction.

2. Review the body systems involved in the regulation and coordination of body movement.

3. Review how the principles of body mechanics and movement are integrated into nursing care.

4. Review the pathological influences on body alignment and mobility, including postural abnormalities; congenital defects; disorders of the bones, joints, and muscles; central nervous system (CNS) damage; and musculoskeletal trauma.
   Ask students to identify specific pathological problems that may be experienced by clients.

5. Explain the general physiological and psychosocial effects of immobility on the client.

6. Ask students to identify specific growth and development factors that may influence mobility status and place the individual at risk for the hazards of immobility.

7. Guide students in the application of the critical thinking model and the nursing process for clients experiencing alterations in mobility.

8. Review the assessment of client mobility in the following areas:
   a. Joint range of motion
   b. Gait
   c. Exercise and activity tolerance
   d. Body alignment

   Ask students what constitutes expected or abnormal findings in the assessment of mobility.

9. Describe the physical assessment of the immobile client to determine the potential for or the presence of physiological, psychosocial, and developmental hazards.

10. Have students identify which assessment technique/equipment should be used to determine the presence of the following:
    a. Muscle atrophy
    b. Orthostatic hypotension
    c. Thrombosis
    d. Urinary retention
    e. Fecal impaction
    f. Atelectasis

11. Ask students what behavioral/psychosocial changes may be experienced by the client, especially a child or an older adult, who is having an adverse response to immobility.

12. Discuss developmentally appropriate nursing measures that may be implemented to reduce/eliminate the negative effects of immobility. Ask students to explain the rationale for these nursing interventions in counteracting the effect of immobility.

13. Have students identify how range-of-motion exercises may be integrated into other nursing care activities.

14. Ask students to identify possible situations in which additional assistance may be needed to position, move, transfer, or ambulate a client.

15. Have students specify the rationale for the use of supports (trochanter rolls, footboard, etc.) for positioning of the client.

16. Invite a physical therapist to speak to the class about measures to prevent the hazards of immobility and appropriate exercises/activities to provide for the immobilized client.

Interactive Exercises

1. Have students identify, orally or in writing, the influences on mobility for the following client problems:
   a. After cerebrovascular accident (CVA), with resultant right-sided hemiparesis
   b. Scoliosis or kyphosis
   c. Multiple fractures
   d. Osteoarthritis
   e. Paraplegia
   f. Parkinson's disease

2. Have students design teaching plans for the following or similar client situations in which mobility may be compromised:
   a. An 8-year-old child with leukemia who is placed on complete bed rest
   b. An 86-year-old who has had a CVA with resultant left-sided hemiplegia
   c. A 32-year-old with advanced multiple sclerosis

Clinical Skills/Techniques

1. Explain and demonstrate (by using simulation mannequin/model or volunteer, appropriate equipment, and educational media, as available) specific nursing interventions that may be implemented to promote proper body alignment and mobility and reduce the hazards of immobility, including:
   a. Lifting (by the nurse)
   b. Range of motion
   c. Positioning and moving a client in bed
   d. Transfer of a client from bed to chair or stretcher
   e. Applying elastic stockings and sequential compression stockings
   f. Assistance with client ambulation, with and without assistive devices

2. Have small groups of students practice the skills to promote body alignment and mobility, by using the appropriate equipment and supplies, and document the procedure and status of the client accordingly. Supervise activities such as client lifting and transfers.

3. Evaluate the students' ability to implement and document selected skills through return-demonstration/skill testing before clinical experience.

Client Care Experiences

1. Assign students to observe and participate in the nursing care of clients in acute, extended, rehabilitation, or home care settings, with focus placed on the promotion of body alignment and mobility.

2. Discuss expectations of students before the experience, specifically emphasizing client safety and requesting assistance in moving clients.

3. Review the students' assessments, strategies used, and evaluation of clients' mobility status after the experience.

4. Have students complete care plans/pathways for an assigned client who is experiencing alterations in physical mobility.

Resource for Student Activity

Immobility and Nursing Interventions

Immobility and Nursing Interventions

	Physiologic Effect of Immobility	Nursing Care to Minimize Effect
Metabolic		
Respiratory		
Cardiovascular		
Musculoskeletal		
Integumentary		
Elimination		
Psychosocial		

Critical Thinking Exercises (from text page 1480)

1. You are caring for a 57-year-old man who has just had a bilateral total knee replacement (TKR) for osteoarthritis. He is 2 days after surgery and beginning to transfer to a chair with help. He is 100 pounds overweight and has a history of deep vein thrombosis. He has compression stockings, continuous passive range of motion, and a heparin/saline lock. Make a list of potential nursing diagnoses.

2. When you are doing a home visit for a 75-year-old woman, the client's granddaughter runs in and says, "Did you show the nurse the sore on your leg that you got from falling yesterday?" What questions about mobility are important to ask the client? How do you begin your assessment?

3. Your clinical experience is in long-term care. You are working in assisted living. The nurse in charge of the assisted living wing asks you to help her with a program titled "Lifestyle Choices: Living Life to Its Fullest." She asks you to participate and discuss how regular exercise can improve overall health and to show how exercise can be incorporated into activities of daily living (ADLs). Develop a content outline and a time frame for your presentation.

4. You are caring for a 75-year-old man who is immobilized after spinal cord trauma from a motor vehicle accident. What potential complications would you be assessing for in this geriatric client?

Suggested Answers

1. Impaired physical mobility related to pain and mobility restrictions secondary to TKR. *Risk for trauma (falling) related to impaired mobility. Risk for altered peripheral tissue perfusion related to altered blood flow secondary to obesity, decreased mobility, and platelet agglutination secondary to TKR.*

2. Begin your assessment by asking Mrs. Miller about the fall, including why she thinks she fell. How did it happen, where did it happen, and has it happened before? Ask her to show you and explain her injuries. Has she done anything to correct the cause for the fall? Has she been checked for osteoporosis? Once assessments are made, then begin to work with Mrs. Miller on any corrective actions needed to be taken, including safety assessment for the home (see Chapter 37 on Safety) and a referral for a check for osteoporosis as necessary.

3. Begin your preparation by reviewing the chapter and paying particular attention to Tables 46-3, 46-4, and 46-10. Spend 10 minutes discussing the positive effects that exercise can have on the skin and the metabolic, respiratory, cardiovascular, musculoskeletal, and urinary systems. Spend 10 minutes with demonstration and return-demonstration of how to include exercises into ADLs. You may plan another session on an introduction to Tai Chi or yoga, depending on the receptivity of the group and the availability of someone to teach class.

4.
1) Neurosensory changes: altered LOC, confusion, decreased movement, strength, sensation, hypo or hyperthermia, and hypo or hyperreflexia
2) Skin and MS changes: skin breakdown, infection, slower wound healing, feeling cold, loss of bone mass, and changes in gait and posture
3) Cardiovascular changes: changes in B/P, decreased cardiac output, congestive heart failure, cardiac dysrhythmias, or DVTs
4) Pulmonary changes: pneumonia, pulmonary embolus, retention of secretions, decreased depth of respirations
5) Gastrointestinal and renal: anorexia, incontinence, constipation, alterations in intake and output, urinary retention, and urinary tract infection

47

$\mathcal{S}$kin Integrity and Wound Care

Instructor Media Resources

Instructor's Resource CD
evolve **Instructor's Resources**

Instructor's Manual
ExamView Test Bank
Image Collection
Power Point Slides
Weblinks
Skills Checklists

Student Media Resources

CD COMPANION

- Review Questions
- Glossary

evolve **WEBSITE**

- Review Questions
- Student Learning Activities
- Glossary

Classroom Discussion

1. Review the anatomy and physiology of the integumentary system.

2. Review the pathogenesis associated with the development of a pressure ulcer. Show photos, slides, and/or videotapes that depict the stages of pressure ulcers.

3. Discuss the prevalence of pressure ulcers in health care settings and the economic consequences of their development.

4. Identify client risk factors that are associated with the development of pressure ulcers.
   Have students provide specific client examples of impaired sensation or motor function, altered level of consciousness, and equipment/treatment (e.g., casts, traction) that may increase the risk for pressure ulcer development.

5. Discuss wound classification, by using photos/illustrations, models, and other available educational media.

6. Describe wound healing by primary and secondary intention. Identify the phases of primary intention healing. Use photos, illustrations, and/or models to differentiate the two types of wound healing.

7. Describe the following complications of wound healing:
   a. Hemorrhage
   b. Infection
   c. Dehiscence/evisceration
   d. Fistula formation

   Have students specify the etiologies and client signs and symptoms for these complications.

8. Explain the assessment tools that may be used to determine a client's risk for pressure ulcer development, including:
   a. Norton scale
   b. Braden scale

   Ask students to compare the tools and identify similarities and differences in their approaches.

9. Discuss factors that influence the development of pressure ulcers and wound healing, including shearing force/friction, moisture, poor nutrition, anemia, cachexia, obesity, infection, impaired peripheral circulation, and the process of aging. Have students provide the rationale for why each factor contributes to pressure ulcer development.

10. Discuss the potential psychosocial impact that wounds may have on an individual.

11. Describe the staging/identification process for pressure ulcers.

12. Review the physical assessment parameters for determination of possible ulcer development as follows:
    a. Skin
    b. Mobility
    c. Nutritional status
    d. Body fluids
    e. Pain

13. Have students identify how the following clients are at risk for pressure ulcer development:
    a. Unconscious client
    b. Client with restraints in place
    c. Client with a full-leg cast
    d. Client with nasal oxygen in place
    e. An incontinent client
    f. A client with hemiplegia or paraplegia

14. Explain the initial and ongoing assessment and treatment of wounds in emergency and stable settings.

15. Discuss the possible characteristics of wound drainage and methods to determine the type and amount of drainage.

16. Identify the nursing measures that may be implemented to prevent pressure ulcer development, including:
    a. Skin care
    b. Positioning
    c. Use of support surfaces
    d. Promotion of nutritional status

17. Discuss the assessment information necessary for the nurse to determine a schedule for positioning and the selection of support surfaces/mattresses.

18. Discuss the newest research and practice of methods to promote pressure ulcer healing, including cleansing, irrigation, and dressings.

19. Invite a nurse who specializes in the treatment of wounds/pressure ulcers to speak to the class about the nurse's role in prevention and promotion of healing.

20. Identify and describe the types of wound-drainage systems (i.e., Penrose, Hemovac).
    Show the students the different types of equipment for evacuation and collection of wound drainage, as available.

21. Discuss the use of sutures and staples for wound closures, by using photos, illustrations, and/or models. Identify the nursing care indicated for the different types of closures.

22. Identify and describe nursing interventions for wound care, including first aid, dressings, use of bandages and binders, irrigations, and application of heat and cold therapy.

23. Discuss and demonstrate different types and uses of dressings.
Ask students to identify which type of dressing may be indicated for the following wounds:
   a. Infected or necrotic wound
   b. Small, superficial wound
   c. Clean, granulating wound
   d. Moderately deep dermal ulcer
   e. Partial-thickness wound
   f. Burn or radiation damage
   g. Clean surgical wound with small amount of drainage

24. Ask students to identify measures that the nurse may implement to promote client comfort before and during wound care.

25. Have students identify situations in which heat and cold therapy may be used, possible complications of the therapy, and factors that may influence an individual's tolerance to the therapy.

26. Invite an infection control nurse to speak to the class about aseptic technique and wound care.

27. Discuss how wound care may be altered from the acute care to the ambulatory care setting. Ask students to identify creative measures that may be implemented for wound care in the home environment, where some equipment and supplies may not be readily available.

28. Guide students in the application of the critical thinking model and the nursing process for clients who are at risk for or are experiencing impaired skin integrity: pressure ulcers and/or wounds .

*I*nteractive Exercises

1. Provide students with examples of types of wounds and ask them to identify, orally and/or in writing, the type of wound and healing process that may be expected.

2. Provide students with photos/illustrations of pressure ulcers and have them identify and document the stage and/or color, with description of size, drainage, etc.
   Use sample agency forms for documentation, as available.

3. Provide examples (photos/illustrations) of the following or similar types of ulcers, and have students determine the types of treatment indicated and/or contraindicated:
   a. Heel ulcer with dry eschar
   b. Clean granulating wound
   c. Infected wound
   d. Deep ulcer with undermining

4. Have students investigate and report back on the types of treatment, equipment, supplies, and medication used in an affiliating agency for pressure ulcer prevention and/or healing.

5. Have the students, working individually or in small groups, design a teaching plan for a family member who will be caring at home for a client who is at risk of developing pressure ulcers. Focus on the areas of skin/hygienic care, nutrition, and/or supportive measures.
   Have students present the teaching plan to the class.

6. Have students design a teaching plan for a client and/or family member who will be responsible for wound care in the home.

7. Have students design a nutritional plan for a client with a risk of developing a pressure ulcer.

8. Have students complete a care plan/pathway for the following client simulation:

   The client is an 82-year-old woman who experienced a cerebrovascular accident (CVA) and has right-sided hemiparesis. She is frequently incontinent of urine and occasionally incontinent of feces. At times she is not fully aware of her surroundings. When not in bed, she spends her day in a wheelchair with a soft jacket restraint. The client was admitted to the extended care facility 1 week ago.

Clinical Skills/Techniques

1. By using volunteers and/or models, simulate different types of wounds and have students practice the assessment and treatment of the wound and the documentation of wound care (use a sample form from an affiliating agency, if available).

2. Explain and demonstrate (by using simulation mannequin/model, appropriate equipment and supplies and available educational media) the following nursing interventions:
   a. Assessment for the risk of pressure ulcer development
   b. Treatment of pressure ulcers
   c. Application of dry and wet-to-dry dressings
   d. Use of vacuum-assisted closure (wound VAC)
   e. Irrigation of wounds
   f. Application of an abdominal or breast binder
   g. Application of an elastic bandage
   h. Application of a hot, moist compress to an open wound
   i. Application of hot and cold therapy

3. Have small groups of students, with supervision, practice and document the selected nursing interventions for the assessment, prevention, and treatment of pressure ulcers and wound care.

4. Evaluate the students' ability, through return-demonstration/skill testing to implement and document the risk assessment, prevention, and treatment of pressure ulcers, and wound care through return-demonstration/skill testing before clinical experience.

Client Care Experiences

1. Assign students to observe and participate in the nursing care of clients who are at risk for or are experiencing impaired skin integrity in the acute, restorative, or home care setting.

2. Discuss client assessment and expectations of nursing interventions before the experience. Review orders for specific supportive measures and wound treatment, as indicated. Review and evaluate students' interventions after the experience, focusing on the implementation of strategies to promote skin integrity.

3. Have students complete a care plan/pathway for clients at risk for an impairment in skin integrity.

4. Assign students to observe and participate in the nursing care of clients in acute and home health care settings, with the focus on wound assessment and implementation of wound-care techniques.

5. Discuss measures for the prevention and treatment of complications of wounds with the group. Have students identify client educational needs regarding wound care. Assist students in the evaluation of wound healing.

6. Have students complete a care plan/pathway for clients who have experienced wounds and/or the complications of wound healing.

Resources for Student Activities

Complications of Wound Healing

Complications of Wound Healing

Complication	Etiology	Signs/Symptoms	Nursing Assessment and Care
Hemorrhage			
Infection			
Dehiscence			
Evisceration			
Fistula Formation			

*C*ritical Thinking Exercises (from text page 1562)

1. When removing a saline-moistened dressing from a sacral pressure ulcer, you note that the gauze is dripping with beige-colored fluid. What assessments should be made, and after the assessment, what should be done next? What could be the possible cause of this drainage?

2. After changing a client's position, you observe redness over the bony prominences. How should this area be assessed?

3. You have just admitted a client from a nursing home to your division. On initial assessment, you assess a stage III pressure ulcer. How do you determine the type of care and dressing to use with this particular pressure ulcer?

4. You are providing care to an older adult incontinent Hispanic man who is bed-bound. How will you assess for pressure ulcers in this client? What measures can you take to prevent his skin from breaking down?

Suggested Answers

1. The assessments that should be made include noting the number of gauze pads that were removed from the wound, as this provide an estimate of the amount of drainage and will provide information for choosing a more effective dressing; noting the presence of odor from the gauze and or wound, as this may indicate the presence of a wound infection; note when the previous dressing was removed to determine if the dressing-change frequency is adequate. It is likely that the wound drainage, because of the abnormal color, is indicative of a wound infection.

2. Assess the reddened area with a gloved finger. Press the gloved finger over the reddened area to determine if this area blanches. If the area does not blanch on palpation, this may be indicative of tissue damage, and a plan should be instituted that decreases the amount of pressure to this area.

3. The client should be evaluated for the cause of the pressure ulcer. This can be done by using the risk-assessment scale, which will provide information on the client's ability to move independently, to sense discomfort, to eat a balanced diet, and will note the presence of moisture, shear, and friction. Once this evaluation is done, a plan to decrease the risk factors can be instituted. Next a wound assessment will provide information on the type of dressing that should be used. Finally, consultation with the client, caregivers, and health care team will provide information on the pressure ulcer plan of care and how this plan will fit into the entire plan of care for the client.

4. Skin assessment is done, noting skin integrity over bony prominences and in the perineal area. Examine the skin in a well-lighted room, using a gloved finger to feel for color changes over at-risk areas. Consider interventions to control moisture, containment devices such as a fecal incontinence pouch or external urinary condom catheter, or protection with a moisture-barrier ointment. Include in the plan of care a support surface that will reduce the pressure, and institute a turning schedule. Assess his ability to maintain an adequate intake of calories and fluid, and work with the health care team to ensure calorie intake.

48

*S*ensory Alterations

Instructor Media Resources

Instructor's Resource CD
Instructor's Resources

Instructor's Manual
ExamView Test Bank
Image Collection
Power Point Slides
Weblinks

Student Media Resources

CD COMPANION

- Review Questions
- Glossary

evolve **WEBSITE**

- Review Questions
- Student Learning Activities
- Glossary

Classroom Discussion

1. Review the anatomy and physiology of the nervous system in respect to the major senses: sight, hearing, touch, smell, taste.

2. Discuss common sensory deficits that the nurse may encounter in client situations.

3. Describe sensory deprivation and overload and its recognition in clients. Ask students to provide examples of possible health care situations that may contribute to sensory deprivation or overload.

4. Discuss factors that influence sensory function.

5. Review the assessment of a client's sensory status, including health promotion behaviors and medical history. Ask students how a client's sensory abilities may be determined through routine observation or communication.

6. Identify clients who are at risk for sensory alterations, including individuals who are older, immobile, engage in particular occupations, have an alteration in mental status, or are isolated.

7. Review the nursing assessment for specific sensory deficits.

8. Discuss health promotion activities for sensory function:
   a. Screening
   b. Safety and prevention
   c. Assistive devices
   d. Stimulation

9. Discuss methods of communication that may be used by individuals experiencing sensory deficits.

10. Have students specify strategies that may be used to interact/communicate with a client experiencing expressive or receptive aphasia or an inability to speak because of a laryngectomy or placement of an endotracheal tube.

11. Invite a speech and/or occupational therapist to speak to the class about promoting the client's self-care activities and communication.

12. Stimulate a discussion on the importance of promoting sensation/stimulation, especially touch, for the older client in a restorative care setting.

Interactive Exercises

1. Have students complete a sensory assessment on a peer or family member/friend, and report and record the findings.

2. Have students investigate and report on available resources within an affiliating agency to facilitate communication with clients.

3. Organize a role-playing experience for the students based on the following or similar scenarios:
   a. Assisting a visually impaired client to ambulate and independently complete activities of daily living (bathing, dressing, eating)
   b. Communicating with a hearing-impaired or aphasic client
   c. Caring for a client in an intensive care or isolation unit
   d. Assisting an older adult client on a medical unit after a right-sided cerebrovascular accident (CVA) with resultant hemiparesis

If possible, have students simulate the sensory deficits that may be present. Be aware that students simulating sensory deficits may experience an anxiety reaction.
   Supervision of these exercises is recommended.

Clinical Skill/Technique

1. Have students modify a simulated client environment to meet optimal safety and stimulation needs. Students should consider the scheduling of client care activities to avoid over- or understimulation.

Client Care Experiences

1. Assign students to observe clients in a health care setting and note the amount and type of stimuli present. If possible, observation in an intensive care, isolation, or burn unit is desirable.

2. Arrange for students to participate in vision and hearing screenings in a community setting, such as a school, clinic, or pediatrician's office.

3. Assign students to observe and participate in the nursing care of clients who may be experiencing sensory/perceptual alterations and/or a risk for injury related to a sensory deficit. Discuss expectations with students before the experience

4. Focus on the assessment of the client's sensory and perceptual status, and the implementation of safety measures, therapeutic communication, and strategies to promote or reduce excessive sensory input.

5. Review and evaluate the students' interactions, noting the degree of sensory stimulation provided and client responses.

6. Have students complete a care plan/pathway for an assigned client with a sensory/perceptual alteration.

Resource for Student Activity

Sensory Assessment/Intervention Chart

Sensory Assessment/Intervention Chart

Senses	Screening Measures	Prevention and Safety Measures	Enhancement and Assistive Devices	Meaningful Stimuli
Vision				
Hearing				
Touch				
Smell				
Taste				

Critical Thinking Exercises (from text page 1590)

1. Mr. Tully is a 54-year-old farmer who is having a physical for insurance purposes. Overall, his health is good. His wife reports that over the past year, he has lost interest in being involved in social gatherings, is more irritable, and often has asked her to repeat what was said. Recently, he complained of a constant buzzing in his ears. What assessment data are needed? What specific interventions may be needed?

2. Mrs. Marfell, 79 years old, is visiting the outpatient cardiac center for a routine checkup. The nurse notices that the client needed help reading the physical forms. She also told the nurse she is having increased difficulty driving at night. What additional assessment data should the nurse gather from Mrs. Marfell?

3. You have an opportunity to speak with a group of parents and students regarding the importance of hearing protection. What information would you share with this varied age group to promote healthy hearing?

Suggested Answers

1. Mrs. Tully is providing a history that correlates with hearing loss. Because Mr. Tully is a farmer, the nurse should gather additional information that relates to noise-induced hearing loss (NIHL), which would result in permanent injury. The nurse should administer the hearing-loss questionnaire and also identify when the tinnitus began, and is it constant and more troublesome at night and in quiet surroundings. The nurse should plan interventions to teach the importance of hearing-protection devices to both Mr. and Mrs. Tully. Teach Mrs. Tully regarding the need to speak more clearly and louder. Educate her regarding the value of offering praise and encouragement for using hearing-protection devices. Because hearing loss exposes one to increased safety risk, the nurse should advise the client to use care to assess surroundings for safety purposes. In addition, Mr. Tully should be referred to an audiologist.

2. The nurse should do a thorough vision assessment. In addition, the nurse should do a home environmental assessment to involve client and family in making the environment safe and to promote functional client independence. Because Mrs. Marfell is having difficulty seeing at night, this is a safety issue, and the nurse should assess the client's need to drive at night. The nurse could assess whether Mrs. Marfell has someone who could drive during fog, haze, rain, and at night. This client may need a referral for a home health nurse to do follow-up assessment related to home safety factors.

3. The nurse should provide information regarding the effect of constant high noise levels on hearing. Explain the factors such as excess exposure to loud music, equipment, firearms, stereo headsets, boats, lawnmowers, and farm equipment. Explain the early symptoms of NIHL such as tinnitus, difficulty hearing some consonants, and hearing sounds that are barrel-like. Explain the value of using hearing-protection devices, and emphasize the importance of family support, which research has shown fosters the use of these devices. Explain the need for consistent use of hearing-protection devices for effective prevention of hearing loss.

49

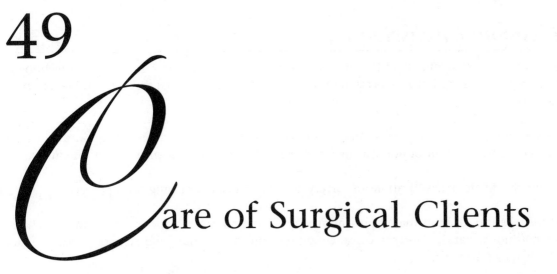

*C*are of Surgical Clients

Instructor Media Resources

Instructor's Resource CD
evolve **Instructor's Resources**

Instructor's Manual
ExamView Test Bank
Image Collection
Power Point Slides
Weblinks
Skills Checklists

Student Media Resources

CD COMPANION

- Review Questions
- Glossary

evolve **WEBSITE**

- Review Questions
- Student Learning Activities
- Glossary

Classroom Discussion

1. Discuss the major highlights of the history of surgical nursing and recent changes in technology (e.g., laser and fiberoptics) and location of surgery (ambulatory centers) that have influenced nursing practice.

2. Ask students how the nursing assessment and its focus may be altered depending on the location of and circumstances surrounding a client's surgery (e.g., same-day or emergency procedures).

3. Discuss the different classifications of surgery and the associated nursing care approaches.

4. Identify client risk factors that, if present, may affect the surgical experience, including the client's age, nutritional status, obesity, medical conditions, pregnancy, fluid and electrolyte balance, and radiotherapy treatment.

5. Describe the components of a comprehensive preoperative nursing assessment of the client, including:
   a. Past medical history
   b. Previous surgeries
   c. Perceptions and understanding of surgery
   d. Medication history
   e. Allergies
   f. Smoking habits
   g. Alcohol/substance abuse
   h. Family support
   i. Occupation
   j. Preoperative pain
   k. Emotional status
   l. Sociocultural background/practices

   Ask students how responses to each area may influence the client's perioperative experience and what the nurse's responsibilities are in relation to follow-up and reporting.

6. Review the physical assessment in relation to preoperative client assessment. Discuss how findings may influence the client's perioperative experience and determine the nurse's interventions, follow-up, and reporting (i.e., elevated temperature, decreased respirations).

7. Discuss preoperative laboratory and diagnostic tests that may be used to determine abnormalities before surgery.

8. Describe the general client preparation and education and nursing responsibilities in the preoperative phase. Ask students how these preoperative preparations and nursing interventions may be altered for clients having ambulatory/same-day surgery.

9. Review the legal parameters and nursing accountability associated with informed consent.
   Ask students what the nurse should do if the client does not demonstrate an understanding of the surgical procedure, or if the client is unconscious and requires an emergency procedure.

10. Identify and describe the purposes and advantages of preoperative teaching for the client and family.

11. Ask students to share personal and/or family perioperative experiences. If the experiences were negative, ask what, if possible, a nurse might have done to improve them.

12. Identify and discuss common expectations of clients in the perioperative phase.

13. Describe common preoperative physical preparation of the client, including promotion of fluid and electrolyte balance, reduction of the risk of surgical wound infection, skin preparation, bowel and bladder preparation, and promotion of rest and comfort. Have students identify any additional specific measures that the nurse may implement to assist the client in the preoperative phase.

14. Review the preparation of the client on the day of surgery, including the following:
    a. Completion of preoperative checklist
    b. Monitoring of vital signs
    c. Provision of hygienic care
    d. Check of hair and cosmetics
    e. Removal/storage of prosthetics and valuables
    f. Preparation of bowel/bladder
    g. Application of antiemboli stockings/compression devices
    h. Implementation of special procedures (i.e., nasogastric [NG] tube insertion)
    j. Administration of preoperative medications
    l. Maintenance of client safety and determination of latex allergy

15. Ask students how the preparation for surgery may differ for clients of different ages, who speak other languages, who have no family support, who have specific spiritual/cultural needs, or who have a psychiatric history.

16. Discuss the nurse's responsibility in client transport to the operating room.

17. Discuss the intraoperative phase of the experience, including the immediate preparation of the client, introduction of anesthesia, client positioning, documentation, and roles and responsibilities of the nurse.

18. Identify and describe the different types of, and the uses, risks, and nursing care associated with anesthesia.

19. Discuss the postoperative phase, including transfer to the postanesthesia care unit (PACU), client monitoring, nursing measures to support vital functions, and documentation. Ask students to indicate specific assessments that the nurse in a PACU may conduct to determine overall client status.

20. Have students identify similarities and differences in postoperative/PACU care for clients after inpatient or ambulatory surgery.

21. Discuss discharge criteria for PACU for clients returning to an acute care unit or to their homes.

22. Discuss postoperative treatment for clients in an acute care setting.

Chapter 49: Care of Surgical Clients 289

23. Identify nursing interventions for clients in the postoperative phase for the promotion and maintenance of respiratory, circulatory, and neurological function; temperature control; fluid and electrolyte balance; nutrition; elimination; skin integrity; wound healing; rest; comfort; self-concept; and self-care abilities.

    Have students identify specific examples of nursing measures that assist clients to attain goals in the postoperative phase (see Resources for Student Activities).

24. Discuss postoperative complications, their recognition, and subsequent nursing interventions.

25. Invite a nurse who practices in an operating room and/or PACU to speak to the class about client assessment, preparation for surgery or discharge, and nursing responsibilities.

26. Have students, by utilizing the following or similar situations, identify interventions that the nurse may implement:
    a. A client who has, on the day of surgery, been found to have no blood work or radiographs completed
    b. A client in the PACU with completely saturated dressings
    c. A client experiencing a rigid, distended abdomen 2 days after surgery
    d. A client who has an elevated temperature on the day of surgery, within 2 days after surgery, or 5 days after surgery
    e. A client with a latex allergy
    f. A client who has a hearing aid, eyeglasses, or religious article

27. Guide students in the application of the critical thinking model and the nursing process for clients in the preoperative, intraoperative, and postoperative phases.

Interactive Exercise

1. Have students role-play the preparation of a client for surgery, including completion of the preoperative checklist.

Clinical Skills/Techniques

1. Explain and demonstrate postoperative exercises. Have students practice along with the demonstration in the classroom or skill laboratory. Evaluate the students' ability to perform/teach the postoperative exercises through return demonstration.

2. Have students prepare a simulated client's room for the postoperative phase.

Client Care Experiences

1. Assign students to accompany clients (as possible) through the intraoperative phase and to observe surgical asepsis, client preparation, and nursing roles. Have students share their observations after the experience in inpatient and/or ambulatory surgery settings.

2. Assign students to observe and/or participate in the care of clients in a PACU. Have students monitor clients' status and provide and document nursing care, with supervision. Have students collaborate with the nursing staff on client discharge from PACU.

3. Assign students to observe and participate in the nursing care of clients on a PACU in an acute care facility. Work with students to prepare and conduct preoperative client teaching. Discuss the assessment of the client and appropriate nursing interventions for the postoperative period, including reinforcement of postoperative exercises.

4. Have students complete a general care plan/pathway for clients undergoing an operative experience. Have students individualize the care plan/pathway for actual clients with specific preoperative and postoperative needs.

Resources for Student Activities

Preoperative Assessment Form
Nursing Interventions for Clients in the Postoperative Phase

Preoperative Assessment

	Assessment Data
Past Medical History	
Previous Surgery	
Medication History	
Allergies	
Smoking Habits	
Alcohol/Substance Abuse	
Family Support	
Occupation	
Preoperative Pain	
Emotional Health	
Sociocultural Factors	

Chapter 49: Care of Surgical Clients   291

Postoperative Nursing Interventions

Client Functions	Nursing Interventions
Respiration	
Circulation	
Temperature Control	
Neurological	
Skin Integrity/Wound Healing	
Genitourinary	
Gastrointestinal	
Fluid/Electrolyte Balance	
Pain Management	

Critical Thinking Exercises (from text page 1642)

1. Your 82-year-old client is admitted after a fall for repair of a fractured hip. What postoperative complications are seen in the older client undergoing this type of surgery?

2. Mr. B. is a 52-year-old client who will have thoracic surgery. He has a 30-year history of smoking one pack of cigarettes per day. What type of pulmonary preventive measures would you expect Mr. B to need postoperatively?

3. Mrs. C. was admitted for ambulatory surgery for an inguinal hernia repair. What discharge criteria would be used for Mrs. C., and what discharge instructions would she require?

4. Your client is scheduled for abdominal hysterectomy at 2:00 PM. Based on nothing-by-mouth (NPO) guidelines, what fasting schedule should you implement in collaboration with the surgeon and anesthesia provider?

Suggested Answers

1. Postoperative complications could include thrombus, embolus, blood loss, atelectasis, dehydration, congestive heart failure (CHF), pneumonia, activity intolerance, and pressure ulcers.

2. Mr. B. would need to deep breathe, cough, and turn a minimum of every 2 hours. More than likely, either incentive spirometry or PEP therapy would be ordered. Aerosol (nebulizer) treatments with a bronchodilator may be indicated, as well as oxygen therapy.

3. Discharge therapy would include the following: the ability to void (if applicable); ability to ambulate (if applicable); alert and oriented; no pain medication for 1 hour; minimal nausea and vomiting; no excess bleeding or drainage; received written postoperative instructions and prescriptions; verbalizes understanding of instructions; and is being discharged with a responsible adult. Discharge instructions would include the following: signs and symptoms of infection; medications, including dose, schedule, purpose, and special instructions; activity restrictions (showering, driving, lifting); diet; wound care; and follow-up appointment.

4. The client should fast from intake of a light meal for 6 or more hours and clear liquids for 2 to 3 hours before surgery. The client can have a light breakfast up until 7:00 to 8:00 AM and no liquids after 12:00 PM. Remove fluids and solid foods from the client's bedside, and post a sign over the bed to alert hospital personnel and family members about fasting restrictions at the designated times.

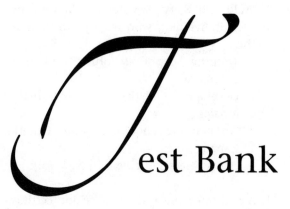

UNIT 1   THE CLIENT AND THE HEALTH CARE ENVIRONMENT

Chapter 1   Nursing Today

1. Contemporary nursing practice is based on knowledge generated through nursing theories. Florence Nightingale's theory introduced the concept that nursing care focuses on:
   1. Health maintenance and restoration
   2. Psychological needs
   3. A maximal level of wellness
   4. Interpersonal interactions with the client

2. Nursing education programs in the United States may seek voluntary accreditation by the appropriate Accrediting Commission Council of the:
   1. American Nurses Association
   2. International Council of Nurses
   3. Congress for Nursing Practice
   4. National League for Nursing

3. For an individual to become a nurse practitioner, specific preparation is required. The minimal educational requirement for a nurse practitioner is:
   1. Diploma in nursing
   2. Baccalaureate in nursing
   3. Master's in nursing
   4. Doctorate in nursing

4. It is important that the interests of nurses be represented within a political framework. A group that lobbies at the state and federal levels for advancement of nursing's role, economic interest, and health care is the:
   1. American Nurses Association (ANA)
   2. State boards of nursing
   3. National Student Nurses' Association
   4. American Hospital Association

5. A nurse moves from Seattle to Boston to begin working in a hospital. The most important factor for the nurse to consider when moving to another state is the:
   1. Standard for nursing practice in Boston
   2. Clinical ladder of mobility in the new hospital
   3. Massachusetts Nurse Practice Act
   4. ANA requirement for continuing education unit (CEU) certification in Massachusetts

6. A nurse is caring for a client who has chronic renal failure. The client is very fatigued and has a knowledge deficit related to the dialysis therapy he will perform at home. The nurse states, "We will do everything possible to return you to the optimal level of self-care." In putting together an approach to best meet the needs of this client, the nurse is fulfilling the role of:
   1. Manager
   2. Educator
   3. Counselor
   4. Communicator

7. Nurses have the opportunity to work in a wide variety of health care agencies around the world. The practice setting, however, where the majority of nurses continue to work is:
   1. Acute care
   2. Home care
   3. Ambulatory care
   4. Long-term care

8. A client is receiving phenytoin (Dilantin) to prevent seizure activity. He seeks employment where his physical challenge will not be a problem. To which allied health care professional should the nurse refer this client?
   1. Respiratory therapist
   2. Physician's assistant
   3. Occupational therapist
   4. Physical therapist

9. The Goldmark Report concluded that:
   1. A theory-based curriculum is necessary for accreditation.
   2. Nursing education programs must be affiliated with universities.
   3. Nursing roles and responsibilities require clarification.
   4. Increased financial support should be provided for nursing education.

10. A number of figures in nursing made significant contributions to the profession and the overall health of the community. Lillian Wald and Mary Brewster (1893) were two such individuals, who were responsible for the:
    1. Training school at Johns Hopkins in Baltimore
    2. Development of the *American Journal of Nursing*
    3. First training school in Toronto, Ontario, Canada
    4. Henry Street Settlement in New York

11. A registered nurse (RN) is seeking certification in a specialty area. To obtain the certification, he or she will have to complete:
    1. An examination and minimal practice requirements
    2. One general examination given to all nurses seeking certification
    3. A graduate degree in nursing
    4. A request for state approval

12. In the ANA Standards of Professional Practice, which one of the following is a specific measurement criterion for "The nurses' decisions and actions on behalf of clients are determined in an ethical manner"?
    1. Acts as client advocate
    2. Participates in data collection
    3. Consults with health care providers for client care
    4. Seeks experiences to maintain clinical skills

13. The nursing students are investigating the origins of professional nursing in the United States. In the 19th century, the growth of nursing was stimulated by:
    1. The Civil War
    2. Federal legislation
    3. Florence Nightingale
    4. The Women's Suffrage Movement

4. An RN who has just received her license is aware of the need to keep current in the field. She recognizes that ongoing education is essential for safe practice. In planning to participate in in-service education, the nurse will attend:
   1. A workshop given at a nursing convention on malpractice
   2. A program on new cardiac medications provided in the hospital where she works
   3. Credit courses in communication offered at the community college
   4. Noncredit courses on nursing issues available through the Internet

5. Nurses need to be aware of current trends in the health care delivery system to respond in educational preparation and practice. A major trend influencing nursing practice today is:
   1. Decreased client acuity
   2. Increased hospital stays
   3. Decreased emphasis on health promotion
   4. Increased incidence of chronic disease

6. Health promotion is an important factor in cost reduction for health care delivery. The nurse assists the client in a health-promotion activity by:
   1. Administering medication
   2. Treating a foot ulcer
   3. Obtaining an operative consent
   4. Discussing exercise and nutrition

Chapter 2 Health Care Delivery System

1. Health care costs increased dramatically from 1965 to 1985 as a result of:
   1. Unrestricted medical prescription
   2. Increased numbers in the work force
   3. Increased incidence of acute disease
   4. A growing birth rate

2. In an attempt to reduce the tremendous increase in health care costs, regulatory or government interventions for cost reduction were initiated. These interventions include:
   1. Prospective payment systems
   2. Federal guidelines for treatment
   3. State limits on health care fees
   4. Court review of insurance coverage

3. Health care professionals are affected by increasing health care costs. Nurses may be most directly influenced by cost control because they:
   1. Constitute a large percentage of the health care budget
   2. Achieve higher salary levels than do other health care professionals
   3. Provide direct client care without reimbursement
   4. Deliver the least cost-effective care

4. Levels of prevention are used by the nurse to provide a framework or guide for nursing interventions. Focus is based on the client's needs and the care or service that is provided. An example of a true health promotion service is a(n):
   1. Immunization clinic
   2. Diabetic support group
   3. Aerobic dance class
   4. Smoking-cessation clinic

5. A wide variety of health care–delivery agencies exist. An example of an agency that provides secondary level care is a:
   1. Home health agency
   2. Hospice
   3. State-owned psychiatric hospital
   4. Nursing home

6. Which of the following fits within the occupational safety and health categories?
   1. Motorcycle helmets
   2. Firearms safety
   3. Swimming lessons
   4. Noise exposure

7. The health care for an employee of a large corporation may be paid, at a discount, through a contractual agreement between a hospital and the corporation. This is an example of a(n):
   1. Preferred Provider Organization (PPO)
   2. Medicare Health Management Organization (HMO)
   3. Fee-for-service plan
   4. Third party payment

8. A client comes to the ambulatory care clinic for management of a chronic condition. While speaking with the nurse, he asks for an explanation as to the difference between Medicare and Medicaid. The nurse tells the client that the Medicaid insurance program is best described as:
   1. A two-part federally funded health care program for older and disabled persons
   2. Acute care hospital insurance for older persons
   3. A state-regulated health care program for persons of low income
   4. A fee-for-service insurance plan that supports preventive health care

9. Quality care management is an innovative approach to delivering health care. The major factor in its success is that it:
   1. Focuses on the process
   2. Uses outcomes to manage the client care
   3. Is used exclusively in the acute care setting
   4. Allows a high degree of flexibility for the nurse delivering the care

10. Case management is one strategy for coordinating health care services. What best describes this caregiving approach?
    1. It is designed for clients requiring minimal to moderate levels of care.
    2. Continuity of care is the primary concern.
    3. The physician is the coordinator of the client care.
    4. This focus of care may be more expensive.

11. The payment mechanism that Medicare uses for its health care financing is:
    1. Capitation
    2. Prospective payment
    3. Fixed payments
    4. Direct contracting

12. A student nurse visiting a nurse-managed clinic should expect to see which of the following services offered?
    1. Same-day surgery
    2. Family support services
    3. Ongoing psychiatric therapy
    4. Physical therapy

13. The client with a disability is being discharged from the medical unit in the hospital but still requires restorative care to return to a prior level of functioning. This client should be referred to a(n):
    1. Assisted living facility
    2. Ambulatory health center
    3. Subacute care unit
    4. Home health care agency

14. Which of the following is an appropriate referral for an older client who requires some assistance with daily activities within a partially protective environment?
    1. Respite care
    2. Rehabilitative care
    3. Assisted living
    4. Extended care

15. The nurse recognizes that discharge planning for clients begins:
    1. After a diagnosis has been established
    2. Once the long-term needs are identified
    3. When the acute care therapies are completed
    4. Immediately on admission to a health care facility

6. A neighbor is asking about what is included in a managed care organization (MCO). He says that he isn't sure how this type of health insurance works. You respond to the neighbor most appropriately by explaining that the MCO:
   1. Allows the individual to go to any physician that he desires
   2. Provides reimbursement for all requested health services
   3. Offers additional coverage for illness-oriented care
   4. Focuses on primary health care for designated members

7. Levels of prevention are used by the nurse to provide a framework or guide for nursing interventions. Focus is based on the client's needs and the care or service provided. An example of the application of the secondary level of prevention is demonstrated by the nurse:
   1. Providing well-baby care
   2. Completing a community health blood pressure screening
   3. Administering a bronchodilating medication
   4. Instructing the client in the cardiac rehabilitation program

Chapter 3   Community-Based Nursing Practice

1. The student nurse is investigating different types of practice settings. In looking at community health nursing, the student recognizes that it:
   1. Requires graduate level educational preparation
   2. Is the same as public health nursing
   3. Focuses on the incidence of disease
   4. Includes direct care and services to subpopulations

2. The community health nurse assumes different roles while working with clients. As an educator assisting the client and family with nutritional needs, the nurse should:
   1. Tell the client the best foods to buy
   2. Purchase foods at the lowest cost for the client
   3. Ask the client and family what they think they should eat
   4. Provide information on food sources and stores with reasonable pricing

3. In community health, the nurse works with clients from different populations who are extremely vulnerable. Which one of the following clients from a vulnerable population currently appears to be at the greatest risk?
   1. A physically abused client in a shelter
   2. An older adult taking medication for hypertension
   3. A schizophrenic client in outpatient therapy
   4. A substance abuser who shares drug paraphernalia

4. A client has a history of a gastrointestinal (GI) disease with eight hospitalizations over the past 21-year period. He eats a well-balanced diet that keeps his GI symptoms suppressed. Which level of prevention corresponds to his dietary management?
   1. Primary prevention
   2. Secondary prevention
   3. Tertiary prevention
   4. Health promotion

5. A client with chronic renal failure receives peritoneal dialysis in his home. He is emotionally upset because of the expenses of his therapy. Which of the following statements from his home health nurse reflects client advocacy in response to the client's concern?
   1. "This peritoneal dialysis is less expensive than hemodialysis in the hospital."
   2. "Have you considered a renal transplant?"
   3. "You must feel awful about this situation, but this is the best course of treatment for you."
   4. "Let's call the regional dialysis center and explore options for reducing the cost of your home dialysis."

6. Community assessments are important for the nurse to understand and respond to the needs of the population. In assessing the structure of the community, the nurse will focus on:
   1. Collecting demographic data on age distribution
   2. Visiting neighborhood schools to review health records
   3. Interviewing clients to determine the cultural makeup of the subgroups
   4. Observing locations where services, such as water sanitation, are provided

7. Change is not always easy for members of a community or a profession. The nurse working as an effective change agent in a community should:
   1. Tell community members how to manage their health needs
   2. Work with clients and groups to select alternative health care sites and treatments
   3. Make decisions for individual clients regarding their health care options
   4. Provide instruction in the way the community should address health issues

8. The client is being discharged from an acute care facility after a total hip replacement. She will need follow-up for her rehabilitation and exercise plan. In addition to a home health care nurse, what referral should be discussed?
   1. Social worker
   2. Dietitian
   3. Physical therapist
   4. Respiratory therapist

9. The nurse recognizes that a greater need exists for comprehensive community health care. Which of the following is the largest contributing factor for the increase in the need for and use of home care?
   1. Government funding of the home care setting has increased greatly.
   2. The existence of more single-income families has increased the need for their elderly relatives to receive care in the home.
   3. Clients are more acutely ill when discharged from the acute care facility.
   4. Seven-days-per-week services are available for the elderly in home care agencies.

10. It is important that critical aspects of *Healthy People 2010* be incorporated into health care delivery in the community. One of the overall goals of this plan is to:
    1. Increase life expectancy
    2. Decrease health care costs
    3. Promote managed care organizations
    4. Establish the credentials of professionals providing services

Chapter 4   Theoretical Foundations of Nursing Practice

1. In preparing to review different theories, the nurse reviews basic information to assist in understanding the material. Theories are defined as:
   1. Statements that describe concepts or connect concepts
   2. Mental formulations of objects or events
   3. Aspects of reality that can be consciously sensed
   4. Concepts or propositions that project a systematic view of phenomena

2. Different types of theories may be used by nurses seeking to study the basis of nursing practice. When the goal of a theory is to speculate on why phenomena occur, it is termed a:
   1. Prescriptive theory
   2. Descriptive theory
   3. Grand theory
   4. Middle-range theory

3. Which one of the four linkages of interest in the nursing paradigm refers to factors in the home or school?
   1. Person
   2. Health
   3. Nursing care
   4. Environment/situation

4. The nurse is working within a health care system that uses Neuman's theory. A client is having difficulty breathing and requires oxygen and medication. Within Neuman's theory, the nurse approaches the client to:
   1. Strengthen the line of defenses at the secondary level of prevention
   2. Promote attainment of biologic self-care requisites
   3. Assist in physiological adaptation to internal changes
   4. Achieve the 14 basic needs

5. Although similarities exist in the different nursing theories, key elements distinguish one from another. The emphasis of Jean Watson's conceptual model is that
   1. Self-care maintains wholeness
   2. Subsystems exist in dynamic stability
   3. Stimuli disrupt an adaptive system
   4. Caring is central to the essence of nursing

6. A community health nurse is working with a variety of clients and decides to use a Systems theory approach to assist them to meet their health care needs. In using the Systems theory, the nurse focuses on the:
   1. Client's interaction with the environment
   2. Hierarchy of the client's human needs
   3. Client's attitudes toward health behaviors
   4. Response of the client to the process of growth and development

7. While working on a postoperative unit, the nurse is applying the elements of the Self-Care theory. The nurse who assists the client to manage or attain self-care in wound management is using the theory developed by:
   1. Florence Nightingale
   2. Virginia Henderson
   3. Dorothea Orem
   4. Imogene King

8. Martha Roger's theory has a framework for practice that includes the:
   1. Twenty-one nursing problems within four major client needs
   2. Manipulation of the client's environment
   3. Seven categories of behavior and behavioral balance
   4. Unitary human being in continuous interaction with the environment

9. If the nurse wanted to apply a theory that focused on stress reduction, a theory proposed by which one of the following individuals should be selected?
   1. Peplau
   2. Orlando
   3. Neuman
   4. Parse

10. A similarity in the theories of Leininger and Benner and Wrubel is:
    1. The Client's adaptation to demands
    2. Caring as a central focus
    3. An emphasis on the maximal level of wellness
    4. Dynamic interpersonal communication

11. The nurse is working with a client with multiple sclerosis to be able to take care of himself in his own home. The nursing theory that best supports this client's situation is:
    1. Henderson's theory
    2. Orem's theory
    3. Abdellah's theory
    4. Neuman's theory

Chapter 5   Nursing Research as a Basis for Practice

1. The nurse may use a number of different types of research approaches when conducting a study. Which of the following is an example of an exploratory type of research?
    1. Establishing facts and relations of past events
    2. Refining a hypothesis on the relations among phenomena
    3. Portraying the characteristics of persons, situations, or groups
    4. Testing how well a program, practice, or policy is working

2. The Health Information Portability and Privacy Act (HIPAA) was implemented in 2003. This newly implemented legislation may influence nursing research in the area of:
    1. The cost of the study
    2. Where the study may be published
    3. What type of study may be conducted
    4. How the data will be obtained and protected

3. As nurses move forward in their education, different roles may be assumed in regard to research. The expected research role for the baccalaureate-prepared nurse is to:
    1. Assume the role of a clinical expert
    2. Identify clinical nursing problems in practice
    3. Develop methods of inquiry relevant to nursing
    4. Acquire funding for research projects

4. A nurse researcher distributed an explanatory information sheet to subjects solicited for participation in her study about the purpose of the study. Which of the following ethical principles that guide research was this researcher using?
    1. Protection of subjects
    2. Freedom from harm
    3. Confidentiality of subjects
    4. Informed consent

5. The nurse takes on ethical responsibilities when conducting research with human subjects. Which of the following violates an ethical responsibility associated with informed consent?
    1. Providing alternatives, including the right of refusal and standard practices
    2. Using data obtained before the initiation of the study
    3. Explaining the possibility of unknown risks when appropriate
    4. Adhering to verbal and written agreements

6. Nurses need to become familiar with the elements of a research publication. A brief explanation of the type of measurement to be used is found in which section of a study?
    1. Introduction
    2. Conclusions
    3. Results
    4. Methods

7. The nurse is conducting a research project on optimal time frames for postoperative ambulation of clients. After identifying the problem, the next step in the research process is to:
1. Select the population
2. Review the literature
3. Identify the instrument to use for data analysis
4. Obtain approval to conduct the study

8. A sample of orthopedic clients varies greatly in requests for postsurgical analgesics. Which type of nursing research would best examine a prospective group of clients in determining what factors affect their alterations in comfort?
1. Historical research
2. Experimental research
3. Correlational research
4. Evaluation research

9. A nurse researcher desires to use the experimental research process instead of the nursing process method. Which of the following best lends itself to this process?
1. The effects of therapeutic touch on a geriatric client with Alzheimer's disease
2. Using humor as an intervention with clients in a sample group who are recovering from orthopedic surgery
3. Determining the blood pressure patterns of a client who recently had a cerebrovascular accident (i.e., stroke)
4. Ranking three nursing diagnoses for a newly admitted client with diabetes mellitus

10. The nurse is looking at different strategies for learning and incorporating new information into practice. A strategy that uses problem solving is demonstrated by:
1. Practicing vital signs over and over until competent
2. Seeking information from the nurse manager on the client's status
3. Reviewing Maslow's Hierarchy in a reference textbook or on the Internet
4. Trying different types of colostomy dressings for maximal effect

11. A nurse researcher has completed a study involving the use of intravenous analgesics for postsurgical discomfort. The description of the 16 clients used for the study would best be written in which part of the research report?
1. Introduction section
2. Methods section
3. Results section
4. Discussion section

12. A nurse works on a neurological nursing unit. She reads about a case study involving the potential positive effects of the early stimulation of clients after head injury. Which of the following questions should be a priority consideration of this nurse before use of the research results?
1. "Were ethical principles maintained?"
2. "What was the cost of the study?"
3. "Were the results of this study published in other journals?"
4. "Are the clients in the study similar to clients on her neurological unit?"

13. The nurse is going to use a predictive type of question as the basis for the research study. An example of a predictive type of question for research is:
1. If guided imagery is used, will stress levels be reduced?
2. How often does the stress reaction occur?
3. What does guided imagery mean to clients?
4. What creates an increase in stress levels?

UNIT 2 CARING THROUGHOUT THE LIFE SPAN

Chapter 6 Health and Wellness

1. There are different ways to look on health and illness. When formulating a definition of "health," a person should consider that health, within its current definition, is:
   1. The absence of disease
   2. A function of the physiological state
   3. A state of well-being involving the whole person
   4. The ability to pursue activities of daily living

2. Which one of the following is one of the main, overreaching goals for *Healthy People 2010*?
   1. Reduction of health care costs.
   2. Elimination of health disparities.
   3. Investigation of substance abuse.
   4. Determination of acceptable morbidity rates.

3. A nurse is using a holistic approach with a client. To incorporate all of the factors that may influence the client, the nurse should respond to the client as follows:
   1. "I would like you to perform this exercise once a day."
   2. "Your physician has left orders for you to follow."
   3. "The laboratory tests reveal the need to reduce your daily percentage of fat grams."
   4. "Adapting your diet and activity will lower your blood glucose levels."

4. The client states, "Heart disease runs in our family. My blood pressure has been high." The nurse determines that this is an example of the client's:
   1. Risk factors
   2. Active strategy
   3. Negative health behavior
   4. Health beliefs

5. A client is discharged from the hospital to his home after a heart attack. The nurse recognizes the restrictions in the client's diet and activity. In using the Stages of Health Behavior Change as a guide, the nurse recognizes that the client is most likely to begin to accept information on diet and exercise during the:
   1. Contemplation stage
   2. Preparation stage
   3. Action stage
   4. Maintenance stage

6. When assessing the external variables that influence a client's health beliefs and practices, the nurse must consider his:
   1. Religious practices
   2. Reaction to the heart disease
   3. Educational background
   4. Income status

7. The client is a paraplegic and is in the hospital for an electrolyte imbalance. Based on the levels of prevention, the client is receiving care at the:
   1. Primary prevention level
   2. Secondary prevention level
   3. Tertiary prevention level
   4. Health promotion level

8. The nurse incorporates the levels of prevention as a basis for the types of client needs that are evident and the nursing care that is provided. Which of the following activities of the nurse is an example of tertiary level preventive caregiving?
    1. Teaching a client how to irrigate a new colostomy
    2. Providing a class on hygiene for an elementary school class
    3. Informing a client that immunizations for her infant are available through the health department
    4. Arranging for a hospice nurse to visit with the family of a client with cancer

9. Client assessment provides the nurse with necessary information for the development of a plan of care. Risk factors are important to identify to assist the client, if possible, to respond and modify his or her lifestyle. Which one of the following assessment findings indicates a lifestyle risk factor?
    1. Obesity
    2. Sunbathing
    3. Overcrowded housing
    4. Industrial-based occupation

10. In the Health Belief Model, the nurse recognizes that the focus is placed on the:
    1. Basic human needs for survival
    2. Functioning of the individual in all dimensions
    3. Relation of perceptions and compliance with therapy
    4. Multidimensional nature of clients and their interaction with the environment

11. The client received a kidney transplant and is now unable to work. She is worried about her husband's stress level because of her illness and the need for him to take over her daily activities in the home. The client is in the process of adapting to a change in:
    1. Body image
    2. Illness behavior
    3. Family dynamics
    4. Self-concept

12. Client assessment provides the nurse with necessary information for the development of an effective plan of care. When determining the influence of an internal variable on the client's health status, the nurse will specifically look for:
    1. Anxiety level present
    2. Family remedies used
    3. Location and type of occupation
    4. Available health insurance coverage

Chapter 7   Caring in Nursing Practice

1. A new graduate is best able to demonstrate caring behavior toward the client by:
    1. Seeking assistance before attempting a new procedure
    2. Attempting to do new treatments as quickly as possible
    3. Being honest and informing clients that he or she has never performed the treatments before on an actual client
    4. Avoiding situations with clients that may be uncomfortable

2. A number of nursing theorists discuss and describe the concept of caring in nursing practice. According to Benner, caring is defined as a:
    1. Central, unifying, and dominant domain necessary for health and survival
    2. New consciousness and moral idea
    3. Nurturing way of relating to a valued other
    4. Person, event, project, or thing that matters to a person

3. The nurse has elected to apply Swanson's concepts of caring. Which one of the following nursing activities is an example of Swanson's "enabling" in the caring process?
    1. Staying with the client before surgery
    2. Performing a catheterization skillfully
    3. Assessing the client's health history
    4. Teaching the client how to do self-injection of insulin

4. Research has been conducted on caring within nursing practice. Riemen's study of nurses' caring behaviors (1986) found which one of the following as a similarity between male and female client's perceptions of nursing caring behaviors?
   1. Physical presence
   2. Promotion of autonomy
   3. Knowledge of injection technique
   4. Speed of treatment completion

5. In relation to caring, the most important aspect for a student nurse to learn in relation to knowing the client is:
   1. Establishing a relationship
   2. Gathering assessment data
   3. Treating discomforts quickly
   4. Assuming emotional needs

6. Caring is evident in many ways in nursing practice. A caring behavior is best demonstrated when the nurse:
   1. Tells the family about the client's problems
   2. Calls the client by his or her first name during the admission interview
   3. Closes the door and covers the client during a bath
   4. Shares personal information about the client with the roommate

7. The nurse manager is not satisfied with the hygienic care that is provided by a particular staff member on the unit. To improve the care provided to the older adult clients on the unit by this staff member, the nurse manager should:
   1. Tell the staff member how to give baths correctly to the clients
   2. Provide the staff member with good resources to read on bathing older clients
   3. Ask another staff member to provide special skin care in the afternoon
   4. Bring the staff member into a client's room and demonstrate a gentle bath

8. A nurse is reading about different theories of caring and wants to adopt Leininger's theory as an approach for his clients. A key element in this theory is that it includes:
   1. Five categories or processes of caring
   2. Connectedness with others
   3. Spiritual dimensions and healing
   4. Transcultural perspectives

Chapter 8   Culture and Ethnicity

1. The nurse recognizes the terminology that applies to culture and ethnicity. Ethnicity differs from race in that ethnicity:
   1. Is a unique factor within a cultural group
   2. Includes more than biologic identification
   3. Refers to subgroups within a race
   4. Is the set of conflicting values between races

2. Within transcultural nursing, sensitivity to social organization is the recognition of the client's:
   1. Language usage
   2. Definition of health and health practices
   3. Status and expected role in the family
   4. Psychological characteristics and coping mechanisms

3. Traditional Western medicine, in contrast to alternative therapy, uses:
   1. Medication administration
   2. Spiritual advising
   3. Acupuncture
   4. Herbal therapy

4. The nurse is completing an assessment of an Asian-American client. Recognizing the commonly seen problems in individuals from this background, the nurse observes for particular signs and symptoms of:
   1. Hypertension
   2. Lactose intolerance
   3. Tuberculosis
   4. Diabetes mellitus

5. In working with clients from other cultural backgrounds, the nurse may find that the client and family are not fluent in English. The nurse recognizes the following as an appropriate strategy for communicating with clients who are not fluent in English:
   1. Speaking in a louder tone of voice
   2. Responding to the client with his or her first name
   3. Interacting with an interpreter for all communication
   4. Incorporating hand gestures and pictures

6. The nurse wants to develop an awareness of the practices of different cultures within the community. One aspect of culture is invisible, or less observable to others. An example of this component of culture is:
   1. Using cotton garments for clothing
   2. Wearing an amulet or charm
   3. Using prayer beads or candles
   4. Believing in supernatural influences

7. Time takes on different meanings from one culture to another. To explore the relation of time to nursing interventions, the nurse should:
   1. Avoid using set times to do procedures, if possible
   2. Maintain a flexible attitude and not become emotionally upset when the client requests procedures to be done at different times
   3. Encourage clients to set their own times when they would like the nurse to perform nursing care activities, regardless of the schedule
   4. Maintain the set times for treatments and inform the client of the schedule

8. The nurse recognizes that changes in demographics have an influence on health care delivery. One of the expectations in the United States by the year 2020 is:
   1. Growth of the European-American population
   2. Reduction of the African-American population by 50%
   3. Equal growth in the Hispanic, Asian, and African-American populations
   4. Increases in the Hispanic and Latino populations

9. The nurse recognizes the terminology that applies to culture and ethnicity and its correct application. A client who goes through the process of acculturation will be:
   1. Identifying with two or more cultures
   2. Giving up his or her own identity in favor of the dominant culture
   3. Socializing within his or her primary cultural group
   4. Adapting to and adopting a new culture

10. The nurse may work with clients from many different cultural backgrounds. Nurses, unfortunately and inadvertently, may impose their own cultural beliefs on clients. An example of a cultural imposition on a client is evident in which of the following examples?
    1. Adaptation of the client's room to accommodate extra family members who are visiting.
    2. Seeking information on gender-congruent care for an Egyptian client.
    3. Holding back more potent pain medication for a client who had a minor procedure.
    4. Encouraging family to assist with the client's care.

11. An older Chinese woman refuses to perform the range-of-motion and breathing exercises after a surgical procedure. She also is hesitant to complete her hygienic care and grooming. The nurse who is culturally aware recognizes that this may most likely be related to:
    1. Dependence on health care providers
    2. Reliance on family members to assist with care
    3. Lack of motivation to participate in self-care
    4. Denial of traditional medical treatment

12. The nurse believes that a client from another cultural background is using herbal remedies along with the prescribed medication to treat her arthritis. The nurse's first action should be to:
    1. Tell the client that herbs will interfere with the prescribed medication
    2. Ask the client why additional remedies are being used
    3. Determine what herbs are being used and their effectiveness
    4. Contact the physician to alert him or her about the herbal remedies

13. Gender-appropriate care is an important factor in nursing practice. The nurse recognizes that clients of different cultures may react differently to health care professionals of the opposite sex. Modesty is an especially important issue for women from the following background:
    1. African-American
    2. Native American
    3. Afghan
    4. Filipino

14. The father is invited into the delivery room as the mother is ready to push. The nurse may find that some men from particular religious or cultural backgrounds will regularly decline the offer to observe the birth. An example is a male individual who is:
    1. Hindu
    2. Hispanic
    3. Korean
    4. Catholic

15. The client is being prepared for surgery later in the afternoon. The nurse observes that the client is wearing a religious charm on a small fabric ribbon around her right wrist. When asked, the client says that she would like it to stay. The nurse's best initial approach is to:
    1. Remove the bracelet
    2. Tape the bracelet in place
    3. Ask the client to remove the item and leave it with family members
    4. Determine if the item may remain in place during the procedure

16. The nurse has been working with a client and family of the Buddhist faith. The client, who was extremely ill, died a few minutes ago. The nurse recognizes that clients from this cultural background will:
    1. Bury the individual before sundown
    2. Refuse to see the individual
    3. Select cremation rather than burial
    4. Not move the body until all warmth is lost

17. A community health screening is being held for residents at the local town hall. The nurse is alert to the biocultural history of clients and aware that individuals with a greater potential for and incidence of hypertension are:
    1. Native Americans
    2. African-Americans
    3. Hispanics
    4. Asians

18. In Western versus non-Western cultures, differences are noted in the cultural contexts of health and illness. The nurse is aware that the overall treatment in Western culture is:
    1. Naturalistic
    2. Herbal
    3. Holistic
    4. Specialty specific

19. In working with individuals from diverse cultural backgrounds, the nurse attempts to anticipate their particular nutritional needs. For a client who is an Orthodox Jew and maintains a kosher diet, the nurse will make sure that the following is not included in the menu:
    1. Beef
    2. Eggs
    3. Milk
    4. Shellfish

20. In working with individuals from diverse cultural backgrounds, the nurse attempts to anticipate their particular nutritional needs. For a client who is a Buddhist and maintains a traditional diet, the nurse will make sure that a sufficient quantity of the following is included in the menu:
    1. Beef
    2. Milk
    3. Fish
    4. Vegetables

Chapter 9   Caring for Families

1. Among a number of changes in the way in which individuals live in today's society, which of the following is a current trend in families or family living?
    1. People marrying earlier
    2. Reduction in the divorce rate
    3. People having more children
    4. More people living alone

2. Certain societal trends or concerns may have an influence on the overall health of families and create a challenge for health care providers. Of the following trends, which represents the greatest current health care challenge to nurses?
    1. "Homelessness"
    2. Single-parent families
    3. "Sandwiched" or middle generation
    4. Alternate relationship patterns

3. When working with families, the nurse may view the family as context or client. Which one of the following examples demonstrates the view of the family as context?
    1. The family's ability to support the client's dietary and recreational needs.
    2. The client's ability to understand and manage his or her own dietary needs
    3. The family's demands on the client based on his or her role performance
    4. The adjustment of the client and family to changes in diet and exercise

4. The nurse is observing for the signs of a healthy family. In an assessment of a healthy family, the nurse expects to find that:
    1. Change is viewed as detrimental to family processes
    2. A passive response exists to stressors
    3. The structure is flexible enough to adapt to crises
    4. Minimal influence is exerted on the environment

5. The nurse is visiting a client and family in the community for the first time. In completing a client's family assessment, the nurse should begin by:
    1. Gathering the health data from all the family members
    2. Testing the family's ability to cope
    3. Evaluating communication patterns
    4. Determining the family's structure and attitudes

6. The nurse is visiting the client and family in the home after the client's discharge from the medical center. The nurse seeks to assist the client to return to the home environment. In implementing family-centered care, the nurse:
    1. Provides his or her own beliefs on how to solve problems
    2. Assists family members to assume dependent roles
    3. Works with clients to help them accept blame for their interactions
    4. Offers information about necessary self-care abilities

7. A client with severe arthritis is returning home after having had a colostomy. The client is unable to perform the colostomy care independently. The nurse should first:
   1. Inform the client that management of the colostomy must be learned
   2. Arrange for a private duty nurse to take care of the client
   3. Investigate whether someone else in the family or neighborhood will be able to assist with the colostomy care
   4. Refer the client to a colostomy self-help support group

8. The nurse is observing the interaction of family members during a home visit. The nurse recognizes that the optimal goal of effective communication within the family is:
   1. Problem solving and psychological support
   2. Role development of individual members
   3. Socialization among individual members
   4. Better financial conditions for the family

9. The nurse has recently been employed in a long-term care facility and must learn gerontologic principles related to families. Which of the following is one of those principles?
   1. Members of later-life families do not have to work on developmental tasks
   2. The caregivers are often not members of the family
   3. Role reversal is usually expected and well accepted by the elderly client
   4. Social support systems are likely to be different from those of clients in younger age groups

10. The nurse makes a home visit to a client living in a nuclear family system. In assessing the roles and power structure of the family, the nurse should specifically ask the client:
    1. "Who decides where to go on vacation?"
    2. "What type of health care insurance do you have?"
    3. "How many people live in your home?"
    4. "What types of activities do you and your family like?"

11. An older adult with two grown children is being discharged home and will need insulin injections and some assistance with activities of daily living. The client's son lives within 2 miles of the client's home. The daughter tells the nurse that she doesn't know how to handle her parent's and her own children's needs. The nurse's initial response is to:
    1. Work with the family on delegating responsibility
    2. Tell the daughter to look into nursing home placement immediately
    3. Arrange for the client to remain in the medical center
    4. Make decisions for the family on how to manage the care at home

12. After visiting the client in the home, the nurse suspects that physical abuse is present. In recognition of the pattern of family violence, the nurse knows that:
    1. Abuse is present primarily in lower-income families
    2. Spouses are the most frequent abusers
    3. Child abuse is declining in frequency
    4. Mental illness is a major cause of abuse

Chapter 10
Developmental Theories

1. A nurse who wants to apply a theory that relates to moral development should read more about:
   1. Kohlberg
   2. Gould
   3. Freud
   4. Erikson

2. The nurse using Erikson's theory to assess a 20-year-old client's developmental status expects to find which of the following behaviors?
   1. Coping with physical and social losses
   2. Enjoyment of a sense of freedom and participation in the community
   3. Applying themselves to learning productive skills
   4. Overcoming a sense of guilt or frustration

3. The nurse recognizes that Freud's theory approaches development by looking at:
   1. Cognitive development
   2. Moral reasoning
   3. Logical maturity
   4. Psychosexual aspects

4. The nurse working in a pediatric clinic uses Piaget's theory for assessment of her client's developmental status. According to Piaget, a preschool child (3 to 5 years old) who comes to the clinic is expected by the nurse to exhibit which of the following behaviors?
   1. Exploration of the environment
   2. Thinking with the use of symbols and images
   3. Cooperation and sharing
   4. Organization of thoughts and far-reaching problem solving

5. Since working in the assisted living facility, the nurse has done a lot of reading on the developmental changes associated with the older adult client. A common behavioral task or critical event for the older adult client is:
   1. Selecting a mate
   2. Rearing children
   3. Finding a congenial social group
   4. Adjusting to decreasing physical strength

6. The nurse working in an adult medical clinic wishes to learn more about a developmental theory that focuses on the adult years. The nurse investigates different possibilities and selects the theory proposed by:
   1. Gould
   2. Piaget
   3. Freud
   4. Chess and Thomas

7. Knowledge of the principles of growth and development is important for the nurse to have the better to understand the behaviors and responses of clients from different age groups. The nurse recognizes that which one of the following statements about growth and development is correct?
   1. Development ends with adolescence.
   2. Growth refers to qualitative events.
   3. Developmental tasks are age-related achievements.
   4. Cognitive theories focus on emotional development.

8. In Kohlberg's Moral Development theory, an individual who reaches Level II, Conventional Thought, is expected to exhibit:
   1. Absolute obedience to authority
   2. Reasoning based on personal gain
   3. Personal internalization of other's expectations
   4. Self-chosen ethical principles, universality, and impartiality

9. According to Piaget, the infant is in the first period of development, which is characterized by:
   1. Sensorimotor intelligence
   2. Concrete operations
   3. Identity versus role confusion
   4. Preoperational thought

10. The nurse in a pediatric health care setting is using Piaget as a developmental model for assessment of the clients. Piaget's stage of cognitive development in which the child understands the concept of ice becoming water is seen in:
    1. Sensorimotor
    2. Preoperational
    3. Concrete operations
    4. Formal operations

11. The nurse in a pediatric health care setting is using Kohlberg's developmental theory for assessment of the clients. The child is evaluated as having reached Level I, the Preconventional Level. He or she:
    1. Makes sure not to be late for school
    2. Cleans the blackboards after school for the teacher
    3. Runs for school council to change policies
    4. Stays away from gangs at school that harass other children

12. In applying Gould's developmental theory, the nurse anticipates that a client will have a greater concern for one's health within the following theme and age group:
    1. First theme (20s)
    2. Second theme (early 30s)
    3. Fourth theme (40s)
    4. Fifth theme (50s)

13. The nurse is working with the parents of a newborn. The mother will require surgery, and the follow-up treatment will interfere with bonding. In applying Freud's theory, the nurse recognizes that the stage of development that is affected is the:
    1. Oral stage
    2. Anal stage
    3. Phallic stage
    4. Latent stage

14. The nurse interacts primarily with middle adult clients in the physician's office. Erikson's developmental theory is applied by the nurse to determine the stages of the clients that are seen. It is expected by the nurse, in accordance with Erikson's theory, that a middle adult client will be involved in the process of:
    1. Developing a sense of identity
    2. Searching for meaning in life
    3. Enhancing one's capability to love others
    4. Expanding personal and social involvement

Chapter 11 Conception through Adolescence

1. A client in her second trimester of pregnancy comes to the prenatal clinic for a checkup. Which of the following is the most important for the nurse to assess in caring for a woman at this stage of her pregnancy?
   1. Detection of fetal movement
   2. Observation that the uterus is below the symphysis pubis
   3. Confirmation of the desire to breast- or bottle-feed
   4. Determination of the presence of morning sickness

2. A 6-month-old child is brought to the clinic for a well-baby examination. The nurse conducting the examination is checking the baby's reflexes. Which one of the following newborn reflexes should the nurse be able to elicit at this visit?
   1. Babinski
   2. Extrusion
   3. Startle
   4. Moro

3. The nurse is aware of the expected growth and development of the infant to determine whether any abnormalities are present. In evaluating the infant's physical status and growth, the nurse expects to find that the:
   1. Birth height increases 1 inch each month for the first 6 months
   2. Anterior fontanel closes 4 to 8 weeks after birth
   3. Chest circumference is larger than head circumference at 12 months
   4. Birth weight triples by 6 months

4. A 6-month-old is seen for a well-baby examination. On evaluation of the infant's developmental status, the nurse expects that the child at this age will be:
   1. Assuming a sitting position independently
   2. Pulling self to a standing position
   3. Rolling completely over
   4. Creeping on all four extremities

5. The nurse works in a pediatric medical day care center. An important aspect of his role is to determine whether the children are achieving developmental milestones. For a 2-year-old child, the cognitive development is characterized by:
   1. Using short sentences to express independence
   2. Initiating play with other children
   3. Recognizing right and wrong
   4. Having a vocabulary of at least 1000 words

6. An 18-month-old child is admitted for a hernia procedure. In planning nursing care for this child, the nurse should know the predominant developmental characteristic of children this age.
   1. Imaginary playmates
   2. Parallel play
   3. Peer pressure
   4. Mutilation anxiety

7. A 5-year-old boy is admitted to the surgical center to have his tonsils removed. In working with children of this age, the nurse plans to:
   1. Allow the child to take responsibility for his own preoperative hygienic care
   2. Leave him alone to relax before the procedure
   3. Allow him to handle and look at the equipment when taking his blood pressure
   4. Provide magazines and puzzles for diversion

8. A parent of a 3-year-old states that she is concerned because he was potty trained long before hospitalization but now refuses to use the toilet. What is the best response by the nurse?
   1. "You may need to include the staff in using discipline because children easily lose the ability to be toilet trained during hospitalization."
   2. "This common behavior is expressed when the child is stressed or anxious."
   3. "Your son was probably not ready to be potty trained, and you may want to continue the training for the next 6 months."
   4. "Your son is probably feeling neglected, and you should make an effort to spend more time with him."

9. A 4½-year-old is crying from pain related to her fractured leg. Which of the following is the most appropriate nursing response to her alteration in comfort?
   1. "Please try to not move your leg, and that will make it feel better."
   2. "I'll give you a shot that will help take the pain away."
   3. "It's OK to cry. I'll get you something to make you feel better. Would you like to hold your favorite doll?"
   4. "Would you like to hold this needle and tell me where you want me to give you your shot?"

10. The nurse is going to teach the parents of a 3-month-old about basic infant safety. The nurse should emphasize:
    1. Placing gates or fences at stairways
    2. Keeping bathroom doors closed
    3. Giving large teething biscuits
    4. Removing bibs at bedtime

11. The parents of a 3-month-old ask the nurse what behavior they should expect. The nurse informs the parents that the child will be able to:
    1. Say Da-da
    2. Smile responsively
    3. Differentiate a stranger
    4. Play peekaboo games

12. A client in her first trimester of pregnancy asks the nurse about how the baby is growing. The nurse responds correctly by telling the client that:
    1. "The organ systems are beginning to develop."
    2. "Fingers and toes are differentiated clearly."
    3. "The sex of the baby can be determined."
    4. "Fine hair covers the body."

13. The nurse assists the family of a 9-year-old with nutritional information. A recommended after-school snack for a child of this age is:
    1. Bite-size candy
    2. Thick milk shakes
    3. Potato chips
    4. Plain popcorn

14. The nurse in the elementary school works closely with the students and is responsible for evaluating each child's overall physical development. During the school-aged years, the nurse anticipates that:
    1. The child will grow an average of 1 to 2 inches per year
    2. The child's weight will almost triple
    3. Few physical differences will be apparent among children at the end of middle childhood
    4. Body fat will gradually increase, which contributes to the child's heavier appearance

15. A 6-year-old is hospitalized for asthma. Which of the following activities would be appropriate to help this child resolve the crisis of hospitalization?
    1. Crayons and a book to color in
    2. A 1000-piece puzzle to complete
    3. A cassette player with soothing tapes to listen to
    4. A nerf football to throw around the room

16. Which one of the following is correct regarding the preadolescence developmental stage?
    1. It appears 2 years earlier in boys than in girls
    2. Intimate feelings about school and friends are confided in the parents
    3. Interest in the opposite sex is still not a factor for this age group
    4. It signals the development of secondary sex characteristics

17. The nurse, aware that suicide is a serious potential in the adolescent age group, is teaching parents about probable warning signs that a teenager is considering suicide and tells them to be alert to:
    1. An increase in appetite
    2. A sudden interest in school activities
    3. A unexplained increase in sleepiness
    4. Verbalization of thoughts about death and personal harm

18. A 14-year-old girl is visiting the county health center for "birth control help." Which of the following is the most appropriate question the nurse could ask her to obtain the most information?
    1. "Have you told your parents that you are sexually active?"
    2. "Are any of your friends participating in sexual behaviors?"
    3. "What can you tell me about your past sexual activities?"
    4. "Have you been protecting yourself with safe sex measures?"

19. The neonate in the delivery room demonstrates a heart rate less than 100 beats per minute, a slow, irregular respiratory effort, some flexion of the extremities, a vigorous cry, and a pink trunk with bluish hands and feet. According this observation, the nurse determines that the neonate's Apgar score is:
    1. 4
    2. 6
    3. 8
    4. 10

20. In the nursery, the nurse is taking the newborn's vital signs. The nurse compares the newborn's measurements with the expected values for this age group, which are:
    1. HR, 140; BP, 72/44; R, 46
    2. HR, 100; BP, 90/50; R, 24
    3. HR, 90; BP, 100/60; R, 20
    4. HR, 80; BP, 100/70; R, 16

21. Folic acid is extremely important during the first trimester of pregnancy. The client asks the nurse to recommend foods high in folic acid so that they may be included in her dietary intake. The nurse informs the client that a rich source of folic acid is:
    1. Ice cream
    2. Beef
    3. Orange juice
    4. Green, leafy vegetables

22. The nurse is caring for the newborn immediately after delivery. To reduce the newborn's loss of heat through evaporation, the nurse should:
    1. Use the radiant warmer
    2. Apply warm blankets
    3. Dry the newborn and provide a cover
    4. Move the newborn quickly to the nursery

23. The nurse works in a pediatric medical day care center. An important aspect of his role is to determine whether the children are achieving developmental milestones. For a 12-month-old child, the nurse anticipates that he or she will just be able to:
    1. Creep on all four extremities
    2. Ambulate independently
    3. Place objects into a container
    4. Use a palm grasp with fingers around an object

24. The nurse in the elementary school is observing a 6-year-old child's level of development. At this stage, the nurse anticipates that the child's gross motor skills will enable this child to:
    1. Hop and jump onto small squares
    2. Catch and throw a ball accurately
    3. Play in an ice hockey game
    4. Perform a standing high jump of 3 feet

25. The nurse is working with a family who has just brought home a newborn. This is their first child, and they have concerns about the baby's nutrition. The nurse will recommend to the parents that they:
    1. Introduce solid foods at 3 months
    2. Provide cereals and fruits after 6 months
    3. Add honey to water to encourage intake
    4. Use cow's milk if the baby is not going to be breast-fed

26. On the pediatric unit, the nurse is taking a preschooler's vital signs. The nurse compares the measurements obtained from this preschooler with the expected values for this age group, which are:
    1. HR, 100; BP, 70/40; R, 40
    2. HR, 90; BP, 100/60; R, 32
    3. HR, 80; BP, 90/50; R, 24
    4. HR, 70; BP, 100/70; R, 16

Chapter 12   Young to Middle Adult

1. A client thinks that she might be pregnant. Which first trimester physiological changes would most likely indicate this?
    1. Amenorrhea and nausea
    2. Braxton-Hicks contractions
    3. Increased urinary frequency
    4. Edematous ankles and dyspnea

2. A 29-year-old single parent of three children comes into the well-child clinic for a prenatal visit. To determine how the client will be able to cope with the pregnancy, the nurse should ask the client:
    1. "Have you ever been married?"
    2. "Where do you work now?"
    3. "Has anyone ever taught you the principles of contraception?"
    4. "Who do you have for support during this pregnancy?"

3. The nurse is performing a physical examination on a 40-year-old adult client. The nurse will most likely find that the client of this age is experiencing which one of the following physiologic changes related to normal aging?
   1. Decreased hearing acuity
   2. Decreased sense of smell
   3. Decreased strength of abdominal muscles
   4. Decreased function of the cranial nerves

4. A 49-year-old client is experiencing problems with depression. She has come to the clinic showing signs of malnutrition and fatigue. Which of the following is the best initial response for the nurse to take in the assessment phase?
   1. "Your depression is somewhat uncommon—can you tell me what has happened recently to cause it?"
   2. "Have you recently been experiencing menopausal symptoms?"
   3. "Depression is something to expect at your age, and with assistance you will get better."
   4. "How much weight have you lost over the past month?"

5. The nurse is aware of the external influences on young and middle adult clients. With this knowledge, the nurse recognizes that an effective strategy to promote positive health habits for this age group is:
   1. Teaching clients to abstain from all alcohol consumption
   2. Demonstrating how to take an accurate blood pressure measurement
   3. Determining an effective daily exercise schedule for stress reduction
   4. Describing the types of medications commonly used for treating depression

6. In reviewing the developmental patterns of young adults, the nurse is aware that individuals at this point in their life are generally expected to:
   1. Continue their physical growth
   2. Experience severe illnesses
   3. Ignore physical symptoms
   4. Seek frequent medical care

7. A nurse is preparing an education program on safety for a young adult group. Based on the major cause of the mortality and morbidity for this age group, the nurse should focus on:
   1. Birth control
   2. Automobile safety
   3. Occupational hazards
   4. Prevention of heart disease

8. The nurse is working in the health office at a local college. Most of the students are young adults. Being aware of the major concerns for this age group, the nurse includes assessment of her clients':
   1. Marital status
   2. Lifestyle and leisure activities
   3. Experience with chronic disease
   4. History of childhood accidents

9. Health problems generally become more prevalent as an individual enters middle adulthood. The middle adult may be influenced by chronic illness that results in:
   1. Decreased health care tasks
   2. Reinforcement of prior family roles
   3. Changed sexual behavior
   4. Improved family relationships

10. The nurse is performing a physical examination on a 58-year-old adult client. The nurse will most likely find that the client of this age is experiencing which one of the following physiological changes related to normal aging?
    1. Reduced pupillary reaction to light
    2. Palpable thyroid lobes
    3. Decreased skin turgor
    4. Increased range of joint motion

11. The nurse is alert to stressors that may have an influence on the young adult client. One example of a common stressor for this age group is:
    1. Occupational pursuits
    2. Health-related matters
    3. Coping with cognitive changes
    4. Caring for older adult parents

12. A client comes to the clinic for a regular checkup. The nurse determines that the client works in a dry-cleaning establishment. Based on this information, the nurse assesses the client for:
    1. Asbestosis
    2. Dermatitis
    3. Tendonitis
    4. Raynaud's phenomenon

13. The nurse is completing a physical examination for a client who has come to the family practice office. In evaluating the observations made during the examination, the nurse recognizes that an expected finding for a client in this age group is:
    1. Hepatomegaly
    2. Visual acuity less than 20/50
    3. A temperature of 39°C
    4. Increased skin turgor and moisture

Chapter 13   Older Adult

1. The nurse is performing a physical examination of an older adult client in an assisted living facility. On completion of the examination, the nurse compares the results with findings expected for individuals in this age group. An expected finding for this client is:
   1. Increased tactile responsiveness
   2. Increased sensitivity to glare
   3. Increased hearing acuity for higher tones
   4. Increased thoracic expansion during ventilation

2. A 70-year-old client is to have her blood pressure checked each shift. She asks the nurse to explain her hypertension. An appropriate response by the nurse is that older clients often experience hypertension because of:
   1. Vascular changes and accumulation of plaque on arterial walls, both of which reduce contractility
   2. Reduction in physical activity
   3. Ingestion of processed foods high in sodium
   4. Myocardial damage

3. In reviewing changes in the older adult, the nurse recognizes that the following statement related to cognitive functioning in the older client is true:
   1. Reversible systemic disorders are often implicated as a cause of delirium
   2. Cognitive deterioration is an inevitable outcome of aging
   3. Delirium is easily distinguished from irreversible dementia
   4. Therapeutic drug intoxication is a common cause of senile dementia

4. A client has been recently diagnosed with Alzheimer's disease. When teaching the family about the prognosis, the nurse must explain that:
   1. It usually progresses gradually with a deterioration of function
   2. Many individuals can be cured if the diagnosis is made early
   3. Diet and exercise can slow the process considerably
   4. Few clients live more than 3 years after the diagnosis

5. For older adults, a number of health-related concerns should be addressed. The nurse incorporates this information to meet the needs of the older adult client. Which of the following statements accurately reflects data that the nurse should use in planning care?
   1. Approximately 50% of adults older than 65 years have two chronic health problems
   2. Cancer is the most common cause of death among older adults
   3. Minimal nutritional needs for older adults are essentially the same as those for younger adults
   4. Adults older than 65 years make up the highest percentage of users of prescription medications

6. Myths exist regarding the older adult population in the United States. The nurse is aware that the majority of older adults:
   1. Live alone
   2. Live in institutional settings
   3. Are unable to care for themselves
   4. Are active and involved in their community

7. The nurse works with elderly clients in a wellness screening clinic on a weekly basis. Which of the following is the best statement made to clients in the older adult age group?
   1. "Your shoulder pain is normal for your age."
   2. "Continue to exercise your joints regularly to your tolerance level."
   3. "Don't worry about taking that combination of medications because your doctor has prescribed them."
   4. "Why don't you begin walking 3 to 4 miles per day, and we'll evaluate how you feel next week."

8. A long-term care facility sponsors a discussion group on the administration of medications. The participants have a number of questions concerning their medications. The nurse responds most appropriately by saying:
   1. "Don't worry about the medication's name if you can identify it by its color and the way it looks."
   2. "Please feel free to ask your physician why you are receiving the medications that are ordered for you."
   3. "Remember that the hepatic system is primarily responsible for the pharmacotherapeutics of your medications."
   4. "Unless you have severe side affects from taking your medications, don't worry about the minor changes in the way you feel."

9. Not all older adult clients respond well to the physical changes associated with the aging process. Some individuals act to deny the effects of aging by:
   1. Reducing cosmetic use
   2. Spending more time with other older adults
   3. Refusing assistance with certain activities
   4. Exaggerating their actual ages

10. In performing a physical assessment for an older adult, the nurse anticipates finding which of the following normal physiological changes of aging?
    1. Increased perspiration
    2. Increased audio pitch discrimination
    3. Increased salivary secretions
    4. Increased airway resistance

11. The nurse recognizes that factors associated with aging influence the musculoskeletal system. The nurse recognizes that:
    1. Older men have a greater problem with osteoporosis
    2. Muscle fibers increase in size and become tight
    3. Exercise reduces the loss of bone mass
    4. Muscle strength does not diminish as much as muscle mass

12. The nurse, preparing to discharge an 81-year-old client from the hospital, recognizes that the majority of older adults:
    1. Require institutional care
    2. Have no social or family support
    3. Are unable to afford any medical treatment
    4. Are capable of taking charge of their own lives

13. To assist older adults to meet their needs for sexuality, the nurse should recognize that:
    1. Therapeutic medications may alter sexual function
    2. Physiological changes do not adversely influence sexual activity
    3. Sexual interest declines and then fades completely with age
    4. Prevention of sexually transmitted diseases is no longer an issue with this age group

14. The nurse is presenting an information session on nutritional guidelines at a senior living center. Incorporated into the discussion are the recommendations for nutritional intake for individuals of this age group, which includes a reduction in:
    1. Fiber
    2. Protein
    3. Vitamin A
    4. Refined sugars

15. The nurse is presenting an information session on nutritional guidelines at a senior living center. Incorporated into the discussion are the recommendations for nutritional intake for individuals of this age group. Which of the following foods meets the recommended nutritional guidelines for older adults?
    1. Grilled chicken
    2. Hamburger and french fries
    3. Hot dog with pickle relish
    4. Baked potato with cheese and bacon bits

16. In the assessment of older adult clients, it is often difficult to discriminate between delirium and dementia. A major difference that the nurse is alert to is that delirium is characterized by:
    1. Lasting months to years
    2. A normal state of alertness
    3. A slow progression
    4. Occurrences at twilight or darkness

*U*NIT 3 CRITICAL THINKING IN NURSING PRACTICE

*C*hapter 14 Critical Thinking in Nursing Practice

1. Which of the following best reflects the philosophy of critical thinking as taught by a nurse educator to a nursing student?
   1. "Don't draw subjective inferences about your client—be more objective."
   2. "Please think harder—I am looking for a single solution."
   3. "Trust your feelings—don't be concerned about trying to find a rationale to support your decision."
   4. "Think about several interventions that you could use with this client."

2. The second component of critical thinking in the "critical thinking model" is:
   1. Competencies
   2. Experience
   3. Specific knowledge
   4. Diagnostic reasoning

3. The nurse enters the room of a client who has a history of heart disease. On looking at the client, the nurse feels that something is "not right" with the client and proceeds to take the vital signs. This is the nurse acting on:
   1. Intuition
   2. Reflection
   3. Knowledge
   4. Scientific methodology

4. The nurse manager has developed a staff protocol for peer evaluation. The nurses on her surgical unit are nervous about using her instrument. If the nurse manager continues to implement the new strategy, which of the following critical thinking attitudes is she portraying?
   1. Accountability
   2. Thinking independently
   3. Risk taking
   4. Humility

5. The nurse is working with a client who has recently had a colostomy. The client is having difficulty using the supplies that are provided for the ostomy care. The nurse investigates the other types of available supplies and works with the client to see which ones are the best. This is an example of the critical thinking strategy of:
   1. Inference
   2. Problem-solving
   3. Management
   4. Diagnostic reasoning

6. Which of the following is an example of a nurse's statement that reflects using the scientific method in the nursing process?
   1. "My instincts tell me that the client is getting depressed."
   2. "The client doesn't look the same today. I think something is wrong."
   3. "The client's husband told me that she is feeling uncomfortable."
   4. "The client seems to be having more pain today than yesterday, and her blood pressure is elevated."

7. The nurse decides to administer tablets of acetaminophen (Tylenol) instead of the intramuscular meperidine (Demerol) she has been giving one of her orthopedic clients, in accordance with the prescriber's order. Which step of the nursing process does this address?
   1. Assessment
   2. Nursing diagnosis
   3. Planning
   4. Implementation

8. The nurse has a multiple client assignment on the surgical unit. When beginning the shift, the nurse needs to determine which postoperative client should be seen first. Of the following, the nurse should go to see the client who:
   1. Is reported as having a BP of 90/50
   2. Received medication for pain 10 minutes ago
   3. Needs to be out of bed and ambulating
   4. Requires instructions for wound care

9. Of the variety of levels of critical thinking, an example of critical thinking at the complex level is:
   1. Following a procedure for catheterization step by step
   2. Giving medication at the time ordered
   3. Discussing alternative pain-management techniques
   4. Reviewing the client's medical records thoroughly

10. The nurse is deciding on the type of dressing to use for a client. Which step of the decision-making process is being used when the nurse observes the absorbency of different dressing brands?
    1. Defining the problem
    2. Considering consequences
    3. Testing possible options
    4. Making final decisions

1. Which one of the following examples demonstrates the critical thinking attitude of responsibility and authority?
   1. Offering an alternative approach
   2. Looking for a different treatment option
   3. Sharing ideas about nursing interventions
   4. Reporting client difficulties

2. Use of the intellectual standard of critical thinking implies that the nurse:
   1. Questions the physician's order
   2. Recognizes conflicts of interest
   3. Listens to both sides of the story
   4. Approaches assessment logically and consistently

3. A client requires urinary catheterization but has difficulty keeping her legs in the usual position. The nurse has worked for many years and adapts the procedure to allow the client to lie on her side. This action is based on the critical thinking element of:
   1. Curiosity
   2. Experience
   3. Perseverance
   4. Scientific knowledge

Chapter 15 Nursing Assessment

1. A client interview consists of three phases. The nurse recognizes that those phases are:
   1. Introduction, assessment, conclusion
   2. Orientation, documentation, database
   3. Introduction, controlling, selection
   4. Orientation, working, termination

2. During the admission history, the client states that he has trouble breathing at night. In obtaining data for a problem-oriented database, the nurse should first question the client about:
   1. The onset and duration of his present breathing problem
   2. His smoking and exercise practices
   3. Any family members who have heart disease
   4. Changes in other body systems

3. The client has come to the emergency department experiencing chest pain. In this situation, the nurse begins the assessment by asking the client about:
   1. A family history of heart problems
   2. Medications taken at home
   3. Concerns about hospitalization
   4. The severity and duration of the chest pain

4. A nurse seeks to organize the data obtained from the client in a logical manner. This organization that identifies relations between factors and symptoms in the database is known as:
   1. Clustering data
   2. Validating data
   3. Formulating a problem statement
   4. Performing a peer review

5. The client recently became febrile and stated he "felt hot." You take the client's temperature and find it to be 38.2° C. In addition, the pulse is 88 beats per minute, and his blood pressure is 168/80. Which of the following is an example of subjective data?
   1. Pulse of 88 beats per minute
   2. Blood pressure of 168/80
   3. The statement regarding his feeling hot
   4. The fact that he became febrile

6. The nurse decides to interview the client by using the open-ended question technique. Which of the following statements reflects this type of questioning?
   1. "Is your pain worse or better than it was an hour ago?"
   2. "Do you believe that your nausea is from the new antibiotic?"
   3. "What do you think has been causing your depression?"
   4. "What effects have you had with the medications, and what have you done to alleviate them?"

7. The nurse is gathering a nursing health history on the client. The client tells the nurse that he just lost his job and that his son has newly diagnosed juvenile-onset diabetes. Which of the following categories best fits the loss of the job?
   1. Family history
   2. Psychosocial history
   3. Environmental history
   4. Biographical history

8. The nurse is going to perform the admission history for the newly admitted client on the medical unit. The optimal time for completion of the history is planned for:
   1. Coordination with the physician's visit
   2. The time that the client's friends and family are visiting
   3. Immediately before the client's magnetic resonance imaging (MRI) testing
   4. After the client has become oriented to the room and completed lunch

9. The nurse has completed an assessment and found that the client has an activity and exercise abnormality. This type of documentation indicates that the following organizing format has been used:
   1. Review of systems
   2. Nursing health history
   3. Gordon's functional health patterns
   4. Biographical information database

10. After visiting with the client, the nurse documents the assessment data. Both objective and subjective information have been obtained during the assessment. Which of the following is classified as objective data?
    1. Pain in the left leg
    2. Elevated blood pressure
    3. Fear of surgery
    4. Discomfort on breathing

11. An alert, oriented client is admitted to the medical center for diagnostic testing. The primary source of information when completing an assessment for this client is the:
    1. Client
    2. Physician
    3. Family member
    4. Experienced nurse on the unit

12. On beginning the process of data collection, the first step the nurse should take is the:
    1. Physical examination
    2. Client interview
    3. Review of medical records
    4. Discussion with other health team members

13. During an interview, the nurse needs to obtain specific information about the signs and symptoms of a health problem. To obtain these data most efficiently, the nurse should use:
    1. Channeling
    2. Open-ended questions
    3. Closed-ended questions
    4. Problem-seeking responses

14. The nurse is conducting an interview with the client and wants to clarify information that the client has shared in the discussion. Which response by the nurse is an example of the clarifying technique of communication?
    1. "I understand how you must feel."
    2. "This medication is used to lower your blood pressure."
    3. "You appear anxious. You're wringing your hands constantly."
    4. "I'm not sure that I understand. Could you give me an example of how the pain feels?"

5. When clustering data according to functional health patterns, the nurse determines that the client is able to ambulate only short distances without becoming fatigued and requires rest periods during AM care. The health pattern that requires intervention is identified by the nurse as:
   1. Respiratory
   2. Activity and exercise
   3. Sleep and rest pattern
   4. Self-care deficit: activities of daily living

6. After visiting with the client, the nurse documents the assessment data. Both objective and subjective information has been obtained during the assessment. Which of the following is classified as subjective data?
   1. "Client appears sleepy"
   2. "No distress noted"
   3. "Abdomen soft and nontender"
   4. "States feels anxious and tense"

Chapter 16   Nursing Diagnosis

1. After completion of the client assessment, the nurse uses nursing diagnoses because they:
   1. Make all client problems become more quickly and easily resolved
   2. Assist the nurse to distinguish medical from nursing problems
   3. Are required for accreditation purposes
   4. Identify the domain and focus of nursing

2. A 53-year-old client is seen at the clinic for a yearly physical examination. In evaluating the client's weight, the nurse also considers the age and height. This is an example of:
   1. Defining the client problem
   2. Recognizing gaps in data assessment
   3. Comparing data with normal health patterns
   4. Drawing conclusions about the client's response

3. Nursing diagnoses must meet specific criteria so they accurately reflect both the client's problem and the possible etiology involved. Of the following statements, which one is an example of an appropriately written nursing diagnosis?
   1. Acute pain related to left mastectomy
   2. Impaired gas exchange related to altered blood gases
   3. Deficient knowledge related to need for cardiac catheterization
   4. Need for high-protein diet related to alteration in nutrition

4. Nursing diagnoses must meet specific criteria so they accurately reflect both the client's problem and the possible etiology involved. Of the following statements, which one is an example of an appropriately written nursing diagnosis?
   1. Cardiac output decreased related to motor vehicle accident
   2. Potential for injury related to improper teaching in the use of crutches
   3. Ineffective airway clearance related to increased secretions
   4. Risk for change in body image related to cancer

5. The nurse has diagnosed the client's problem as altered elimination. From the database, the nurse identifies all the following as appropriate etiologies for this diagnosis *except*:
   1. Poor fiber intake
   2. Limited fluid intake
   3. Total hip replacement
   4. Lower abdominal discomfort

6. The nurse is concerned that atelectasis may develop as a postoperative complication. Which of the following is an appropriate diagnostic label for this problem should it occur?
   1. Ineffective airway clearance
   2. Impaired gas exchange
   3. Decreased cardiac output
   4. Impaired spontaneous ventilation

7. The nurse recognizes that which one of the following statements is true with regard to the formulation of nursing diagnoses?
   1. The etiology of the diagnosis must be within the scope of the health care team's practice.
   2. The diagnosis must remain constant during the client's hospitalization.
   3. The diagnosis should include the problem and the related contributing conditions.
   4. The diagnosis should identify a "cause and effect" relation.

8. When completing a client assessment and determining nursing diagnoses, the nurse may make an error. A diagnostic error can influence the application of the nursing care plan. A likely source for a nursing diagnosis error is if the nurse:
   1. Validates the assessment information in the database
   2. Uses the North American Nursing Diagnosis Association (NANDA) list of diagnoses as a source
   3. Formulates a diagnosis too closely resembling a medical diagnosis
   4. Distinguishes the nursing focus instead of other health care disciplines

9. Identify the defining characteristics in the following nursing diagnosis: *Altered speech related to recent neurological disturbance, as evidenced by inability to speak in complete sentences*:
   1. "Altered speech"
   2. "As evidenced by"
   3. "Recent neurological disturbances"
   4. "Inability to speak in complete sentences"

10. The nurse recognizes that the primary purpose of a nursing diagnosis is to:
    1. Support the medical plan of care
    2. Provide a standardized approach for all clients
    3. Recognize the client's response to an illness or situation
    4. Offer the nurse's subjective view of the client's behaviors

11. Nursing diagnoses must meet specific criteria to reflect accurately both the client's problem and the possible etiology involved. Which one of the following is an appropriate etiology for a nursing diagnosis?
    1. Abnormal blood gas levels
    2. Myocardial infarction
    3. Increased airway secretions
    4. Cardiac catheterization

12. Nursing diagnoses must meet specific criteria to reflect accurately both the client's problem and the possible etiology involved. Which of the following is an appropriate etiology for a nursing diagnosis?
    1. Incisional pain
    2. Poor hygienic practices
    3. Need to use bedpan frequently
    4. Inadequate prescription of medication by the physician

13. Nursing diagnoses must meet specific criteria to reflect accurately both the client's problem and the possible etiology involved. Of the following statements, which one is an example of an appropriately written nursing diagnosis?
    1. Diarrhea related to food intolerance
    2. Alteration in comfort related to pain
    3. Risk for impaired skin integrity related to poor hygiene habits
    4. Potential complications related to insufficient vascular access

14. Nursing diagnoses must meet specific criteria to reflect accurately both the client's problem and the possible etiology involved. Of the following statements, which one is an example of an appropriately written nursing diagnosis?
    1. Chronic pain related to insufficient use of medication
    2. Pain related to difficulty ambulating
    3. Anxiety related to cardiac monitor
    4. Bedpan required frequently as a result of altered elimination pattern

15. The nurse is working with a client who has abnormal breath sounds, dyspnea, an intermittent cough, and variable respiratory rate. Based on this information, the nurse identifies the most appropriate nursing diagnosis as:
    1. Risk for injury
    2. Excess fluid volume
    3. Ineffective airway clearance
    4. Impaired spontaneous ventilation

16. In selecting a nursing diagnosis, the nurse elects to use the recommended labels from NANDA. Which one of the following is a NANDA nursing diagnosis label?
    1. Risk for impaired parenting
    2. Abnormal hygienic care practices
    3. Coughing and dyspnea
    4. Frequent urination

Chapter 17   Planning Nursing Care

1. The nurse is working with a client who is being prepared for a diagnostic test this afternoon. The client tells the nurse that she wants to have her hair shampooed. Which of the following is the most appropriate label with regard to assigning a priority for her request?
    1. Low priority
    2. An unmet need
    3. Intermediate priority
    4. A safety and security need

2. The client is a tailor who was admitted for eye surgery. Assuming that all of the following are realistic, a long-term goal for this client should include:
    1. Returning to sewing
    2. Preventing ocular infection
    3. Performing independent hygienic care in hospital
    4. Administering eye drops on time in the hospital

3. The nurse writes the following goal for a client who is hypertensive: "Client will maintain a blood pressure within acceptable limits." Which of the following would be the most appropriate outcome criterion?
    1. Client will request pain medication as needed.
    2. Client will identify at least two things that cause stress.
    3. Client will have a 7 AM blood pressure reading less than 140/90.
    4. Client will experience no headache or dizziness.

4. Nursing interventions may be categorized based on the degree of nursing autonomy. Which of the following nursing interventions is considered as physician or prescriber initiated?
    1. Teaching a client to administer his or her insulin injection
    2. Assisting a new mother with breast-feeding
    3. Notifying the nutritionist of a client's dietary preferences
    4. Giving an enema in preparation for radiological testing

5. Nursing interventions should be documented according to specific criteria so that they are clearly understood by other members of the nursing team. The intervention statement "Nurse will apply warm, wet soaks to the patient's leg while the patient is awake" lacks which of the following components?
    1. Method
    2. Quantity
    3. Frequency
    4. Qualifications of the person who will perform the action

6. The nurse recognizes that client goals or outcomes should be documented according to specific criteria so that they are clear and easily understood by other members of the health care team. Of the following, the outcome statement that best meets the established criteria is:
   1. Client will describe activity restrictions.
   2. Client will understand treatments.
   3. Client will ambulate in hallway 3 times each day.
   4. Client's respiratory rate will remain within 20 to 24 breaths per minute by 9/24.

7. The client is receiving postural drainage from physical therapy and intermittent breathing treatments from respiratory therapy. Which type of care plan would be the ideal method to document interventions for this client?
   1. Nursing Kardex
   2. Computerized care plan
   3. Critical pathway
   4. Standardized care plan

8. The nurse is involved in requesting a management consultation for personnel-related issues. Which of the following is true regarding the consultation process in which the nurse is involved?
   1. The problem area is usually identified by another member of the health care team.
   2. Consultation is often used when the exact problem remains unclear.
   3. Detailed feelings about the problem should be described to the consultant by the nurse.
   4. The problem area should be totally delegated to the consultant.

9. In completing an assessment on an assigned client, the nurse obtains important information for planning nursing care. Which of the following client needs should take priority?
   1. An impending divorce
   2. A nutritional deficit
   3. Difficulty breathing
   4. Financial problems

10. The nurse recognizes that client goals or outcomes should be documented according to specific criteria so that they are clear and easily understood by other members of the health care team. Of the following, the outcome statement that best meets the established criteria is:
    1. Vital signs will return to normal.
    2. Nursing assistant will ambulate the client in the hallway 3 times each day.
    3. Lungs will be clear to auscultation, and respiratory rate will be 20 breaths per minute
    4. Urinary output will be at least 100 ml per hour within 24 hours

11. In goal setting, the nurse is aware that the factor that is associated with available client resources and motivation is:
    1. Client-centered
    2. Observable
    3. Measurable
    4. Realistic

12. Nursing interventions may be categorized based on the degree of nursing autonomy. An example of a nurse-initiated intervention is:
    1. Providing client teaching
    2. Administering medication
    3. Ordering a computed tomography (CAT) scan
    4. Referring a client to physical therapy

13. Nursing interventions may be categorized based on the degree of nursing autonomy. Which of the following nursing interventions is considered as physician or prescriber initiated?
    1. Taking vital signs
    2. Providing support to a family
    3. Changing a dressing 2 times each day
    4. Measuring intake and output each shift

14. Which one of the following interventions selected by the nurse is classified as Level 2, Domain 2 (Physiological: complex)?
    1. Maintaining regular bowel elimination
    2. Promoting the health of the family
    3. Managing restricted body movement
    4. Restoring tissue integrity

15. In documentation of nursing care plans, critical pathways differ from traditional nursing care plans in their:
    1. Multidisciplinary approach
    2. Nursing interventions
    3. Client outcomes
    4. Client assessment

16. Nursing interventions should be documented according to specific criteria so that they are clearly understood by other members of the nursing team. The most appropriate of the following intervention statements is:
    1. Offer fluids to the client q2h
    2. Observe the client's respirations
    3. Change the client's dressing daily
    4. Irrigate the nasogastric tube q2h with 30 ml normal saline

17. Nursing interventions should be documented according to specific criteria so that they are clearly understood by other members of the nursing team. The most appropriate of the following intervention statements is:
    1. Apply dry dressing with two 4 × 4-inch gauze pads tid
    2. Turn client in bed as needed
    3. Take vital signs
    4. Refer client to a therapist

18. Care plans for students usually differ from those that are completed by nurses working on client units. An aspect of the plan that is usually included in the student's care plan, but not in the client's record, is:
    1. Nursing diagnoses
    2. Client outcomes
    3. Nursing interventions
    4. Scientific rationales

19. A nurse may use a concept map when implementing a plan of care. The purpose and distinction of a concept map is for:
    1. Quality assurance in the health care facility
    2. Multidisciplinary communication
    3. Provision of a standardized format for client problems
    4. Identification of the relation of client problems and interventions

20. A client is newly diagnosed with diabetes mellitus. The nurse identifies a nursing diagnosis of *Knowledge deficient related to new diagnosis and treatment needs*. The most appropriate outcome statement based on the established criteria is:
    1. Client will perform glucose measurements often
    2. Client will appear less anxious about diagnosis
    3. Urinary output will reach normal levels
    4. Client will independently perform subcutaneous insulin injection by 8/31.

Chapter 18
Implementing Nursing Care

1. The nurse is working with postoperative clients on a surgical unit. One aspect of care is manipulation of the client's environment. This involves the nurse:
    1. Delegating ambulation of clients to the nursing assistant
    2. Providing pain medication to the client before a dressing change
    3. Removing clutter from the client's room
    4. Repositioning the client q2h

2. The client is given an injection of an antibiotic. Shortly afterward, she says that she has hives and is itchy. The nurse administers an antihistamine to counteract the effect of the antibiotic. The nurse is using which one of the following intervention methods?
   1. Preventive measures
   2. Assisting with activities of daily living (ADLs)
   3. Preparing for special procedures
   4. Compensation for adverse reactions

3. The client is scheduled to receive warfarin (Coumadin, an anticoagulant) at 9:00 AM. His morning laboratory results show him to have a high partial thromboplastin time (PTT). His nurse decides to withhold the warfarin. Which step of the implementation process is she using?
   1. Reassessing the client
   2. Modifying the nursing care plan
   3. Revising the nursing diagnosis
   4. Stating an expected outcome

4. The nurse notes that a narcotic is to be administered "per epidural cath." The nurse, however, does not know how to perform this procedure. Which aspect of the implementation process should be followed?
   1. Seek assistance
   2. Reassess the client
   3. Use interpersonal skills
   4. Critical decision making

5. The nurse recognizes the discharge needs of a client after a hip replacement. This is an example of which type of nursing skill?
   1. Cognitive
   2. Interactive
   3. Psychomotor
   4. Communication

6. The nurse uses a variety of skills in the application of the nursing process. An example of a cognitive nursing skill is:
   1. Providing a soothing bed bath
   2. Communicating with the client and family
   3. Giving an injection to the client per the physician's orders
   4. Recognizing the potential complications of a blood transfusion

7. An enterostomal nurse shows a client's significant other how to assist with the supplies for and manipulation of the ostomy equipment. The nurse in demonstrating the technique to the client is using what type of nursing skill?
   1. Cognitive
   2. Interactive
   3. Affective
   4. Psychomotor

8. For a client with a nursing diagnosis of *Impaired physical mobility related to bilateral arm casts*, the nurse should select which of the following methods of nursing intervention?
   1. Counseling
   2. Teaching
   3. Compensating for adverse reactions
   4. Assisting with ADLs

9. A number of different types of nursing interventions may be incorporated into the plan of care. An example of a specific lifesaving measure that the nurse may implement is:
   1. Restraining a violent client
   2. Administering analgesics
   3. Initiating stress-reduction therapy
   4. Teaching the client how to take his or her pulse

Chapter 19   Evaluation

1. The client smokes two packs of cigarettes per day. The nurse works with the client, and they agree that he will smoke one cigarette less each week until he is down to one pack per day. In 3 weeks, the client is smoking two and a half packs of cigarettes per day. This is an example of:
   1. A realistic goal
   2. A compliant client
   3. A negative evaluation
   4. A nonmeasurable goal

2. The client is seen in the clinic for her first prenatal visit. The nurse formulates a diagnosis of *Knowledge deficit related to complications of pregnancy*. One outcome criterion is that the client can state five symptoms that indicate a possible problem that should be reported. The client is able to tell the nurse three symptoms. The evaluation statement would be:
   1. Goal met; client able to state three symptoms
   2. Goal partially met; client able to state three symptoms
   3. Goal not met; client unable to list five symptoms
   4. Goal not met; client able to list three symptoms

3. The nurse begins to auscultate the client's lungs. While listening, the nurse notices fresh bloody drainage oozing from the abdominal dressing. The nurse stops auscultating and applies direct pressure to the wound site. This is an example of:
   1. Performing a nursing assessment
   2. Reorganizing the nursing diagnoses
   3. Setting realistic goals and implementing nursing interventions
   4. Critically analyzing the data and effectively implementing the safest nursing action

4. The client is able to ambulate without signs or symptoms of shortness of breath. Which statement by the nurse is the best example of an objective evaluation of the client's goal attainment?
   1. "Client has no pain after ambulating."
   2. "Client has no manifestations of nausea while up in hall."
   3. "Client has no evidence of respiratory distress when ambulating."
   4. "Client walked well and did not have any problem when up."

5. The client's status has changed significantly over the past few days. The nurse recognizes the need to update the plan of care. When modifying a care plan to meet a client's changing needs, the nurse should:
   1. Re-do the entire care plan
   2. Focus only on the nursing diagnoses and goals that have changed
   3. Perform a complete reassessment of all client factors
   4. Add more nursing interventions from a standardized plan of care

6. The nurse has determined an outcome criterion of: Client will independently complete necessary assessments before administration of digoxin (cardiotonic). Based on this outcome, the nurse will evaluate the client's ability to:
   1. Assess the respiratory rate during exercise
   2. Palpate the radial pulse
   3. Review dietary habits
   4. Inspect the color of the skin

7. The nurse has determined an outcome for a client with a skin impairment that identifies: Erythema will be reduced in 3 days. Evaluation will specifically focus on:
   1. Measurement of the diameter of the ulceration daily
   2. Notation of the odor and color of drainage
   3. Inspection of the color and condition of the area
   4. Selection of appropriate wound care

8. The client has a nursing diagnosis of *Impaired gas exchange* as a result of excess secretions. An outcome for the client is that the airways will be free of secretions. A positive evaluation will focus on the client's:
   1. Ability to perform incentive spirometry
   2. Lungs clear bilaterally on auscultation
   3. Complaint of chest pain
   4. Respiratory rate

Chapter 20   Managing Client Care

1. It is necessary for the new nurse manager to delegate tasks to the staff. What is a requirement for the nurse manager in this delegation process?
   1. Obtaining the employee's voluntary acceptance of the task
   2. Communicating the work assignment in understandable terms
   3. Functioning from a laissez-faire style of leadership
   4. Working alongside the staff to evaluate their care

2. To be able to meet the needs of assigned clients and the responsibilities associated with the position, nurses must be aware of time-management techniques. The time-management skills for the nurse include:
   1. Meeting all of the client's needs in the early morning hours
   2. Anticipating possible interruptions by therapists and visitors
   3. Doing each of the client's assessments and treatments individually at separate times throughout the day
   4. Leaving each day unplanned to allow adaptations in treatments

3. In anticipation of a nursing shortage, the nursing management in a facility are investigating a nursing care delivery model that involves the division of tasks, with one nurse assuming the responsibility for particular tasks. This model is called
   1. Total patient care
   2. Functional nursing
   3. Team nursing
   4. Primary nursing

4. The medical center has changed its overall management philosophy from centralized to decentralized management. One advantage of a decentralized management structure for the nursing units over a centralized structure is that:
   1. Staff are not responsible for defining their roles.
   2. Managers handle the difficult decisions.
   3. Communication pathways are simplified.
   4. Each staff member is accountable for evaluating the plan of care.

5. The determination of indicators in a Quality Improvement program that evaluate the manner in which care is delivered are:
   1. Structure indicators
   2. Team indicators
   3. Process indicators
   4. Client indicators

6. A threshold of 90% is identified for an outcome indicator in the Quality Improvement program. Which of the following situations indicates a need for further review of the quality improvement plan?
   1. The waiting time for clinic appointments has decreased 96%.
   2. Clients with renal dialysis expressed a 95% satisfaction with their care.
   3. In 93% of clients, subjective expressions of postoperative pain have decreased.
   4. Wound infections are evident in 92% of clients after care of intravenous (IV) access ports.

7. In anticipation of a nursing shortage, the nursing management in a facility are investigating a nursing care delivery model that involves staff members working under the direction of a registered nurse leader. This model is called
   1. Team nursing
   2. Primary nursing
   3. Functional nursing
   4. Total patient care

8. Accountability is a critical aspect of nursing care. An example of a specific decision-making process of accountability is demonstrated by:
   1. Selecting the medication schedule for the client
   2. Implementing discharge teaching plans that meet individual needs
   3. Evaluating the client's outcomes after implementation of care
   4. Promoting participation of all staff members in unit meetings

9. The student nurse is seeking to learn skills associated with priority setting. In discussing different priorities of care, an example of a second-order priority is:
   1. An obstructed airway
   2. The need to urinate
   3. The side effects of a medication
   4. Activities of daily living in the home environment

0. The nurse on the unit is determining what activities may be delegated to assistive personnel. A number of factors are included in the nurse's decision. Assuming that the nurse assistant is competent, which one of the following activities may be safely delegated by the registered nurse?
   1. Vital signs on a stable client
   2. An admission history on a new client
   3. Initial transfer of a postoperative client
   4. Administration of medications prepared by the nurse

UNIT 4 PROFESSIONAL STANDARDS IN NURSING PRACTICE

Chapter 21   Ethics and Values

1. The client states that she needs to exercise regularly, watch her weight, and reduce her fat intake. This demonstrates that the client:
   1. Believes she will have a heart attack
   2. Values health promotion activities
   3. Believes she will not become sick
   4. Has unrealistic expectations for herself

2. A client has actively picketed for gun control. During a robbery of his business, he was shot in the leg. As the nurse assists him with morning care, which statement would the nurse expect him to make that coincides with his values?
   1. "Individuals should arm themselves for protection."
   2. "Firearms may have a place in our society."
   3. "Prosecution should be the maximum for that felon."
   4. "Protection is a necessary evil for the good guy."

3. A secondary-school teacher with advanced multiple sclerosis insists on teaching from a wheelchair and being treated the same as other colleagues. The teacher is demonstrating which of the following?
   1. Prizing her choice
   2. Choosing from alternatives
   3. Considering all consequences
   d. Acting with a pattern of consistency

4. The nurse recognizes that values-clarification interventions are beneficial for the client when:
   1. The client and nurse have different beliefs
   2. The client is experiencing a values conflict
   3. The nurse is unsure of a client's values
   4. The client has rejected normal values

5. The nurse is working with the client and trying to clarify the client's values regarding his care. Which of the following statements reflects an example of the type of response a nurse should use in a values-clarification situation?
   1. "Your questions were pretty blunt."
   2. "Tell me what you're thinking right now."
   3. "I've felt that way before; I'd be upset, too."
   4. "You seem concerned about your tests. Let me explain them."

6. A nurse's use of ethical responsibility can best be seen in which of the following ways?
   1. Delivery of competent care
   2. Formation of interpersonal relationships
   3. Application of the nursing process
   4. Evaluation of new computerized technologies

7. A student nurse realizes that she has administered the wrong dose of medication to a patient. She immediately informs her clinical instructor. This student nurse is best described professionally as:
   1. Confident
   2. Trustworthy
   3. Compliant
   4. Accountable

8. The physician has informed a client that she has cancer. The client tells the nurse and physician that she is not sure if she wants her family to know. The nurse encourages the client to consider sharing the information with her family so they can support her through the decisions she will need to make regarding her care. The nurse is using the principle of:
   1. Confidentiality
   2. Fidelity
   3. Veracity
   4. Justice

9. The nurse is investigating the process for resolution of an ethical problem. The correct sequence for resolving ethical problems is:
   1. Examine one's own values, evaluate, identify the problem
   2. Evaluate the outcomes, gather data, consider actions
   3. Gather facts, verbalize the problem, consider actions
   4. Recognize the dilemma, evaluate, gather information

10. A nurse is ambivalent as to the need to provide suction vigorously to a terminal client in a comatose state. Which of the following is an appropriate statement by the nurse in regard to processing an ethical dilemma?
    1. "I need to know the legalities of the living will of this client."
    2. "My spiritual beliefs mandate that I continue to provide all the interventions in my scope of practice."
    3. "I cannot figure out what's right in this situation. I need to collect more data."
    4. "I just feel as if I should not suction this client."

11. Which of the following statements best illustrates the deontological ethical theory?
    1. "I believe this disease was allowed by a supreme being."
    2. "He has become a stronger individual through experiencing the loss of his father."
    3. "It would never be right for a person to stop cardiopulmonary resuscitation (CPR) efforts."
    4. "The chemotherapy did not cure this person, but it provided a better life for him."

12. A nurse stopped at an accident scene and began to provide emergency care for the victims. Her actions are best labeled ethically as:
    1. Respect for persons
    2. Beneficence
    3. Nonmaleficence
    4. Triage

13. The nurse is aware that an ethics committee in a health care facility serves to:
    1. Interview all persons involved in a case
    2. Illustrate circumstances that demonstrate malpractice
    3. Serve as a resource for specific situations that may occur
    4. Examine similar previous instances for comparison of outcome decisions

14. A client in the emergency department believes that she has been waiting longer than the other individuals because she has no insurance. The ethical principle that is involved in this particular situation is:
    1. Justice
    2. Autonomy
    3. Beneficence
    4. Nonmaleficence

15. An example of the nurse's use of the specific ethical principle of autonomy in a client situation is:
    1. Learning how to do a procedure safely and effectively
    2. Returning to speak to a client at an agreed-on time
    3. Preparing the client's room for comfort and privacy
    4. Supporting a client's right to refuse therapy

16. The nurse always tries to maintain ethical principles in clinical practice. Which of the following statements reflects application of the specific ethical principle of confidentiality?
    1. "I'm concerned that decreased funding may affect the outpatient program."
    2. "I'm going to make sure that client understands the instructions."
    3. "I cannot share that information with you about the client."
    4. "I need to get more information about the client's health history."

17. The client has been diagnosed with malignant bone cancer. Treatment involves chemotherapy on an outpatient basis. Over the course of the treatment, the client becomes very ill, is experiencing tremendous side effects from the therapy, and has a severe reduction in the quality of life. The specific ethical principle that is in question in this situation is:
    1. Veracity
    2. Fidelity
    3. Justice
    4. Nonmaleficence

Chapter 22   Legal Implications in Nursing Practice

1. The client has an order for intramuscular (IM) morphine sulfate as needed for pain. A nurse accidentally administers an incorrect dosage of the morphine sulfate to the client. Which source of law best addresses this situation?
   1. Civil law
   2. Criminal law
   3. Common law
   4. Administrative law

2. On admission to the hospital, a terminal cancer patient says he has a living will. This document functions to state the client's desire to:
   1. Receive all means of technical assistance and equipment used to prolong his life
   2. Have his wife make decisions regarding his care
   3. Be allowed to die without life-prolonging techniques
   4. Have a lethal injection administered to relieve his suffering

3. A junior nursing student prepares to give her client an injection. What standard of care applies to the student nurse's conduct when providing care normally performed by a registered nurse (RN)? The student is held to:
   1. A standard of care of an unlicensed person
   2. The same standard of care as an RN
   3. A standard similar to but not the same as the staff nurse with whom she is assigned to work
   4. No special standard of care because her faculty member is responsible for her conduct

4. The nurse has just obtained a license to practice and is determining whether individual malpractice insurance is necessary. Which of the following is the most important factor in a nurse's deciding whether to carry malpractice insurance?
   1. The amount of the malpractice insurance provided by the employer
   2. The evaluation of whether the nurse works in a critical area of nursing where clients have higher morbidity and mortality rates
   3. The time frames and individual liability of the employer's malpractice coverage
   4. The nurse's knowledge level of Good Samaritan laws

5. An unconscious client with a head injury needs surgery to live. His wife speaks only French, and the health care providers are having a difficult time explaining his condition. Which of the following is the most correct answer regarding this situation?
   1. Two licensed health care personnel should witness and sign the preoperative consent indicating their hearing an explanation of the procedure given in English.
   2. An institutional review board must be contacted to give their emergency advice on the situation.
   3. A friend of the family could act as an interpreter, but the explanation could not provide details of the client's accident, because of confidentiality laws.
   4. The health care team should continue with the surgery after providing information in the best manner possible.

6. A physician asks a family nurse practitioner to prescribe a medication that the nurse practitioner knows is incompatible with the current medication regimen. If the nurse practitioner follows the physician's desire, which of the following is the most correct answer?
   1. The nurse practitioner will be liable for the action.
   2. Good Samaritan laws will protect the nurse.
   3. If the nurse practitioner has developed a good relationship with the client, there will probably not be a problem.
   4. This type of situation is why nurse practitioners should have malpractice insurance.

7. A registered nurse interprets a scribbled medication order by the attending physician as 25 mg. The nurse administers 25 mg of the medication to a client and then discovers that the dose was incorrectly interpreted and should have been 15 mg. Who would ultimately be responsible for the error?
   1. Attending physician
   2. Assisting resident
   3. Pharmacist
   4. Nurse

8. Because of an influenza epidemic among nursing staff, a nurse has been moved from the eye unit to a general surgical floor. The nurse recognizes that he is inexperienced in this specialty. The nurse's initial recourse is to:
   1. Politely refuse to move, take a leave-of-absence day, and go home
   2. Ask to work with another general surgery nurse
   3. Fill out a report noting his dissatisfaction
   4. Notify the state board of nursing of the problem

9. The nurse recognizes that issues concerning death and dying may influence nursing practice. Which of the following is true concerning the legalities of death and dying issues?
   1. Passive euthanasia is illegal in all states.
   2. Assisted suicide is a constitutional right.
   3. Organ donation must be attempted if it will save the recipient's life.
   4. Feedings may be refused by competent individuals who are unable to feed themselves.

10. As per the standards of care of the Joint Commission on Accreditation of Healthcare Organizations (JCAHO), an institution is required to have:
    1. Limits of professional liability
    2. Educational standards for nurses
    3. A delineated scope of practice for health professionals
    4. Written nursing policies and procedures for care

11. Under specific circumstances that are outlined in the state's nurse practice act, a nurse's license may be suspended or revoked. In the event that a nursing license is revoked, which of the following is correct?
    1. The hearings are usually held in court.
    2. Due process rights are waived by the nurse.
    3. Appeals may be made regarding the decisions.
    4. The federal government becomes involved in the procedures.

12. In the course of practice, a nurse may be liable for actions that constitute an unintentional tort. Which one of the following is an example of an unintentional tort?
    1. Restraining a client who refuses care
    2. Taking photos of a client's surgical wounds
    3. Leaving the side rails down, and the client falls and is injured
    4. Talking about a client's history of sexually transmitted diseases

13. The nurse must be aware of individuals who are able to give consent for procedures and treatments. Which one of the following individuals may legally give informed consent?
    1. A 16-year-old for her newborn child
    2. A sedated 42-year-old client
    3. The friend of an 84-year-old married client
    4. A 56-year-old who does not understand the proposed treatment plan

14. A client is to have a surgical procedure tomorrow morning, and the nurse has gone into the room to obtain the consent form. The nurse's signature as a witness on an informed consent indicates that the client:
    1. Fully understands the procedure
    2. Agrees with the procedure to be done
    3. Has voluntarily signed the form
    4. Has authorized the physician to continue with the treatment

15. In working with clients who have DNR (do not resuscitate) orders, the nurse recognizes that these orders:
    1. Are legally required for terminally ill clients
    2. May be written by the physician without client consent if resuscitation is futile
    3. Are maintained throughout the client's stay in an acute or long-term facility
    4. Follow nationally consistent standards for implementation

16. The nurse understands the implications of the Patient Self-Determination Act. This legislation requires that:
    1. Clients designate a power of attorney
    2. DNR orders for clients meet a standard criterion
    3. Organ donation is required on death, if possible
    4. Information be provided to the client regarding rights for refusal of care

17. The nurse is investigating legislation that may have an effect on nursing practice. The nurse finds that the newly enacted Health Insurance Portability and Accountability Act (HIPAA) of 2003 requires:
    1. Insurance coverage for all clients
    2. Policies on how to report communicable diseases
    3. Limits on information and damages awarded in court cases
    4. Safeguards to protect written and verbal information about clients

18. The nurse enters the room and tells the client that he has to take the medication, including an injection. The client refuses the medication, but the nurse continues to administer the medications. This action is an example of the intentional tort of:
    1. Assault
    2. Battery
    3. Invasion of privacy
    4. Malpractice

19. The nurse is working with a client who has been diagnosed with acquired immunodeficiency syndrome (AIDS). On the way downstairs in the elevator, the nurse shares the client's name and diagnosis with a co-worker. Unknown to the nurse, a friend of the client also is on the elevator and hears the entire story. The nurse who shared the information may be held liable for:
    1. Slander
    2. Assault
    3. Malpractice
    4. Invasion of privacy

Chapter 23
Communication

1. The nurse has provided the client with information regarding the treatment plan for the diagnosis. The client tells the nurse that he understands most of the information, but still has questions concerning the medication. This response is an example of:
   1. Referent
   2. Receiver
   3. Channel
   4. Feedback

2. The nurse is in the process of conducting an admission interview with the client. At one point in the discussion, the client has provided information that the nurse would like to clarify. The nurse uses the technique of clarification, as indicated by the response:
   1. "I'm not sure that I understand what you mean by that statement."
   2. "The electrocardiogram (ECG) records information about your heart's electrical activity."
   3. "Let's look at the problem you have had with your medication at home."
   4. "What's your biggest concern at the moment?"

3. The faculty member is reviewing a process recording with the student nurse. The student has been working with a client who has had an amputation of the lower left leg and is emotionally fragile. The student receives positive feedback from the faculty member for the following response made to the client:
   1. "Why are you so upset today?"
   2. "I'm sure that everything will be all right."
   3. "You shouldn't cry. The wound will heal soon."
   4. "It must be very difficult to have this happen to you."

4. The client draws back when the nurse reaches over the side rails to take his blood pressure. To promote effective communication, the nurse should first:
   1. Tell the client that the blood pressure can be taken at a later time
   2. Rotate the nurses who are assigned to take the client's blood pressure
   3. Continue to perform the procedure quickly and quietly
   4. Apologize for startling the client, and explain the need for contact

5. Active listening and body language work together. The nurse actively listens to the client and:
   1. Sits facing the client
   2. Keeps the arms and legs crossed
   3. Leans back in the chair away from the client
   4. Avoids eye contact as much as possible

6. During the assessment phase of the nursing process, the nurse may uncover data that help to identify communication problems. An example of this information is:
   1. Extreme dyspnea or shortness of breath
   2. Urinary frequency and pain
   3. Chronic stomach pain
   4. Lack of appetite

7. A nurse tells an advanced nurse practitioner that the client is "slipping a little" in reference to hemodynamic pressures. The nurse is using:
   1. Brevity
   2. Relevance
   3. Pacing and control
   4. Connotative meaning.

8. A client is admitted for a computed tomography (CAT scan; diagnostic test) of the cranium. As the nurse explains this diagnostic test, the client moves away from the nurse. This is an example of what influencing factor in communication?
   1. Gender
   2. Environment
   3. Space and territoriality
   4. Sociocultural background

9. The nurse will often display empathy in communication with clients. Of the following responses by the nurse, which one best conveys empathy?
   1. "Good morning. How did you sleep last night?"
   2. "I can understand your concern about learning to inject yourself."
   3. "Do you mean you would like to talk to the new family nurse practitioner?"
   4. "Can you describe what the pain in your abdomen feels like?"

10. In working with a client who is newly diagnosed with diabetes mellitus, the nurse provides feedback to the client on her progress in learning the treatment regimen. Of the following, the nurse demonstrates the use of therapeutic communication by stating:
    1. "I believe that you have come a long way in learning how to manage your care."
    2. "It didn't look as if you were ever going to be able to get the injection technique."
    3. "You really need to be checking your blood sugar more often unless you want to come back here to the hospital."
    4. "You don't appear to have any interest in your dietary intake."

11. A parent tells the pediatric nurse practitioner, "I've never told anyone this information about my son." This is an example of:
    1. Identifying problems and goals
    2. Building trust
    3. Clarifying roles
    4. Revealing

12. Discussing the client's follow-up dietary needs immediately after the surgery when the client is experiencing discomfort is an error in:
    1. Pacing
    2. Intonation
    3. Timing and relevance
    4. Denotative meaning

13. The nurse is aware of the client's zones of personal space when planning interactions. The zone of personal space and touch that extends the greatest amount from an individual is the:
    1. Personal zone
    2. Social zone
    3. Consent zone
    4. Vulnerable zone

14. Communication is used throughout the nursing process. In the evaluation phase, the nurse specifically uses communication to:
    1. Delegate activities to other staff members
    2. Validate the client's health needs
    3. Acquire verbal and nonverbal feedback
    4. Document expected outcomes and planned interventions

15. A number of variables may influence the client's communication with the health care team. Which of the following is an example of an interpersonal variable?
    1. Postoperative discomfort
    2. An extremely warm room
    3. A talkative roommate
    4. A loud television

16. The nurse is establishing a helping relationship with the client. In addressing the client, the nurse should:
    1. Use the client's first name
    2. Touch the client right away to establish contact
    3. Sit far enough away from the client
    4. Knock before entering the client's room

17. In using communication skills with clients, the nurse evaluates which response as being the most therapeutic?
    1. "Why don't you stick to the special diet?"
    2. "I noticed that you didn't eat lunch. Is something wrong?"
    3. "I think you need to find another physician that's better than this one."
    4. "We can't continue talking about your financial problems right now. It's time for your bath."

18. Communication skills are adapted by the nurse for pediatric clients. What communication technique may be used most effectively with toddlers or preschoolers?
    1. Using analogies to explain health-related ideas
    2. Allowing manipulation of equipment to be used
    3. Moving quickly and minimizing contact to avoid distress
    4. Focusing on what other children have done

19. Communication skills are adapted for clients with special needs. For a client with aphasia, the nurse may enhance communication by:
    1. Using visual cues
    2. Speaking loudly
    3. Using open-ended questions
    4. Using a speech therapist to communicate with the client

Chapter 24 Client Education

1. The client has been informed that he can be discharged once he can irrigate his colostomy independently. The client requests the nurse to observe his irrigation technique. Which of the following learning motives is the client displaying?
   1. Physical need
   2. Social activity
   3. Task mastery
   4. Evaluation stance

2. An industrial nurse is planning to give an informative talk on hypertension to employees in honor of Heart Month. He plans to teach individuals how to take their blood pressures. Which information is important for him to ask the planning committee before this presentation?
   1. Specific ages of all of the people involved
   2. Names of employees who are married
   3. Number of employees with high blood pressure
   4. Type of room available and number of participants

3. The nurse established an objective for the client who was unable to void: The client's intake will be at least 1000 ml between 7 AM and 3:30 PM. Feedback indicating success is indicated by the client:
   1. Voiding at least 1000 ml during the shift
   2. Verbalizing abdominal comfort without pressure
   3. Having adequate intake and output
   4. Drinking 240 ml of fluid, 5 or 6 times during the shift

4. The nurse selects a variety of teaching methods to use with clients. For a toddler, the nurse should use:
   1. Role playing
   2. Problem solving
   3. Independent learning
   4. Simple explanations and pictures

5. The nurse has important information to share with a parent who has brought his child to the emergency department. The nurse discovers that the parent, who appears very anxious, has just learned his son will require surgery. The most effective teaching approach in this situation is:
   1. Telling
   2. Entrusting
   3. Participating
   4. Group teaching

6. A client is taught the clinical manifestations of inflammation to allow early detection of a complication of a surgical wound. The client states, "I will look at the wound 4 times a day and tell my surgeon if it looks red or swollen." Her statement is an example of:
   1. Attitudes
   2. Application
   3. Analysis
   4. Evaluation

7. The client continues to ask questions about a surgical wound. The client states, "I think I would like help the first time I look at my wound." This is an example of:
   1. Guided response
   2. Adaptation
   3. Perception
   4. Organizing

8. The nurse assesses the client's readiness to learn insulin injection sites. Many factors are assessed before teaching, but the most important factor for the nurse to assess first is the:
   1. Previous knowledge level of the client
   2. Willingness of the client to want to learn the injection sites
   3. Financial resources available to the client for the equipment
   4. Intelligence and developmental level of the client

9. The nurse is demonstrating to the client how to put on antiembolytic stockings. In the middle of the lesson, the client asks, "Why have my feet been swelling?" The nurse stops and responds to the client. Which of the following is the teaching principle that the nurse should adhere to?
   1. Timing
   2. Setting priorities
   3. Building on existing knowledge
   4. Organizing teaching materials

10. The nurse is evaluating the responses of clients to teaching sessions. An example of an evaluation of a psychomotor skill is:
    1. Client is able to state side effects of medication.
    2. Client responds appropriately to eye contact.
    3. Client planned an exercise program.
    4. Client uses the cane correctly.

11. Different topics are presented in the information sessions that are held in the outpatient clinic. In planning for a session on health maintenance/illness prevention, the nurse should select a topic on:
    1. Use of assistive devices, such as canes
    2. Self-help devices for post-CVA (cerebrovascular accident) clients
    3. Stress-management techniques for working parents
    4. Environmental alterations for clients in wheelchairs

12. The nurse is evaluating the responses of clients to teaching sessions. An example of an evaluation of a client's attainment of a cognitive skill is:
    1. Client explains that the medication should be taken with meals.
    2. Client looks at the surgical incision without prompting.
    3. Client uses crutches appropriately to go up and down stairs.
    4. Client dresses self after breakfast.

13. The nurse evaluates which of the following statements as an indication that the client is not ready to learn at this time.
    1. "I need to understand more about the reason for the colostomy."
    2. "I will find out when the support group meets."
    3. "There's no sense in showing me. I'm too sick right now."
    4. "Tell me if I am doing this correctly."

14. In planning to teach an older adult client, the nurse should incorporate which teaching method or principle into the plan?
    1. Keep teaching sessions short.
    2. Teach in the early morning or late evening.
    3. Put as much as possible into each teaching session.
    4. Focus on teaching a family member instead.

15. The nurse has completed an assessment of the client and identified the following nursing diagnoses. Which one of the following nursing diagnoses indicates a need to postpone teaching that was planned?
    1. Knowledge deficit regarding impending surgery
    2. Activity intolerance related to pain
    3. Ineffective management of treatment regimen
    4. Noncompliance with prescribed exercise plan

16. The nurse recognizes that a variety of teaching methods may be implemented to meet the client's needs. Which teaching method is best applied to a cognitive learning need?
    1. Computer-assisted instruction
    2. Demonstration of a procedure
    3. Modeling of behavior
    4. Discussion of feelings

17. For a functionally illiterate client, the nurse particularly focuses on:
    1. Using intricate analogies and examples
    2. Avoiding return demonstrations
    3. Incorporating familiar terminology
    4. Spending less time with the client

18. In preparing a teaching plan for adult clients in a cancer support group, the nurse incorporates evidence-based information. The nurse recognizes that evidence obtained about adult learners identified that this group preferred:
    1. Computer-assisted instruction
    2. Traditional classroom settings
    3. Long sessions with lots of technical information
    4. Interesting personal communication techniques

19. The nurse is teaching the client about management of his heart disease. A strategy that is implemented to promote learning in the affective domain is demonstrated by the nurse:
    1. Asking the client what he believes he needs to know about the diagnosis
    2. Providing brochures on current exercises and nutrition guidelines
    3. Encouraging the client to discuss his feelings about his health status
    4. Having the client return demonstrate self-measurement of his blood pressure

20. The nurse is preparing to present a teaching session on skin protection for a group of older adults at a senior center. A principle that has been found to be most effective in teaching older adults is:
    1. Moving the group along at a predetermined pace
    2. Providing information in longer teaching sessions
    3. Speaking very slowly and in a louder tone of voice
    4. Beginning and ending each session with important information

Chapter 25
Documentation

1. The nurse is preparing the information that will be provided to the staff on the next shift. Which of the following should the nurse include in the intershift report to nursing colleagues?
    1. Audit of client care procedures
    2. The client's diagnosis-related group
    3. All routine care procedures required by the client
    4. Instructions given to the client in a teaching plan

2. The client climbed over the side rails and fell to the floor. An incident report is to be completed. The correct reporting of an incident involves which of the following:
   1. The nurse witnessing the event completes the report.
   2. Details of the incident are subjectively described.
   3. An explanation of the possible cause for the incident is entered.
   4. A notation is included in the medical record that an incident report was prepared.

3. Guidelines should be followed when documenting client care. The nurse recognizes that the following is the most appropriate notation:
   1. 1230 Client's vital signs taken
   2. 0700 Client drank adequate amount of fluids
   3. 0900 Meperidine (Demerol) given for lower abdominal pain
   4. 0830 Increased intravenous (IV) fluid rate to 100 ml per hour according to protocol

4. The nurse makes a late entry in a client's record. Which of the following is the best example of how to document this type of situation?
   1. "8:30 AM: Client received aspirin and oxycodone (Percodan; 1 tablet) PO an hour before going to radiology"
   2. "12:15 PM: I gave the client morphine 10 mg IM at 11:10 AM, but did not document it then"
   3. "2:45 PM: Acetylsalicylic acid (ASA) gr X given for temperature of 38.1°C"
   4. "8:30 PM: Abdominal dressing change at 7:30 PM. No s/s of infection, and wound edges approximating well"

5. "Client is wheezing and experiencing some dyspnea on exertion." This is an example of:
   1. The "S" in SOAP documentation
   2. FOCUS documentation
   3. The "P" of PIE
   4. The "R" in DAR documentation

6. Recording a nurse's description of the teaching provided to the client on performance of self-medication administration is found in a(n):
   1. Kardex
   2. Incident report
   3. Nursing history form
   4. Discharge summary form

7. The nurse is documenting on the client's record and notes that she has made an error. The action that the nurse should take is to:
   1. Draw a straight line through the error and initial it.
   2. Erase the error and write over the material in the same spot.
   3. Use a dark color marker to cover the error and continue immediately after that point.
   4. Footnote the error at the bottom of the page.

8. The charge nurse is evaluating the documentation of the new staff nurse. On review of the charting, the charge nurse notes that appropriate documentation is evident when the new staff nurse:
   1. Uses a pencil to make the entries
   2. Uses correction fluid to correct written errors
   3. Identifies an error made by the attending physician
   4. Dates and signs all of the entries made in the record

9. It is late at night on the medical unit in the hospital, and the physician calls to leave orders for one of his clients. The licensed practical nurse (LPN) answers the phone and appropriately responds:
   1. "Let me get the registered nurse on the phone."
   2. "I am unable to take the order at this time. Please call in the morning."
   3. "Please repeat the order for me so I can make sure it is written correctly."
   4. "Let me have your phone number, and I will have the supervisor call you back."

10. A slight hematoma developed on the client's left forearm. The nurse labels the problem as an infiltrated intravenous (IV) line. The nurse elevates the forearm. The client states, "My arm feels better." What is documented as the "R" in FOCUS charting?
    1. "My arm feels better."
    2. "Slight hematoma on left forearm"
    3. "Infiltrated IV line"
    4. "Elevation of left forearm"

11. Which of the following is evaluated as a legally appropriate notation?
    1. "Dr. Green made an error in the amount of medication to administer."
    2. "Verbalized sharp, stabbing pain along the left side of chest."
    3. "Nurse Williams spoke with the client about the surgery."
    4. "Client upset about the physical therapy."

12. To avoid legal risks and possible lack of confidentiality associated with computerized documentation, many programs currently have:
    1. All nursing staff use the same access code
    2. Only centralized medical records use the client dat 1
    3. Thumbprint identification restrictions
    4. Periodic changes in staff passwords

Chapter 26 Self-Concept

1. The client has just learned that his motorcycle accident has resulted in his left leg being amputated. When helping this client form goals and strategies for realistic goals, the nurse needs to assess the client's:
    1. Interests and past accomplishments
    2. Intellectual and spiritual strengths
    3. Involvement with significant others
    4. Ideal and perceived self-concept

2. The nurse is working with a client who is manifesting behaviors that are consistent with a negative self-concept. The nurse has observed that the client maintains:
    1. Frequent eye contact
    2. A passive attitude
    3. Independence in self-care
    4. An interest in the surroundings

3. A 76-year-old client who recently lost his wife is admitted for surgery. The nurse is using Erikson as a psychosocial framework for client assessment. Which of the following behaviors would alert the nurse that the client has an alteration in the integrity stage of his psychosocial development?
    1. Accepting his own limitations
    2. Verbalizing fear about the surgery
    3. Expressing his thoughts about his care
    4. Demanding excessive assistance from his daughter

4. A client has been hospitalized for an extended time while receiving therapies for lung cancer. The client has become very depressed, refuses to participate in personal grooming, and does not want visitors. To assist in achieving resolution of the client's problem, the nurse should have the client:
    1. Get washed and dressed independently
    2. Think positively instead of negatively
    3. Contact a support group and explore a psychological consultation
    4. Become more independent and return to prior activities

5. The client is on the orthopedic unit after back surgery. He states, "I feel like I can't do anything anymore—and I won't be able to continue my landscaping business." This is predominantly an example of a problem in which of the following components of self-concept?
    1. Body image
    2. Self-esteem
    3. Identity
    4. Role

6. A recently divorced client comes to the clinic. She has custody of her two teenagers and is an established lawyer. She states, "I can't keep working so hard and raise my children the way I would like." This is an example of:
   1. Role ambiguity
   2. Role strain
   3. Role conflict
   4. Gender role stereotype

7. A prostitute, with human immunodeficiency syndrome (HIV) and severe complications, is being cared for on a medical unit. The nurse is seeking to develop a therapeutic relationship with the client. Which of the following statements best reflects the nurse's attempt to support the client's self-exploration?
   1. "What type of support do you feel you need?"
   2. "Don't be embarrassed by your former occupation."
   3. "On what type of schedule do you think you could realistically eat your meals without being nauseated?"
   4. "The people who work here are professionals, and we'll try not to judge your past actions."

8. A school-aged client has just been diagnosed with juvenile diabetes. The client is very angry about the new disease. Which of the following statements is most appropriate for the nurse counselor working with this client?
   1. "Try not to be angry because you are receiving the best care possible."
   2. "It is all right to be angry with your friends, but try not be angry with your parents."
   3. "You appear upset about the diagnosis. Let's talk about your feelings."
   4. "You learn quickly and will probably handle the difficult treatments very well."

9. A client is most concerned about the interactions that she has with her family, and she is in the process of establishing a positive view of herself. This client is meeting the developmental needs of the:
   1. 12- to 20-year-old age group
   2. Early 20s to mid-40s age group
   3. Mid-40s to mid-60s age group
   4. Late 60s and older age group

10. In developing role behavior, the child learns which of the following through substitution?
    1. Engaging in an acceptable behavior instead of another unacceptable one
    2. Avoiding unacceptable behavior because it is punished
    3. Internalizing beliefs and values of role models
    4. Refraining from behavior even though tempted

11. The nurse recognizes that self-concept develops throughout an individual's lifetime. Which developmental task associated with self-concept is expected in an assessment of an individual from the 12- to 20-year-old age group?
    1. Identifying with a gender
    2. Exploring goals for the future
    3. Distinguishing oneself from the environment
    4. Feeling positive about one's life achievements

12. The nurse is working with a client and wants to learn about the individual's perception of identity. What question should the nurse use to assess this?
    1. "What changes would you make in your appearance?"
    2. "What activities do you enjoy doing?"
    3. "How would you describe yourself?"
    4. "What is your usual day like?"

13. The client has just been laid off from his job and is very upset about the loss of his position. In establishing a plan of care for the client, the nurse determines that an appropriate outcome for this client with situational low self-esteem is:
    1. Client will recognize his inability to make decisions.
    2. Client will respond to anxiety with decreased amounts of stress.
    3. Client will use therapeutic communication skills to discuss his needs.
    4. Client will discuss a minimum of two areas in which he is functioning well.

Chapter 27 Sexuality

1. The nurse is aware that sexuality is part of growth and development. The preschooler's interest in gender sexuality is characterized by an interest in:
    1. His or her genitalia
    2. Learning how and why his or her anatomy differs from that of other children
    3. Playing and developing friendships with children of the opposite sex
    4. Spending most of his or her time with the parent of the opposite sex

2. A female nurse is working with a male client. During the administration of medications, the male client acts out sexually to the female nurse who is caring for him. The nurse should:
    1. Have a male nurse assume care for this client
    2. Immediately report the incident to the client's physician
    3. Tell the client that his behavior is offensive and leave the room
    4. Review and define the professional relationship for the client

3. A client states that she is afraid that she and her husband will not be able to maintain a healthy sexual relationship now that they have a baby in the house. To assist these clients, it would be most helpful for the nurse to know:
    1. If they have similar parenting beliefs
    2. How long they have been married
    3. How comfortable they are in communicating their feelings to each other
    4. The level of knowledge they have regarding healthy sexual relationships

4. On completion of an assessment of a client in the medical clinic, the nurse documents that the client has dyspareunia based on the client's experience of:
    1. Delay or absence or an orgasm
    2. Deficient or absent sexual desire
    3. Involuntary constriction of the vagina
    4. Recurrent genital pain during intercourse

5. An adolescent female student, who is sexually active, visits the office of the school nurse. Which of the following statements best reflects her understanding of the effective use of contraception devices?
    1. "My boyfriend is able to withdraw before ejaculation, and that prevents me from getting pregnant."
    2. "I take my temperature every morning, and when it goes down for at least 2 days, we have unprotected sex."
    3. "We use 'foam' before each time that we have sex, and I haven't gotten pregnant yet."
    4. "I use a diaphragm and contraceptive cream."

6. A school nurse is responsible for teaching adolescents about sexually transmitted diseases (STDs). When discussing chlamydia, the nurse instructs the students that it is:
    1. A viral infection that cannot be cured
    2. Treated with a full course of antibiotics
    3. Contracted via blood-borne exchange
    4. Prevented with the use of spermicidals

7. The nurse is conducting a sexual history with a client who is scheduled for cardiac surgery. The client tells the nurse that he is nervous about resuming sexual activities. The nurse uses therapeutic communication with the client when responding:
   1. "You can have sexual intercourse after your surgery, but there are serious risks."
   2. "Your partner will be nervous about resuming sexual activities, but that is normal."
   3. "Don't worry. In about 2 months you will be able to return to your normal sexual patterns."
   4. "You are expressing a very normal concern—perhaps we could discuss your feelings further."

8. The nurse is teaching sexuality to a group of senior adults. Which of the following comments by a participant reflects that he or she has an understanding of the changes in sexuality that occur with aging?
   1. "So sexual intercourse will be more painful for my wife, and we should have sex less frequently?"
   2. "We have recently seen the need to begin using a lubricant. That's because we make love less often."
   3. "My orgasms seem to not last as long, but my husband and I are probably more satisfied now than when we were younger."
   4. "It's natural not to have sex anymore. People our age shouldn't still have those feelings."

9. The nurse has completed an assessment on an adult male client and finds that he has difficulty having an erection and has less interest in sex. The nurse notes that the client has recently been given an antihypertensive medication. A nursing diagnosis of *Sexual dysfunction related to side effects of antihypertensive* is identified by the nurse. An appropriate outcome for this client is:
   1. Client will avoid taking medication before intercourse.
   2. Client will relate renewed interest in sex within 1 month.
   3. Client will be seen by a sexual therapist immediately.
   4. Client will seek out other activities or hobbies.

10. A 58-year-old woman asks the nurse what she can do to promote healthy sexual relations. Based on the client's age, the nurse responds by saying:
    1. "Continue what you've been doing. Nothing should have changed."
    2. "I will refer you to a sexual therapist the better to assist you."
    3. "Using a water-based lubricant may be helpful."
    4. "Reducing the frequency of intercourse may help you."

11. In preparing a presentation on the prevention of sexual abuse, the nurse incorporates the following information:
    1. Intensity is generally increased during pregnancies.
    2. Sexual abuse is found primarily in lower socioeconomic groups.
    3. Abusers fit into easily identified, classic profiles.
    4. Most of the incidents occur with strangers or unknown assailants.

12. To increase the tone and sensation of the pelvic floor for a female client, the nurse teaches:
    1. Sensate focus exercises
    2. Kegel exercises
    3. Vaginal dilation
    4. Stop/start techniques

Chapter 28 Spiritual Health

1. When working with adolescent clients and discussing spirituality, the nurse is aware that clients in this age group often:
   1. Have a good concept of a supreme being
   2. Question religious practices and values
   3. Fully accept the higher meaning of their faith
   4. Give themselves over to spiritual tasks

2. The nurse's knowledge about spirituality begins with the nurse:
   1. Researching all popular religions
   2. Looking at his or her own beliefs
   3. Sharing his or her faith with the clients
   4. Providing prayers and religious articles for clients

3. The client experienced a near-death experience (NDE) and was successfully resuscitated. The nurse wants to provide the opportunity for the client to discuss the NDE. The most appropriate response by the nurse is:
   1. "This is a common experience that is easily explained."
   2. "That must have been an awful experience for you."
   3. "Have you ever heard of other persons having NDEs?"
   4. "What was your experience like, and how did it make you feel?"

4. A 76-year-old client has just been admitted to the nursing unit with terminal cancer of the liver. The nurse is assessing the client's spiritual needs and responds best by saying:
   1. "I notice you have a Bible—is that a source of spiritual strength to you?"
   2. "What do you believe happens to your spirit when you die?"
   3. "We would allow members of your church to visit you whenever you desire."
   4. "Has your terminal condition made you lose your faith or beliefs?"

5. A client with diabetes is being cared for in the home, with the assistance of a home health nurse and a family member. The client asks you if eating a vegetarian diet will conflict with the disease. The nurse anticipates that the client will follow a vegetarian diet because he is a member of the following religion:
   1. Hinduism
   2. Judaism
   3. Islam
   4. Sikhism

6. Hope may be used effectively with clients who have terminal diseases. Hope provides a:
   1. Relationship with a divinity
   2. System of organized beliefs
   3. Cultural connectedness
   4. Meaning and purpose

7. While working with a client to assess and support spirituality, the nurse should first:
   1. Refer the client to the agency chaplain
   2. Assist the client to use faith to get well
   3. Provide a variety of religious literature
   4. Determine the client's perceptions and belief system

8. If a client is identified as following traditional health care beliefs of Judaism, the nurse should prepare to incorporate the following into care:
   1. Observance of the Sabbath
   2. Faith healing
   3. Ongoing group prayer
   4. Regular fasting

9. The nurse is conferring with the nutritionist about the needs of a Native American. The nurse anticipates that the client will:
   1. Follow a strict vegetarian diet
   2. Avoid the use of alcohol and tobacco
   3. Avoid pork products
   4. Follow a diet according to individual tribal beliefs

10. The nurse has identified the following nursing diagnoses for his assigned clients. Of the following diagnoses, which one indicates the greatest potential need to plan for the client's spiritual needs?
    1. Altered health maintenance
    2. Ineffective individual coping
    3. Impaired memory
    4. Decreased adaptive capacity

11. The nurse is working in the labor and delivery area with parents who are members of the Shinto and Buddhist religions. The nurse expects that after the birth of the child:
    1. Baptism will be performed immediately.
    2. Special prayers will be said over the child.
    3. Special preparations will be made for the umbilical cord and placenta.
    4. No particular rituals will usually be performed in the immediate postpartum period.

12. The nurse may incorporate similarities of nutritional needs into the plan of care for clients who are Mormon and Buddhist. Members of these religions both:
    1. Follow vegetarian diets
    2. Avoid alcohol and tobacco
    3. Avoid dairy products
    4. Fast on Fridays

13. The nurse anticipates the gender-related needs of the clients and tries to accommodatethose needs whenever possible. A female nurse is arranged for the female client who practices:
    1. Sikhism
    2. Judaism
    3. Hinduism
    4. Buddhism

14. The nurse working in the labor and delivery area is aware that special care is provided for the umbilical cord after the child's birth for the clients who are:
    1. Catholic
    2. Navajo
    3. Shinto
    4. Hindu

Chapter 29   The Experience of Loss, Death, and Grief

1. The nurse is discussing future treatments with a client who has a terminal illness. The nurse notes that the client has not been eating and responds to the nurse's information by saying, "What does it matter?" The most appropriate nursing diagnosis for this client is:
   1. Social isolation
   2. Spiritual distress
   3. Denial
   4. Hopelessness

2. The nurse recognizes that anticipatory grieving can be most beneficial to a client or family because it can:
   1. Be done in private
   2. Be discussed with others
   3. Promote separation of the ill client from the family
   4. Help a person progress to a healthier emotional state

3. A newly graduated nurse is assigned to his first dying patient. The nurse is best prepared to care for this client if he:
   1. Completed a course dealing with death and dying
   2. Is able to control his own emotions about death
   3. Experiences the death of a loved one
   4. Has developed a personal understanding of his own feelings about death

4. An identified outcome for the family of a client with a terminal illness is that they will be able to provide psychological support to the dying client. To assist the family to meet this outcome, the nurse plans to include in the teaching plan:
   1. Demonstration of bathing techniques
   2. Application of oxygen devices
   3. Recognition of client needs and fears
   4. Information on when to contact the hospice nurse

5. The nurse is assigned to a client who was recently diagnosed with a terminal illness. During morning care, the client asks about organ donation. The nurse should:
   1. Have the client first discuss the subject with the family
   2. Suggest the client delay making a decision at this time
   3. Assist the client to obtain the necessary information to make this decision
   4. Contact the physician so consent can be obtained from the family

6. A client has been diagnosed with terminal cancer of the liver and is receiving chemotherapy on a medical unit. In an in-depth conversation with the nurse, the client states, "I wonder why this happened to me?" According to Kübler-Ross, the nurse identifies that this stage is associated with:
   1. Anxiety
   2. Denial
   3. Confrontation
   4. Depression

7. A client who is Chinese-American has just died on the unit. The nurse is prepared to provide after-death care to the client and anticipates that the probable preferences of a family from this cultural background will include:
   1. Pastoral care
   2. Preparation for organ donation
   3. Time for the family to bathe the client
   4. Preparation for quick removal from the hospital

8. Which of the following is the primary concern of the nurse for providing care to a dying client? The nurse should:
   1. Promote optimism in the client and be a source of encouragement
   2. Intervene in the client's activities of daily living and promote as near normal functions as possible
   3. Allow the client to be alone and expect isolation on the part of the dying person
   4. Promote dignity and self-esteem in as many interventions as possible

9. Hospice nursing care has a different focus for client. The nurse is aware that client care provided through a hospice is:
   1. Designed to meet the client's individual wishes, as much as possible
   2. Usually aimed at offering curative treatment for the client
   3. Involved in teaching families to provide postmortem care
   4. Offered primarily for hospitalized clients

10. The nurse is preparing to assist the client in the end stage of her life. To provide comfort for the client in response to anticipated symptom development, the nurse plans to:
    1. Decrease the client's fluid intake
    2. Limit the use of analgesics
    3. Provide larger meals with more seasoning
    4. Determine valued activities and schedule rest periods

11. The nurse is working with a client on an inpatient hospice unit. To maintain the client's sense of self-worth during the end of life, the nurse should:
    1. Leave the client alone to deal with final affairs
    2. Call on the client's spiritual advisor to take over care
    3. Plan regular visits throughout the day
    4. Have a grief counselor visit

12. A nursing intervention to assist the client with a nursing diagnosis of *Sleep pattern disturbance related to the loss of spouse and fear of nightmares* should be to:
    1. Administer sleeping medication per order
    2. Refer the client to a psychologist or psychotherapist
    3. Have the client complete a detailed sleep-pattern assessment
    4. Sit with the client and encourage verbalization of feelings

13. To promote comfort for the terminally ill client specific to nausea and vomiting, the nurse should:
    1. Provide prompt mouth care
    2. Offer high-protein foods
    3. Increase the fluid intake
    4. Offer a high-residue diet

14. A nurse-initiated or independent activity for promotion of respiratory function in a terminally ill client is to:
    1. Limit fluids
    2. Position the client upright
    3. Reduce narcotic analgesic use
    4. Administer bronchodilators

15. The nurse is using Bowlby's phases of mourning as a framework for assessing the client's response to the traumatic loss of her leg. During the "yearning and searching" phase, the nurse anticipates that the client may respond by:
    1. Crying off and on
    2. Becoming angry at the nurse
    3. Acting stunned by the loss
    4. Discussing the change in role that will occur

Chapter 30   Stress and Coping

1. A recommended intervention for a lifestyle stress indicator and reduction in the incidence of heart disease is:
    1. Regular physical exercise
    2. Attendance at a support group
    3. Self-awareness skill development
    4. Time management

2. The nurse is involved in crisis intervention with a family in which the father has just lost his job and is experiencing periods of depression. The mother has a chronic debilitating illness that has put added responsibilities on the adolescent child, who is having behavioral problems. The nurse intervenes specifically to focus the family on their feelings by:
    1. Pointing out the connection between the situation and their responses
    2. Encouraging the use of the family's usual coping skills
    3. Working on time-management skills
    4. Discussing past experiences

3. A child and his mother have gone to the playroom on the pediatric unit. His mother tells him he cannot have a toy another child is playing with. The child cries, throws a block, and runs over to kick the door. This child is using a mechanism known as:
    1. Displacement
    2. Compensation
    3. Conversion
    4. Denial

4. Clients undergoing stress may undergo periods of regression. The nurse assesses this regressive behavior in the situation in which:
    1. An adult client exercises to the point of fatigue
    2. An 8-year-old child sucks his thumb and wets the bed
    3. An adult client avoids speaking about health concerns
    4. An 11-year-old child experiences stomach cramps and headaches

5. During the end-of-shift report, the nurse notes that a client had been very nervous and preoccupied during the evening and that no family visited. To determine the amount of anxiety that the client is experiencing, the nurse should respond:
   1. "Would you like for me to call a family member to come support you?"
   2. "Would you like to go down the hall and talk with another client who had the same surgery?"
   3. "How serious do you think your illness is?"
   4. "You seem worried about something. Would it help to talk about it?"

6. A 23-year-old who recently had a head injury from a motor vehicle accident (MVA) is in a state of unconsciousness. Which of the following physiological adaptations is primarily responsible for his level of consciousness?
   1. Medulla oblongata
   2. Reticular formation
   3. Pituitary gland
   4. External stress response

7. Nurses in the medical center are working with clients experiencing post-traumatic stress disorder (PTSD) after the World Trade Center bombing. An approach that is appropriate and should be incorporated into the plan of care is:
   1. Suppression of anxiety-producing memories
   2. Reinforcement that the PTSD is short term
   3. Promotion of relaxation strategies
   4. Focus on physical needs

8. The nurse is working with clients in an outpatient health care setting. One of the clients is experiencing job-related stress. The nurse believes this client is dissociated as a result of observing the client:
   1. Avoiding discussion of job problems
   2. Acting like another colleague on the job
   3. Experiencing chronic headaches and stomachaches
   4. Sitting quietly and not interacting with any of the staff

9. A 72-year-old client is in a long-term care facility after having had a cerebrovascular accident. The client is noncommunicative, enteral feedings are not being absorbed, and respirations are becoming labored. Which of the stages of the GAS is the client experiencing?
   1. Resistance stage
   2. Exhaustion stage
   3. Reflex pain response
   4. Alarm reaction

10. A client recently lost a child in a severe case of poisoning. The client tells the nurse, "I don't want to make any new friends right now." This is an example of which of the following indicators of stress?
    1. Emotional indicator
    2. Spiritual indicator
    3. Sociocultural indicator
    4. Intellectual indicator

11. A corporate executive works 60 to 80 hours per week and is experiencing some physical signs of stress. The practitioner teaches the client to "include 15 minutes of biofeedback." This is an example of which of the following health promotion interventions?
    1. Guided imagery
    2. Relaxation technique
    3. Time management
    4. Regular exercise

12. The client is assessed by the nurse as experiencing a crisis. The nurse plans to:
    1. Allow the client to work through independent problem solving
    2. Complete an in-depth evaluation of stressors and responses to the situation
    3. Focus on immediate stress reduction
    4. Recommend ongoing therapy

13. While working with clients who are experiencing a significant degree of stress, the nurse is aware that a priority assessment area is:
    1. The client's primary physical needs
    2. What else is happening in the client's life
    3. How the stress has influenced the client's activities of daily living
    4. Whether the client is thinking about harming himself or others

14. The nurse recognizes that the response to stress for older adults may be manifested differently from that in younger adults. For the older adult client, the nurse is aware that:
   1. Losses are more stress provoking
   2. Anxiety disorders are most prevalent
   3. Psychosocial factors are the greatest threats
   4. Timing of stress-inducing events is not significant

$\mathcal{U}$NIT 6   SCIENTIFIC BASIS FOR NURSING PRACTICE

$\mathcal{C}$hapter 31   Vital Signs

1. Pneumonia has developed in a client, and his temperature has increased to 37.7° C. The client is shivering and "feels uncomfortable." The nurse should:
   1. Apply a hypothermia mattress
   2. Apply hot packs to the axilla and groin
   3. Wrap the client's extremities
   4. Restrict fluids

2. The client comes to the emergency department after having been in the sun for an extended period. The nurse also determines that the client is taking a diuretic. Heat stroke is suspected, and the nurse observes for:
   1. Diaphoresis
   2. Confusion
   3. Temperature of 36° C
   4. Decreased heart rate

3. A construction worker is seen in the emergency department with low blood pressure, normal pulse, diaphoresis, and weakness. These are clinical signs of:
   1. Heat exhaustion
   2. Heat stroke
   3. Heat cramp
   4. Hypothermia

4. The nurse is ready to take vital signs on a 6-year-old child. The child has just enjoyed a grape popsicle. An appropriate action would be to:
   1. Take the rectal temperature
   2. Take the oral temperature as planned
   3. Have the child rinse out the mouth with warm water
   4. Wait 20 minutes and take the oral temperature

5. The client is seen in the emergency department for heat exhaustion as a result of exposure. The nurse anticipates that treatment will include:
   1. Replacement of fluid and electrolytes
   2. Antibiotic therapy
   3. Hypothermia wraps
   4. Alcohol baths

6. The nurse is aware that the appropriate site for taking a pulse on 2-year-old is:
   1. Radial
   2. Apical
   3. Femoral
   4. Pedal

7. The client appears to be breathing faster than before. The nurse should:
   1. Ask the client if there have been any stressful visitors
   2. Have the client lie down
   3. Count the rate of respirations
   4. Take the radial pulse

8. A client complains of pain and asks the nurse for pain medication. The nurse first assesses vital signs and finds them to be as follows: Blood pressure, 134/92; pulse, 90; and respirations, 26. The nurse's most appropriate action is to:
   1. Give the medication
   2. Ask if the client is anxious
   3. Check the client's dressing for bleeding
   4. Recheck the client's vital signs in 30 minutes

9. The client has bilateral casts on the upper extremities, so the nurse will be measuring the blood pressure in the leg. The nurse expects the diastolic pressure to be:
   1. 10 to 40 mm Hg higher than in the brachial artery
   2. 20 to 30 mm Hg lower than in the brachial artery
   3. 50 mm Hg higher than in the brachial artery
   4. Essentially the same as that in the brachial artery

10. An 84-year-old diabetic client is admitted for insulin regulation. Which of the following blood pressure, pulse, and respiration measurements, respectively, is considered to be within the expected limits for a client of this age?
    1. BP, 138/88; P, 68; R, 16
    2. BP, 94/52; P, 68; R, 30
    3. BP, 108/80; P, 112; R, 15
    4. BP, 132/74; P, 90; R, 24

11. The student nurse is assessing the vital signs of a 10-year-old client. The expected values for a client of this age are:
    1. P, 140; R, 50; BP, 80/50
    2. P, 100; R, 40; BP, 90/60
    3. P, 80; R, 22; BP, 110/70
    4. P, 60; R, 12; BP, 160/90

12. The nurse has just taken vital signs for the 30-year-old client. Based on the results, the nurse will report the following finding that is out of the expected range for a client of this age:
    1. T, 37.4° C
    2. P, 110
    3. R, 20
    4. BP, 120/76

13. In teaching a client at home to assess accurately the axillary temperature of a 11/2-year-old child with a glass thermometer, the nurse should tell the parent to:
    1. Hold the thermometer at the bulb end
    2. Clean the thermometer in hot water
    3. Leave the thermometer in place for 3 to 5 minutes
    4. Let the child hold the thermometer

14. The postoperative vital signs of an average-size adult client are BP, 110/68; P, 54; R, 8. The client appears pale, disoriented, and has minimal urinary output. The nurse should:
    1. Re-take the vital signs in 30 minutes
    2. Continue with care as planned
    3. Administer a stimulant
    4. Notify the physician

15. A client has just gotten out of bed to go to the bathroom. As the nurse enters the room, the client says, "I feel dizzy." The nurse should:
    1. Go for help
    2. Take the client's blood pressure
    3. Assist the client to sit down
    4. Tell the client to take deep breaths

16. The nurse explains to the nurse assistant that a false high blood pressure reading may be assessed if the assistant:
    1. Wraps the cuff too loosely around the arm
    2. Deflates the cuff too quickly
    3. Repeats the BP assessment too soon
    4. Presses the stethoscope too firmly in the antecubital fossa

17. The client is febrile, and the temperature must be reduced. The nurse anticipates that treatment will include:
    1. An alcohol and water bath
    2. Ice packs to the axillae and groin
    3. Cool, plain water sponges
    4. A cooling blanket

18. The nurse is alert to which of the following factors that lowers the blood pressure?
    1. Anxiety
    2. Heavy alcohol consumption
    3. Cigarette smoking
    4. Diuretic administration

19. While the nurse is taking the client's blood pressure, the client asks if the reading is high. In accordance with the newest guidelines, the nurse informs the client that a blood pressure measurement that is consistent with hypertension is:
    1. 120/70
    2. 130/84
    3. 120/78
    4. 118/80

20. The nurse obtains the following results after measuring the client's vital signs: Blood pressure, 180/100; pulse, 82; R, 16; and rectal temp, 37.5° C. The nurse should:
    1. Re-take the blood pressure
    2. Re-take the temperature
    3. Report all of the findings immediately
    4. Record the findings as within normal limits

21. The client is identified by the nurse as having a remittent fever. The student asks what that means, and the nurse explains that a remittent fever is:
    1. A constant body temperature above 100.4° F with little fluctuation
    2. Spikes in temperature that are interspersed with normal temperatures at least once within 24 hours
    3. Spikes and falls in temperature, but not back down to normal
    4. Periods of febrile episodes interspersed with normal temperatures

22. The nurse is working in the newborn nursery. In planning for temperature measurement, the nurse will obtain the reading on the infants by using the:
    1. Rectal site
    2. Oral site
    3. Tympanic site
    4. Axillary site

23. A mercury-in-glass thermometer is being used to measure a client's temperature in the extended care facility. While taking the client's temperature, the thermometer falls and breaks on the floor without coming in contact with the nurse or client. The nurse's first action is to:
    1. Remove the client from the area
    2. Remove the client's clothing
    3. Wash his or her hands and bathe the client
    4. Notify the environmental services department

24. The nurse enters the room of a client who is being monitored with pulse oximetry. Oon review of the following factors, the nurse suspects that the values will be influenced by the:
    1. Placement of the sensor on the extremity
    2. Client's diagnosis of peripheral vascular disease
    3. Reduced amount of light in the room
    4. Increased temperature of the room

25. An individual contacts the emergency room of the local hospital to ask what to do for a skiing partner who appears to be suffering from hypothermia. The victim is alert and able to respond to questions. The nurse instructs the individual who has called to have the victim:
    1. Take sips of brandy
    2. Drink warm soup
    3. Drink a cup of very hot coffee
    4. Run the affected extremities under hot water

26. The visiting nurse is evaluating the measurement of the client's blood pressure by his spouse. The nurse determines that additional teaching is required if the spouse is observed:
    1. Deflating the cuff at 2 mm Hg per second
    2. Having the client sit down for the measurement
    3. Using the same time each day for the measurement
    4. Taking the blood pressure after the client comes back from a walk

27. The client has bilateral casts on the upper extremities, so the nurse will be measuring the blood pressure in the leg. The nurse palpates the pulse before the measurement at the:
1. Popliteal fossa behind the knee
2. Inner side of the ankle below the medial malleolus
3. Top of the foot between the extension tendons of the great toe
4. Inguinal ligament midway between the symphysis pubis and the anterior superior iliac spine

28. The student is preparing to take the client's apical pulse. The nurse instructs the student to place the stethoscope along the left clavicular line at the:
1. Second to third intercostal space
2. Third to fourth intercostal space
3. Fourth to fifth intercostal space
4. Fifth to sixth intercostal space

29. The nurse enters the room to measure the client's pulse rate. The nurse recognizes that the client's rate may be increased as a result of:
1. A febrile condition
2. Administration of digoxin
3. The client's athletic conditioning
4. Unrelieved severe postoperative pain

30. On entering the room, the nurse notes that the client has an irregular respiratory rate, with periods of apnea and increases in respiration, followed by a reversal of the pattern. The nurse reports this respiratory assessment as:
1. Biot's respirations
2. Kussmaul's respirations
3. Hyperpneic respirations
4. Cheyne-Stokes respirations

Chapter 32   Health Assessment and Physical Examination

1. The position that maximizes the nurse's ability to assess the client's body for symmetry is:
1. Sitting
2. Supine
3. Prone
4. Dorsal recumbent

2. The nurse is examining a client with dark skin. In assessing for pallor, the nurse will specifically look at the:
1. Buccal mucosa of the mouth
2. Dorsal surface of the hands
3. Ear lobe
4. Sclera

3. A female client is seen in the outpatient clinic for numerous cuts, bruises, and apparent burns. In a discussion with the client, the nurse finds that the injuries are inconsistent with the stated cause. The client also states that she is having trouble sleeping, and she appears anxious. Based on these findings, the nurse suspects that the client may be experiencing:
1. Substance abuse
2. Domestic violence
3. Vascular disease
4. Mental illness

4. A client in the clinic has been having severe headaches and some visual disturbances. The nurse performs an eye examination. Which of the following is true concerning the procedure for this assessment?
1. To evaluate the lower eyelids, the nurse uses a syringe with sterile water.
2. The client's lacrimal apparatus is best assessed by using a dull object to stimulate her normal reflex conditions.
3. Accommodation is tested by asking the client to comply with the nurse's requests.
4. The red reflex should be assessed with the ophthalmoscope.

5. In preparing to conduct a physical examination on a client, the nurse plans to:
   1. Perform painful procedures at the end of the examination
   2. Take long, detailed notes of all the findings during the examination
   3. Keep the TV or radio on to distract the client throughout the examination
   4. Assess only the dominant side of the body in the examination

6. The client has an enlarged thyroid gland and is currently admitted to a medical nursing unit. Which of the following is accurate regarding the procedure for a thyroid assessment for this client?
   1. Deep palpation should be used anterior and posterior
   2. Swallowing sips of water causes the isthmus of the thyroid gland to rise
   3. The posterior approach is used with the fingers placed over the trachea
   4. The diaphragm of the stethoscope is best for auscultation of bruits

7. The nurse is auscultating the client's lungs and notes normal vesicular sounds as:
   1. Medium-pitched blowing sounds with inspiration equaling expiration
   2. Loud, high-pitched, hollow sounds with expiration longer than inspiration
   3. Soft, breezy, low-pitched sounds with longer inspiration
   4. Sounds created by air moving through small airways

8. The nurse could best auscultate the point of maximum impulse (PMI) in an 8-year-old at the:
   1. Fourth intercostal space, left of the midclavicular line
   2. Fifth intercostal space, left of the midclavicular line
   3. Second intercostal space, right of the midclavicular line
   4. Third intercostal space, right of the midclavicular line

9. The nurse suspects that the client may have vascular disease. During the examination, the nurse is alert to the client's complaint of:
   1. Headache, dizziness, and tingling of body parts
   2. Diplopia, floaters, and headaches
   3. Leg cramps, numbness of extremities, and edema
   4. Pain and cramping in the lower extremities relieved by walking

10. A 21-year-old woman asks when she should perform a breast self-examination during the month. The nurse should inform the client:
    1. "Any time you think of it."
    2. "At the same time each month."
    3. "On the first day of your menstrual period."
    4. "Two to three days after your menstrual period."

11. During an assessment of the client's integument, the nurse notes a flat, nonpalpable change in skin color that is smaller than 1 cm. This finding is documented by the nurse as a:
    1. Macule
    2. Papule
    3. Vesicle
    4. Nodule

12. The nurse asks a client to explain the meaning of the phrase, "Every cloud has a silver lining." This part of the examination is designed to measure:
    1. Knowledge
    2. Judgment
    3. Association
    4. Abstract thinking

13. Measurement of the client's ability to differentiate between sharp and dull sensations over the forehead tests which cranial nerve?
    1. Optic
    2. Facial
    3. Trigeminal
    4. Oculomotor

14. Assessment of the client's skin reveals a fluid-filled circumscribed elevation of 0.4 cm. The nurse identifies this as a:
    1. Nodule
    2. Macule
    3. Vesicle
    4. Wheal

15. The expected appearance of the oral mucosa in a light-skinned adult is:
    1. Pinkish-red, smooth, and moist
    2. Light pink, rough, and dry
    3. Cyanotic, with rough nodules
    4. Deep red, with rough edges

16. In the assessment of a 90-year-old client, the nurse documents an exaggeration of the posterior curvature of the thoracic spine as:
    1. Lordosis
    2. Osteoporosis
    3. Scoliosis
    4. Kyphosis

17. If a low-pitched murmur is suspected with prior assessment, the best position for the client to auscultate the apical site is:
    1. Sitting up
    2. Standing
    3. Lying on the left side
    4. Dorsal recumbent

18. As part of the examination, the nurse will be assessing the client's balance. The test that should be administered is the:
    1. Weber test
    2. Allen test
    3. Romberg test
    4. Rinne test

19. Part of the neurological examination is evaluating the response of the cranial nerves. To test cranial nerve VIII, the nurse should:
    1. Ask the client to read printed material
    2. Assess the directions of the gaze
    3. Assess the client's ability to hear the spoken word
    4. Ask the client to say "ah"

20. A student nurse is working with a client who has asthma. The primary nurse tells the student that wheezes can be heard on auscultation. The student expects to hear:
    1. Coarse crackles and bubbling
    2. High-pitched musical sounds
    3. Dry, grating noises
    4. Loud, low-pitched rumbling

21. The nurse instructs the male client that the protocol for testicular self-examination is to:
    1. Perform the examination annually after age 35 years
    2. Use both hands to roll the testicles and feel the consistency
    3. Perform the examination before bathing or showering
    4. Contact the physician if a cordlike structure is felt on the top and back of the testicle

22. The nurse uses olfaction in the client's assessment. If a sweet, fruity smell is noticed in the oral cavity, the nurse suspects:
    1. Diabetic acidosis
    2. Gum disease
    3. Stomatitis
    4. Malabsorption syndrome

23. A physical examination is to be performed by the nurse on a client that has cardiopulmonary disease. Knowing this about the client, the nurse is alert when checking the nails for the presence of:
    1. Clubbing
    2. Paronychia
    3. Beau's lines
    4. Splinter hemorrhages

24. During the physical examination, the client tells the nurse that he has been told he has myopia. The nurse expects to find that the client:
    1. Is near-sighted
    2. Has decreased peripheral vision
    3. Has diminished night vision
    4. Experiences more glare, flashes, and floaters

25. The school-age child is brought to the school nurse after experiencing a nosebleed during a softball game. The appropriate intervention is for the nurse to:
    1. Have the child lean backward
    2. Apply pressure to the anterior nose
    3. Apply a warm cloth to the area
    4. Have the child close his mouth and blow his nose

26. An older adult client is visiting the physician's office for a checkup. The client asks the nurse how often the influenza and pneumonia vaccines should be taken. The nurse responds to the client that these vaccinations should be done:
    1. Every 6 months
    2. Annually
    3. Every 5 years
    4. Every 7 years

27. A pregnant client is seen by the nurse in the antenatal clinic. On inspection, the nurse expects that this client's breasts will have:
    1. Softer tissue
    2. Flatter nipples
    3. Darkened areolae
    4. Diminished superficial veins

28. A client with vascular insufficiency is seen regularly in the medical clinic. The nurse notes that the client requires further instruction about her condition if the client:
    1. Walks regularly
    2. Wears knee-length stockings
    3. Elevates the feet when sitting
    4. Alternates periods of sitting and standing

29. During the physical examination, the nurse should assess the client's glands by using the:
    1. Dorsum of the hand
    2. Pads of the fingers
    3. Palmar surface of the hand
    4. Fingertip grasp of the tissue

30. The nurse is evaluating the client for conduction deafness in the right ear. In using Weber's test, the nurse appropriately places the tuning fork and confirms this type of deafness when:
    1. Sound is not heard in either ear
    2. Sound is heard best by the client in the left ear
    3. Sound is heard best by the client in the right ear
    4. Sound is reduced and heard longer through air conduction

31. An inspection of the lower extremities is being performed. The presence of arterial insufficiency is suspected when the nurse observes:
    1. Increased hair growth
    2. Cooler skin temperatures
    3. Marked edema
    4. Brown pigmentation

32. In the auscultation of the thorax, the nurse notes that the sounds heard over the trachea are expected to be:
    1. Soft, low-pitched, and breezy
    2. Loud, high-pitched, and hollow
    3. Moist, crackling, and bubbling
    4. High-pitched and musical

33. During the neurological component of the physical examination, the nurse tests the function of the client's cranial nerves. In testing cranial nerve III, the nurse determines the client's ability to:
    1. Smile and frown
    2. Read printed material
    3. Identify sweet and sour tastes
    4. React to light with changes in pupil size

Chapter 33 Infection Control

1. The client has a 6-inch laceration on his right forearm, and an infection develops. Which of the following is a sign of an acute inflammatory process?
   1. A blanching of the skin
   2. A decrease in temperature at the site
   3. A decrease in the number of white blood cells
   4. A release of histamine that adds to the pain response

2. A female client has been undergoing diagnostic testing since admission to the medical unit in the hospital. The results of blood testing are sent back to the unit. On reviewing the results, the nurse will report the following abnormal finding to the physician:
   1. Erythrocyte sedimentation rate (ESR), 35 mm/hr
   2. White blood cells (WBCs), 8000/mm^3
   3. Neutrophils, 65%
   4. Iron, 75 g/100 ml

3. The nurse is observing the new staff member work with the client. Of the following activities, which one has the greatest possibility of contributing to a nosocomial infection and requires correction?
   1. Washing hands before applying a dressing
   2. Taping a plastic bag to the bed rail for tissue disposal
   3. Placing a Foley catheter bag on the bed when transferring a client
   4. Using alcohol to cleanse the skin before starting an intravenous line

4. Droplet precautions will be instituted for the client admitted to the infectious disease unit with:
   1. Streptococcal pharyngitis
   2. Herpes simplex
   3. Pertussis
   4. Measles

5. The nurse works in a small rural hospital with a wide variety of clients. Of the clients admitted this afternoon, the nurse recognizes that the individual with the highest susceptibility to infection is the individual with:
   1. Burns
   2. Diabetes
   3. Pulmonary emphysema
   4. Peripheral vascular disease

6. The nurse shows an understanding of the psychological implications for a client on isolation when planning care to control the risk of:
   1. Denial
   2. Aggression
   3. Regression
   4. Isolation

7. The nurse uses surgical aseptic technique when:
   1. Inserting an intravenous catheter
   2. Placing soiled linen in moisture-resistant bags
   3. Disposing of syringes in puncture-proof containers
   4. Washing hands before changing a dressing

8. The client has a large, deep abdominal incision that requires a dressing. The incision is packed with sterile half-inch packing and covered with a dry 4 × 4-inch gauze. When changing the dressing, the nurse accidentally drops the packing onto the client's abdomen. The nurse should:
   1. Add alcohol to the packing and insert it into the incision
   2. Throw the packing away, and prepare a new one
   3. Pick up the packing with sterile forceps, and gently place it into the incision
   4. Rinse the packing with sterile water, and put the packing into the incision with sterile gloves

9. A client has a viral infection. Which of the following is typical of the illness stage of the course of her infection?
   1. No longer are any acute symptoms observed.
   2. An oral temperature reveals a febrile state.
   3. The client was first exposed to the infection 2 days ago but has no symptoms.
   4. The client "feels sick" but is able to continue her normal activities.

10. The nurse recognizes that special care must be taken in the handling of which of the following to prevent the transmission of hepatitis A?
    1. Blood
    2. Feces
    3. Saliva
    4. Vaginal secretions

11. The parent of a preschool child asks the nurse how chickenpox (varicella zoster) is transmitted. The nurse identifies that the virus is:
    1. Carried by a vector organism
    2. Carried though the air in droplets after sneezing or coughing
    3. Transmitted through person-to-person contact
    4. Acquired through contact with contaminated objects

12. While working with clients in the postoperative period, the nurse is very alert to the results of laboratory tests. Which one of the following results is indicative of an infectious process?
    1. Iron, 80 g/100 ml
    2. Neutrophils, 65%
    3. White blood cells (WBCs), 18,000/mm^3
    4. Erythrocyte sedimentation rate (ESR), 15 mm/hr

13. The nurse is aware that it is important to break the chain of infection. An example of a nursing intervention that is implemented to reduce a reservoir of infection for a client is:
    1. Covering the mouth and nose when sneezing
    2. Wearing disposable gloves
    3. Isolating client's articles
    4. Changing soiled dressings

14. The single most important technique to prevent and control the transmission of infections is:
    1. Hand hygiene
    2. The use of disposable gloves
    3. The use of isolation precautions
    4. Sterilization of equipment

15. A client with active tuberculosis is admitted to the medical center. The nurse recognizes that admission of this client to the unit will require the implementation by the staff of:
    1. Airborne precautions
    2. Droplet precautions
    3. Contact precautions
    4. Reverse isolation

16. The nurse recognizes the appropriate procedures for sterile asepsis. Of the following, which action is consistent with sterile asepsis?
    1. Clean forceps may be used to move items on the sterile field.
    2. Sterile fields may be prepared well in advance of the procedures.
    3. The first small amount of sterile solution should be poured and discarded.
    4. Wrapped sterile packages should be opened starting with the flap closest to the nurse.

17. The nurse suspects that an older adult client may be experiencing hypostatic pneumonia. Older adult clients may react differently to infectious processes, so the nurse is alert to atypical signs and symptoms, such as:
    1. Hypotension
    2. Confusion
    3. Erythema
    4. Chills

18. A nursing assistant is learning how to use protective equipment when caring for a client in isolation. The nursing assistant is instructed in the correct sequence for putting on the protective equipment which is to:
    1. Wash her hands, apply the mask and eyewear, put on the gown, and then apply gloves
    2. Apply the mask and eyewear, put on the gown, wash her hands, and then apply gloves
    3. Wash her hands, put on the gown, apply the mask and eyewear, then apply the gloves
    4. Put on the gown, apply the mask and eyewear, wash her hands, and then apply gloves

19. A client requires a sterile dressing change for a midabdominal surgical incision. An appropriate intervention for the nurse to implement in maintaining sterile asepsis is to:
    1. Put sterile gloves on before opening sterile packages
    2. Discard packages that may have been in contact with the area below waist level
    3. Place the cap of the sterile solution well within the sterile field
    4. Place sterile items on the very edge of the sterile drape

20. The nurse is preparing to assist with a sterile procedure in the surgical suite. An appropriate technique that the nurse includes in the surgical scrub is to:
    1. Keep the hands below the elbows throughout the scrub
    2. Use a brush on the palms and dorsal surface of the hands
    3. Maintain the scrub for at least 2 to 5 minutes
    4. Wash well around all jewelry

21. A client is found to have methicillin-resistant *Staphylococcus aureus* (MRSA). An appropriate isolation procedure for the nurse to implement when working with this client is to:
    1. Leave all linen in the client's room
    2. Place specimen containers in plastic bags for transport
    3. Wipe the stethoscope before removing it from the room
    4. Remove the mask and goggles first when leaving the client's room

22. A client is found to have a bacterial infection of *Escherichia coli*. The nurse, recognizing the effects of these bacteria, anticipates that the client will demonstrate:
    1. Diarrhea
    2. Coughing
    3. Cold sores around the mouth
    4. Discharge from the eyes

Chapter 34   Medication Administration

1. A client is nauseated, has been vomiting for several hours, and needs to receive an antiemetic (antinausea) medication. The nurse recognizes that which of the following is accurate?
    1. An enteric-coated medication should be given.
    2. Medication will not be absorbed as easily because of the nausea.
    3. A parenteral route is the route of choice.
    4. A rectal suppository must be administered.

2. The client receiving an intravenous infusion of morphine sulfate begins to experience respiratory depression and decreased urine output. This effect is described as:
    1. Therapeutic
    2. Toxic
    3. Idiosyncratic
    4. Allergic

3. The client is to receive a medication via the buccal route. The nurse plans to implement the following action:
   1. Place the medication inside the cheek
   2. Crush the medication before administration
   3. Offer the client a glass of orange juice after administration
   4. Use sterile technique to administer the medication

4. The physician orders a grain and a half of sodium quinalbarbitone (Seconal) to help a client sleep. The label on the medication bottle reads, Seconal, 100 mg. How many capsules should the nurse give the client?
   1. ½
   2. 1
   3. 1½
   4. 2

5. The physician has ordered 6 mg morphine sulfate every 3 to 4 hours prn for a client's postoperative pain. The unit dose in the medication dispenser has 15 mg in 1 ml. How much solution should the nurse give?
   1. ⅕ ml
   2. ⅓ ml
   3. ⅖ ml
   4. ¼ ml

6. To determine proper drug dosages for children, calculations are most precisely made on the basis of the child's:
   1. Weight
   2. Height
   3. Age
   4. Body surface area

7. The nurse is documenting administration of a medication that is given at 10:00 AM, 2:00 PM, and 6:00 PM. The medication that the nurse is documenting is:
   1. Morphine sulfate, 10 mg q4h prn
   2. Propranolol (Inderal), 10 mg po bid
   3. Diazepam, 5 mg po tid
   4. Cephalexin (Keflex), 500 mg po q8h

8. The nurse is working on the pediatric unit. In preparing to give medications to a preschool-age child, and appropriate interaction by the nurse is:
   1. "Do you want to take your medication now?"
   2. "Would you like the medication with water or juice?"
   3. "Let me explain about the injection that you will be getting."
   4. "If you don't take the medication now, you will not get better."

9. In preparing two different medications from two vials, the nurse must:
   1. Inject fluid from one vial into the other
   2. Uncap the syringe and wipe the needle with an alcohol preparation before inserting into either vial
   3. Discard the medication from vial number two if medication from vial number one is pushed into it
   4. Insert air into the first vial, but not the second vial

10. The nurse is teaching the client how to prepare 10 units of regular insulin and 5 units of NPH insulin for injection. The nurse instructs the client to:
    1. Inject air into the regular insulin, then into the NPH
    2. Withdraw the regular insulin first
    3. Inject air into and withdraw the NPH immediately
    4. Inject air into both vials and withdraw the regular insulin first

11. A client has a prescription for a medication that is administered via an inhaler. To determine whether the client requires a spacer for the inhaler, the nurse will determine the:
    1. Dosage of medication required
    2. Coordination of the client
    3. Schedule of administration
    4. Use of a dry powder inhaler (DPI)

12. The student nurse reads the order to give a 1-year-old client an intramuscular injection. The appropriate and preferred muscle to select for a child is the:
    1. Deltoid
    2. Dorsogluteal
    3. Ventrogluteal
    4. Vastus lateralis

13. The nurse administers the intramuscular medication of iron by the Z-track method. The medication was administered by this method to:
    1. Provide faster absorption of the medication
    2. Reduce discomfort from the needle
    3. Provide more even absorption of the drug
    4. Prevent the drug from irritating sensitive tissue

14. The client is ordered to have eyedrops administered daily to both eyes. Eyedrops should be instilled on the:
    1. Cornea
    2. Outer canthus
    3. Lower conjunctival sac
    4. Opening of the lacrimal duct

15. After the administration of ear drops to the left ear, the client should be positioned:
    1. Prone
    2. Upright
    3. Right lateral
    4. Dorsal recumbent with hyperextension of the neck

16. The order is for eye medication, ii gtts OD. The nurse administers:
    1. 2 ml to the right eye
    2. 2 drops to the left eye
    3. 2 drops to the right eye
    4. 2 drops to both eyes

17. The most effective way in the acute care environment to determine the client's identity before administering medications is to:
    1. Ask the client's name
    2. Check the name on the chart
    3. Ask the other caregivers
    4. Check the client's name band

18. An order is written for meperidine (Demerol), 500 mg IM q3-4h prn for pain. The nurse recognizes that this is significantly more than the usual therapeutic dose. The nurse should:
    1. Give 50 mg IM as it was probably intended to be written
    2. Refuse to give the medication, and notify the nurse manager
    3. Administer the medication, and watch the client carefully
    4. Call the prescriber to clarify the order

19. An order is written for 80 mg of a medication in elixir form. The medication is available in 80 mg/tsp strength. The nurse prepares to administer:
    1. 2 ml
    2. 5 ml
    3. 10 ml
    4. 15 ml

20. The client is to receive a Mantoux test for tuberculosis. This test is administered via an intradermal injection. The nurse recognizes that the angle of injection that is used for an intradermal injection is:
    1. 15 degrees
    2. 30 degrees
    3. 45 degrees
    4. 90 degrees

21. The nurse prepares to administer an intradermal injection for the administration of medication for:
    1. Pain
    2. Allergy sensitivity
    3. Anticoagulant therapy
    4. Low-dose insulin requirements

22. The nurse is evaluating the integrity of the ventrogluteal injection site. The nurse finds the site by locating the:
    1. Middle third of the lateral thigh
    2. Greater trochanter, anterior iliac spine, and iliac crest
    3. Anterior aspect of the upper thigh
    4. Acromion process and axilla

23. The client is to receive heparin by injection. The nurse prepares to inject this medication in the client's:
    1. Scapular region
    2. Vastus lateralis
    3. Posterior gluteal
    4. Abdomen

24. A medication is prescribed for the client and is to be administered by intravenous (IV) bolus injection. A priority for the nurse before the administration of medication via this route is to:
    1. Set the rate of the IV infusion
    2. Check the client's mental alertness
    3. Confirm placement of the IV line
    4. Determine the amount of IV fluid to be administered

25. A client on the medical unit receives regular insulin at 7:00 AM. The nurse is alert to a possible hypoglycemic reaction by:
    1. 7:30 AM
    2. 10:00 AM
    3. 4:00 PM
    4. 8:00 PM

26. A priority for the nurse in the administration of oral medications and prevention of aspiration is:
    1. Checking for a gag reflex
    2. Allowing the client to self-administer
    3. Assessing the ability to cough
    4. Using straws and extra water for administration

27. The nurse is to administer several medications to the client via the nasogastric (NG) tube. The nurse's first action is to:
    1. Add the medication to the tube feeding being given
    2. Crush all tablets and capsules before administration
    3. Administer all of the medications mixed together
    4. Check for placement of the NG tube

28. The nurse is administering an injection at the ventrogluteal site. On aspiration, the nurse notices blood in the syringe. The nurse should:
    1. Inject the medication
    2. Pull the needle back slightly, and inject the medication
    3. Move the skin to the side, and inject the medication slowly
    4. Discontinue the injection, and prepare the medication again

29. A 3-year-old child is to receive an iron preparation orally. The nurse should:
    1. Give the child a straw
    2. Administer the medication by injection
    3. Mix the medication in water
    4. Ask the pharmacy to send up a pill for the child to swallow

30. The client has an order for 30 U of U-500 insulin. The nurse is using a U-100 syringe and will draw up and administer:
    1. 5 U
    2. 6 U
    3. 10 U
    4. 30 U

Chapter 35
Complementary and Alternative Therapies

1. In selecting alternative therapies, the nurse recognizes that therapeutic touch may be most effective with a:
    1. Premature infant
    2. Headache sufferer
    3. Pregnant woman
    4. Psychiatric client

2. The nurse is preparing a presentation on alternative therapies for a community group. The nurse should identify that herbal therapies are:
   1. Approved by the Food and Drug Administration, under the Food, Drug, and Cosmetic Act
   2. Sold as medicines in most stores because they lack major side effects
   3. Allowed to be packaged as dietary supplements if they are without health claims
   4. Consistent in their standards for concentrations of major ingredients and additives

3. The client asks the nurse about different herbal therapies that may promote physical endurance and reduce stress. Based on the client's request, the nurse provides information on:
   1. Ginseng
   2. Ginger
   3. Echinacea
   4. Chamomile

4. The nurse recognizes that which one of the following statements is correct concerning complementary and alternative medicine?
   1. One third to half of the U.S. population uses one or more forms of alternative therapy.
   2. Insurance coverage is available at the same amount as for traditional medicine.
   3. Use of alternative therapies is still not incorporated into medical journals.
   4. Use of alternative therapies is primarily by those who are less educated or in a lower socioeconomic group.

5. The nurse is aware of the positive responses that may be obtained with the use of alternative therapies. A benefit that the client can gain from relaxation therapy is a decrease in:
   1. Receptivity
   2. Peripheral skin temperature
   3. Oxygen consumption
   4. Alpha brain activity

6. In selecting an appropriate alternative therapy, the nurse knows that the client who may benefit the most from the passive type of relaxation is one who is experiencing:
   1. Hypertension
   2. Terminal cancer
   3. Work-related stress
   4. Dysfunctional grieving

7. In selecting an appropriate alternative therapy, the nurse knows that the client who has Raynaud's disease with intermittent peripheral ischemia may benefit the most from:
   1. Relaxation therapy
   2. Imagery
   3. Biofeedback
   4. Acupuncture

8. A nurse must be alert to possible negative responses to biobehavioral therapies. Clients who have reacted negatively have most often experienced:
   1. Aggressive behaviors
   2. Delusions
   3. Insomnia
   4. Loss-of-control sensations

9. A practitioner or client who uses traditional Chinese medicine bases the therapy on the primary concept of:
   1. Yin/yang
   2. Meridians
   3. Six evil senses
   4. Acupoints

10. The nurse is preparing to assist the client with meditation and breathing. In preparing to implement this therapy, the first step is to:
    1. Position the client
    2. Provide a warm environment
    3. Have the client close his or her eyes
    4. Note areas of tension or pain

11. During the admission history, the client informs the nurse that she follows a macrobiotic diet. The nurse knows that the client's diet includes:
    1. Increased meats and other proteins
    2. A protein/carbohydrate/fat ratio of 30%:40%:30%
    3. Increased intake of vitamin C and beta-carotene
    4. Whole grains, vegetables, and fish

12. The client has a history of gastrointestinal problems and has used herbal remedies in the past. The nurse expects that this client will be taking:
    1. Chamomile
    2. St. John's wort
    3. Echinacea
    4. Gingko biloba

13. A client at the clinic informs the nurse during an examination that he has been taking chaparral as an anticancer agent. The client asks if there is any reason why this remedy should not be taken. The nurse responds accurately when telling the client that chaparral:
    1. Should not be taken with coffee or other caffeinated beverages
    2. May induce veno-occlusive disease
    3. Contains a carcinogenic substance
    4. Is associated with liver toxicity

UNIT 7   BASIC HUMAN NEEDS

Chapter 36   Activity and Exercise

1. A client has been on bed rest for a prolonged period. Specifically to promote the use of resistive isometric exercise for the client, the nurse will initiate:
   1. Quadriceps setting
   2. Gluteal muscle contraction
   3. Moving the arms and legs in circles
   4. Pushing against a footboard

2. The nurse is assessing the body alignment of an alert and mobile client. The first action that the nurse should take is to:
   1. Observe gait
   2. Put the client at ease
   3. Determine activity tolerance
   4. Determine range of joint motion

3. An average size male client has right-sided hemiparesis. The nurse helps this client to walk by:
   1. Standing at his left side and holding his arm
   2. Standing at his left side and holding one arm around his waist
   3. Standing at his right side and holding his arm
   4. Standing at his right side and holding one arm around his waist

4. The nurse is working with a client who has left-sided weakness. After instruction, the nurse observes the client ambulate to evaluate the use of the cane. Which action indicates that the client knows how to use the cane properly?
   1. The client keeps the cane on the left side
   2. Two points of support are kept on the floor at all times.
   3. A slight lean to the right occurs when the client is walking.
   4. After advancing the cane, the client moves the right leg forward.

5. A client with a fractured left femur has been using crutches for the past 4 weeks. The physician tells the client to begin putting a little weight on the left foot when walking. Which of the following gaits should the client be taught to use?
   1. Two-point
   2. Three-point
   3. Four-point
   4. Swing-through

6. The client needs to use crutches at home and will have to manage going up and down a short flight of stairs. The nurse evaluates the use of an appropriate technique if the client:
   1. Uses a banister or wall for support when descending
   2. Uses one crutch for support while going up and down
   3. Advances the crutches first to ascend the stairs
   4. Advances the affected leg after moving the crutches to descend the stairs

7. While ambulating in the hallway of a hospital, the client complains of extreme dizziness. The nurse, alert to a syncopal episode, should first:
   1. Support the client and walk quickly back to the room
   2. Lean the client against the wall until the episode passes
   3. Lower the client gently to the floor
   4. Go for help

8. Nurses must implement appropriate body mechanics to prevent injury to themselves and clients. Which principle of body mechanics should the nurse incorporate into client care?
   1. Flex the knees, and keep the feet wide apart
   2. Assume a position far enough away from the client
   3. Twist the body in the direction of movement
   4. Use the strong back muscles for lifting or moving

9. The nurse is presenting a teaching session on exercise for a group of corporate executives. An appropriate recommendation is that:
   1. Continuous activity is required for the exercise to be worthwhile.
   2. 3000 to 4000 calories may be easily expended each week.
   3. Lower-intensity activities need to be done more often for value.
   4. Only formal exercise activities are counted in a regular plan.

10. After an assessment of the client, the nurse identifies the nursing diagnosis: *Activity intolerance related to increased weight gain and inactivity.* An outcome identified by the nurse should be:
    1. Resting heart rate will be 90 to 100 beats per minute.
    2. Blood pressure will be maintained between 140/80 and 160/90.
    3. Exercise will be performed 3 to 4 times over the next 2-week period.
    4. Achievement of a rating of 3 for activity endurance

Chapter 37 Client Safety

1. The nurse has investigated safety hazards and recognizes that which one of the following statements is accurate regarding safety needs?
   1. Bacterial contamination of foods is uncontrollable.
   2. Fire is the greatest cause of unintentional death.
   3. Carbon dioxide levels should be monitored in home settings.
   4. Temperature extremes seldom affect the safety of clients in acute care facilities.

2. An ambulatory client is admitted to the extended care facility with a diagnosis of Alzheimer's disease. In using a Fall Assessment tool, the nurse knows that the greatest indicator of risk is:
   1. Confusion
   2. Impaired judgment
   3. Sensory deficits
   4. History of falls

3. An inservice program is being offered in the hospital on bioterrorism and the response of the health care agency. During the program, the mitigation phase is described. The nurse is informed that this phase includes:
   1. Determination of hazard vulnerability and the impact of the emergency situation
   2. Steps taken to manage the effects of the event and an inventory of available resources
   3. Steps taken by staff to perform triage for victims
   4. Restoration of essential services

4. An inservice program is being offered in the hospital on bioterrorism and the response of the health care agency. An important aspect of the program is the recognition of the signs and symptoms of bacterial and viral infections. A practice drill is held, and the nurse recognizes that the clients admitted with possible anthrax will demonstrate:
   1. Abdominal cramping, diarrhea, drooping eyelids, jaw clench, and difficulty swallowing
   2. Flu-like symptoms, gastrointestinal distress, and papular lesions
   3. Fever, cough, chest pain, and hemoptysis
   4. Vesicular skin lesions on the face and extremities

5. A 1-year-old child is scheduled to receive an intravenous (IV) line. The most appropriate type of restraint to use for this client to prevent removal of the IV line would be a(n):
   1. Wrist restraint
   2. Jacket restraint
   3. Elbow restraint
   4. Mummy restraint

6. A 79-year-old resident in a long-term care facility is known to "wander at night" and has fallen in the past. Which of the following is the most appropriate nursing intervention?
   1. An abdominal restraint should be placed on the client during sleeping hours.
   2. The client should be checked frequently during the night.
   3. A radio should be left playing at the bedside to assist in reality orientation.
   4. The client should be placed in a room away from the activity of the nursing station.

7. The workmen cause an electrical fire when installing a new piece of equipment in the intensive care unit. A client is on a ventilator in the next room. The first action the nurse should take is to:
   1. Pull the fire alarm
   2. Attempt to extinguish the fire
   3. Call the physician to obtain orders to take the client off the ventilator
   4. Use an Ambu bag and remove the client from the area

8. In a nursing home, an elderly client drops his burning cigarette in a trash can and starts a fire. The most appropriate type of fire extinguisher for the nurse to use is the:
   1. Type A
   2. Type B
   3. Type C
   4. Type D

9. A visiting nurse completes an assessment of the ambulatory client in the home and determines the nursing diagnosis of *Risk for injury related to decreased vision*. Based on this assessment, the client will benefit the most from:
   1. Installing fluorescent lighting throughout the house
   2. Becoming oriented to the position of the furniture and stairways
   3. Maintaining complete bed rest in a hospital bed with side rails
   4. Applying physical restraints

0. Which one of the following statements by the parent of a child indicates that further teaching by the nurse is required?
    1. "Now that my child is 2 years old, I can let her sit in the front seat of the car with me."
    2. "I make sure that my child wears a helmet when he rides his bicycle."
    3. "I have spoken to my child about safe sex practices."
    4. "My child is taking swimming classes at the community center."

1. The nurse assesses that the client may need a restraint and recognizes that:
    1. An order for a restraint may be implemented indefinitely until it is no longer required by the client.
    2. Restraints may be ordered on an as-needed basis.
    3. No order or consent is necessary for restraints in long-term care facilities.
    4. Restraints are to be periodically removed to have the client re-evaluated.

2. On entering the client's room, the nurse sees a fire burning in the trash can next to the bed. The nurse removes the client and calls in the fire. The next action of the nurse is to:
    1. Extinguish the fire
    2. Remove all of the other clients from the unit
    3. Close all the doors of client rooms
    4. Move the trash can into the bathroom

13. A mother of a young child enters the kitchen and finds the child on the floor. A bottle of cleanser is next to the child, and particles of the substance are around the child's mouth. The parent's first action should be to:
    1. Call the Poison Control unit
    2. Provide ipecac syrup
    3. Check the child's airway and breathing
    4. Remove the particles of cleanser from the mouth

Chapter 38   Hygiene

1. The client has a red, raised skin rash. During the bath, the priority action of the nurse is to:
    1. Assess for further inflammatory reactions
    2. Discuss the body-image problems created by the presence of the rash
    3. Wash the skin thoroughly with hot water and soap
    4. Moisturize the skin to prevent drying

2. The nurse is caring for a client who has right-sided paralysis after a CVA (stroke). Which of the following factors would be most likely to result in pressure ulcer formation for this client?
    1. Poor nutrition
    2. Immobility
    3. Reduced hydration
    4. Skin secretions

3. The nurse delegates the hygienic care of a male client to the nursing assistant. In reviewing the client assignment, the nurse instructs the assistant to make sure to use an electric razor to shave the client with:
    1. Thrombocytopenia
    2. Congestive heart failure
    3. Osteoarthritis
    4. Pneumonia

4. The nurse delegates morning care to a new certified nursing assistant. Which of the following actions by the assistant would be evaluated as appropriate?
    1. Placing dentures in a tissue while not worn
    2. Cutting the clients' nails with scissors
    3. Using soap to cleanse the eye orbits
    4. Washing the client's legs with long strokes from the ankle to the knee

5. A 61-year-old with diabetes mellitus has physician's orders for meticulous foot care. Which of the following is the best rationale for the order?
   1. The aging process causes increased skin breakdown.
   2. Increased neuropathy occurs with this pathology and places the client at risk.
   3. The client probably has a history of poor hygienic care.
   4. The lower extremities are difficult to see and therefore hard to maintain with good hygiene.

6. The nurse is instructing the client with peripheral vascular disease about daily foot care. The nurse's instruction for the client includes:
   1. Soaking the feet 5 to 10 minutes each day
   2. Filing the nails into a curve shape
   3. Using commercial corn removers if needed
   4. Applying lamb's wool between the toes

7. To administer oral care to a semicomatose client, the nurse should place the client in which of the following positions?
   1. Reverse Trendelenberg
   2. High Fowler's with the head to the side
   3. Side-lying with the head turned toward the nurse
   4. Supine with the neck slightly forward

8. The client is unable to perform self-care for the hair. The nurse is aware that which of the following is accurate when performing hair care?
   1. Brushing the hair distributes the natural oils evenly.
   2. Using a hot comb may be very helpful for straight and oily hair.
   3. Very tight braids keep the hair in good condition.
   4. Shampooing should be done daily.

9. A client has recently experienced difficult hearing out of both ears. Which of the following is the best nursing response to the client?
   1. "Let's irrigate your ears with cool water."
   2. "Can you turn your head toward me when I am talking to you?"
   3. "Your hearing aid should not need a new battery for at least 3 months."
   4. "Try to avoid putting a Q-Tip (cotton tipped applicator) into your ears."

10. An adolescent client with acne should be taught by the nurse to:
    1. Apply moisturizing lotions or creams
    2. Wash the face and hair daily with very warm water and soap
    3. Use a depilatory to remove excess hair
    4. Add moisture to the air with the use of a humidifier

11. A client has severe right-sided weakness and is unable to complete bathing and grooming independently. Based on this observation, the nurse identifies a nursing diagnosis of:
    1. Powerlessness
    2. Self-care deficit
    3. Tissue integrity impairment
    4. Knowledge deficit of hygiene practices

12. A different approach to traditional hygienic care is the "bag bath." The best rationale for using this approach is that it:
    1. Is less expensive than the traditional method
    2. Takes less time to complete
    3. Leaves the skin softer
    4. Reduces the risk of infection

13. The nurse is preparing to assist the adult female client with perineal care. The position of choice for this client is:
    1. Dorsal recumbent
    2. Side-lying
    3. Supine
    4. Prone

14. A client who is suspected of having vascular insufficiency to the lower extremities is assessed by the nurse to have a(n):
    1. Increased hair growth on the legs and feet
    2. Dull appearance of the skin
    3. Erythema on elevation of the feet
    4. Diminished pedal pulses

15. The nurse is completing a bed bath for a dependent adult male client. During the perineal care, the client has an erection. The nurse should:
    1. Continue with the perineal care
    2. Tell the client it's okay and just to relax
    3. Ask the client to try and do the care as well as he can
    4. Defer the care until a little later in the bath

16. A client on chemotherapy is experiencing stomatitis. The nurse advises the client to use:
    1. A commercial mouthwash
    2. An alcohol and water mixture
    3. Normal saline rinses
    4. A firm toothbrush

Chapter 39   Oxygenation

1. The nurse has reviewed information about the cardiovascular system before caring for a client with heart disease. The nurse knows that which following statement is true concerning the physiology of the cardiovascular system?
    1. Stimulating the parasympathetic system would cause the heart rate to go up.
    2. When a person has heart muscle disease, the heart muscles stretch as far as is necessary to maintain function.
    3. The QRS interval on the electrocardiogram represents the electrical impulses passing through the ventricles.
    4. When stroke volume decreases, a resultant decrease in heart rate occurs.

2. The nurse is working on a respiratory care unit in the hospital. On entering the room of a client with emphysema, it is noted that the client is experiencing respiratory distress. The nurse should:
    1. Instruct the client to breathe rapidly
    2. Provide 20% oxygen at 2 L per minute via nasal cannula
    3. Place the client in the supine position
    4. Go to contact the physician

3. A 64-year-old client is seen in the emergency department for palpitations and mild shortness of breath. The ECG reveals a normal P wave, PR interval, and QRS complex with a regular rhythm and rate of 108. The nurse should recognize this cardiac dysrhythmia as:
    1. Sinus dysrhythmia
    2. Sinus tachycardia
    3. Supraventricular tachycardia
    4. Ventricular tachycardia

4. A client recently fractured his spinal cord at the C3 level and is at great risk for developing pneumonia, primarily because the:
    1. Resulting paralysis immobilizes him, and secretions will increase in his lungs
    2. Innervation to the phrenic nerve is absent, preventing chest expansion
    3. Resulting abnormal chest shape disallows efficient ventilatory movement
    4. Trauma decreases the ability of his red blood cells to carry oxygen

5. The client has experienced a myocardial infarction, resulting in damage to the left ventricle. A possible complication the client may experience that the nurse is alert to is:
    1. Jugular neck vein distention
    2. Pulmonary congestion
    3. Peripheral edema
    4. Liver enlargement

6. On admitting a client, the nurse finds a history of myocardial ischemia. The most disconcerting dysrhythmia for electrocardiography to reveal is:
   1. Sinus bradycardia
   2. Sinus dysrhythmia
   3. Ventricular tachycardia
   4. Atrial fibrillation

7. Acute renal failure and a resulting metabolic acidosis develop in a client. The nurse recognizes that the respiratory system compensates through:
   1. Hypoventilation and increase of bicarbonate in the bloodstream
   2. Alternating periods of deep versus shallow breaths to maintain homeostasis of the serum pH
   3. Hyperventilation to decrease the serum CO_2 and thereby increase the pH
   4. Expansion of the lung tissues to their fullest, which increases the inspiratory reserve volumes to provide more oxygen to the tissues

8. A client is brought to the emergency department with a suspected narcotic (heroin) overdose. The nurse anticipates that assessment findings will reveal:
   1. Agitation
   2. Hyperpnea
   3. Restlessness
   4. Decreased level of consciousness

9. The nurse identifies that the client is unable to cough to produce a sputum specimen and must be suctioned. Which suctioning route is preferred for obtaining this specimen?
   1. Nasopharyngeal
   2. Nasotracheal
   3. Oropharyngeal
   4. Orotracheal

10. The nurse is checking the client's overa[ll] oxygenation. In assessment of the presenc[e] of central cyanosis, the nurse will inspect th[e] client's:
    1. Palms and soles of the feet
    2. Nail beds
    3. Earlobes
    4. Tongue

11. A client has recently had a mitral valv[e] replacement. To prevent excess serosan[-] guinous fluid buildup, the nurse anticipate[s] that care will include:
    1. Increased oxygen therapy
    2. Frequent chest physiotherapy
    3. Incentive spirometry on a regularl[y] scheduled basis
    4. Chest tube placement in the thoracic cav[-] ity

12. The client is admitted to the emergenc[y] department with a pneumothorax. Th[e] nurse anticipates that the client will be expe[-] riencing:
    1. Dyspnea
    2. Eupnea
    3. Fremitis
    4. Orthopnea

13. The client with a chronic obstructive respira[-] tory disease is receiving oxygen via a nasa[l] cannula. The nurse plans to include the fol[-] lowing intervention in the client's care:
    1. Assess nares for skin breakdown ever[y] 6 hours
    2. Check patency of the cannula ever[y] 2 hours
    3. Inspect the mouth every 6 hours
    4. Check oxygen flow every 24 hours

14. All of the following clients are experiencing increased respiratory secretions and require intervention to assist in their removal. Chest percussion is indicated and appropriate for the client experiencing:
    1. Thrombocytopenia
    2. Cystic fibrosis
    3. Osteoporosis
    4. Spinal fracture

15. The nurse is working on a pulmonary unit at the local hospital. The nurse is alert to one of the early signs of hypoxia in the clients, which is:
    1. Cyanosis
    2. Restlessness
    3. A decreased respiratory rate
    4. A decreased blood pressure

16. It is suspected that the client's oxygenation status is deteriorating. The nurse is aware that the abnormal assessment finding that represents the most serious indication of the client's decreased oxygenation is:
    1. Poor skin turgor
    2. Clubbing of the nails
    3. Central cyanosis
    4. Pursed-lip breathing

17. In teaching a client about an upcoming diagnostic test, the nurse identifies that which one of the following uses an injection of contrast material?
    1. Holter monitor
    2. Echocardiography
    3. Cardiac catheterization
    4. Exercise stress test

18. At a community health fair, the nurse informs the residents that the influenza vaccine is recommended for clients:
    1. Only older than 65 years
    2. Aged 40 to 60 years
    3. In any age group who have a chronic disease
    4. In any age group who are currently experiencing flu-like symptoms

19. The unit manager is orienting a new staff nurse and evaluates which of the following as an appropriate technique for nasotracheal suctioning?
    1. Placing the client in a supine position
    2. Preparing for a clean or nonsterile technique
    3. Suctioning the oropharyngeal area first, and then the nasotracheal area
    4. Applying intermittent suction for 10 seconds during catheter removal

20. The client has chest tubes in place after thoracic surgery. In working with a client who has a chest tube, the nurse should:
    1. Clamp off the tubes except during client assessments
    2. Remove the tubing from the connection to check for adequate suction power
    3. Milk or strip the tubes every 15 to 30 minutes to maintain drainage
    4. Coil and secure excess tubing next to the client

21. The client has supplemental oxygen in place and requires suctioning to remove excess secretions from the airway. To promote maximal oxygenation, an appropriate action by the nurse is to:
    1. Suction continuously for 30-second intervals
    2. Replace the oxygen and allow rest between suctioning passes
    3. Increase the amount of suction pressure to 200 mm Hg
    4. Complete a number of suctioning passes until the catheter comes back clear

22. A client with a chest tube in place is being transported by stretcher to another room closer to the nurse's station. During the transport, the collection unit bangs against the wall and breaks open. The nurse immediately:
    1. Clamps the tube
    2. Tells the client to hyperventilate
    3. Raises the tubing above the client's chest level
    4. Places the end of the tube in a container of sterile water

23. The client is experiencing a sinus dysrhythmia with a pulse rate of 82 beats per minute. On entering the room, the nurse expects to find the client:
    1. Extremely fatigued
    2. Complaining of chest pain
    3. Experiencing a "fluttering" sensation in the chest
    4. Having no clinical signs based on the assessment

24. The electrical activity of the client's heart is being continuously monitored while he is on the coronary care unit. Suddenly, the nurse finds that the client is experiencing ventricular fibrillation. The nurse will:
    1. Administer atropine
    2. Prepare for cardiopulmonary resuscitation (CPR)
    3. Prepare the client for surgical placement of a pacemaker
    4. Instruct the client to perform the Valsalva maneuver

25. The client is admitted to the medical center with a diagnosis of right-sided heart failure. In assessment of this client, the nurse expects to find:
    1. Dyspnea
    2. Confusion
    3. Dizziness
    4. Peripheral edema

26. The nurse is preparing to teach a group of adult women about the signs and symptoms of a myocardial infarction (heart attack). The nurse will include in the teaching plan the results of research that demonstrate that women may experience specific symptoms, such as:
    1. Visual difficulties
    2. Epigastric pain
    3. Loss of motor function unilaterally
    4. Right scapular discomfort and stiffness

27. The nurse is reviewing the results of the client's diagnostic testing for pulmonary function. Of the following results, the finding that falls within expected or normal limits is:
    1. SpO_2, 88%
    2. pH 7.52
    3. $PaCO_2$, 40 mm Hg
    4. Decreased peak expiratory flow rate (PEFR) from prior assessment

28. The nurse is completing a physical examination for an anemic client. In assessing the client's eyes, a sign assessed by the nurse that is consistent with the diagnosis is:
    1. Xanthelasma
    2. Petechiae
    3. Corneal arcus
    4. Pale conjunctiva

Chapter 40 Fluids, Electrolytes, and Acid-Base Balances

1. When an excess of body fluid exists in the intravascular compartment, all of the following signs can be expected *except*:
    1. Crackles
    2. A bounding pulse
    3. Engorged peripheral veins
    4. An elevated hematocrit level

2. A homeless client is brought into the emergency department with indications of extremely poor nutrition. Arterial blood gases are assessed, and the nurse anticipates that this client will demonstrate the following results:
    1. pH, 7.3; $PaCO_2$, 38 mm Hg; HCO_3 19 mEq/L
    2. pH, 7.5; $PaCO_2$, 34 mm Hg; HCO_3 20 mEq/L
    3. pH, 7.35; $PaCO_2$, 35 mm Hg; HCO_3 24 mEq/L
    4. pH, 7.52; $PaCO_2$, 48 mm Hg; HCO_3 28 mEq/L

3. When a client's serum sodium level is 120 mEq/L, the priority nursing assessment is to monitor the status of which body system?
   1. Neurological
   2. Gastrointestinal
   3. Pulmonary
   4. Hepatic

4. An 8-year-old is admitted to the pediatric unit with pneumonia. On assessment, the nurse notes that the child is warm and flushed, is lethargic, has difficulty breathing, and crackles noted on auscultation. The nurse determines that the child has:
   1. Metabolic acidosis
   2. Respiratory acidosis
   3. Respiratory alkalosis
   4. Metabolic alkalosis

5. Arterial blood gases are obtained for the client. The client's results of pH, 7.48; CO_2, 42; HCO_3, 32; indicate which one of the following acid-base imbalances?
   1. Metabolic acidosis
   2. Respiratory acidosis
   3. Respiratory alkalosis
   4. Metabolic alkalosis

6. The nurse is aware that the compensating mechanism that is most likely to occur in the presence of respiratory acidosis is:
   1. Hyperventilation to decrease the CO_2 levels
   2. Hypoventilation to increase the CO_2 levels
   3. Retention of HCO_3 by the kidneys to increase the pH level
   4. Excretion of HCO_3 by the kidneys to decrease the pH level

7. Of all of the following clients, the nurse recognizes that the individual who is most at risk for a fluid volume deficit is:
   1. A 6-month-old learning to drink from a cup
   2. A 12-year-old who is moderately active in 80° F weather
   3. A 42-year-old with severe diarrhea
   4. A 90-year-old with frequent headaches

8. A client experiences a loss of intracellular fluid. The nurse anticipates that the IV therapy that will be used to replace this type of loss is:
   1. 0.45% normal saline (NS)
   2. 10% dextrose
   3. 5% dextrose in lactated Ringer's
   4. Dextrose 5% in ½ NS

9. The client has been experiencing right flank and lower back pain. Which of the following laboratory values would be most desirable for the nurse to obtain based on the client's assessment?
   1. Serum potassium
   2. Serum sodium
   3. Serum magnesium
   4. Serum calcium

10. The physician orders 1000 ml of D5RL with 20 mEq KCl to run for 8 hours. With an infusion set with a drop factor of 15 gtt/ml, the nurse calculates the flow rate to be:
    1. 12 drops per minute
    2. 22 drops per minute
    3. 32 drops per minute
    4. 42 drops per minute

11. The nurse will be starting a new intravenous infusion and needs to select the site for the insertion. In selection of a site, the nurse should:
    1. Start with the most proximal site
    2. Look for hard, cordlike veins
    3. Use the dominant arm
    4. Inspect sites on the extremity away from a dialysis graft

12. A client has intravenous therapy for the administration of antibiotics and is stating that the "IV site hurts and is swollen." Which of the following information assessed on the client indicates the presence of phlebitis, as opposed to infiltration?
    1. Intensity of the pain
    2. Warmth of integument surrounding the IV site
    3. Amount of subcutaneous edema
    4. Skin discoloration of a bruised nature

13. A client complains of a headache and nausea and vomiting during a blood transfusion. Which one of the following actions should the nurse take immediately?
    1. Check the vital signs.
    2. Stop the blood transfusion.
    3. Slow the rate of blood flow.
    4. Notify the physician and blood bank personnel.

14. For a client with a nursing diagnosis of *Fluid volume excess*, the nurse is alert to which one of the following signs and symptoms?
    1. Weak, thready pulse
    2. Hypertension
    3. Dry mucous membranes
    4. Flushed skin

15. A client is currently taking furosemide (Lasix) and digoxin. As a result of the medication regimen, the nurse is alert to the presence of:
    1. Cardiac dysrhythmias
    2. Severe diarrhea
    3. Hyperactive reflexes
    4. Peripheral cyanosis

16. A rapid infusion of citrated blood has been given to the client. The nurse observes for:
    1. Diaphoresis
    2. Anxiety
    3. Chvostek's sign
    4. Nausea and vomiting

17. For a child who has ingested the remaining contents of an aspirin bottle, is breathing rapidly, and has a blood pH of 7.47, the nurse suspects signs and symptoms consistent with:
    1. Metabolic acidosis
    2. Metabolic alkalosis
    3. Respiratory acidosis
    4. Respiratory alkalosis

18. The single best indicator of fluid status is the nurse's assessment of the client's:
    1. Skin turgor
    2. Intake and output
    3. Serum electrolyte levels
    4. Daily body weight.

19. An IV of 125 ml is to be infused over a 1-hour period. A microdrip infusion set will be used. The nurse calculates the infusion rate as:
    1. 32 gtt/min
    2. 60 gtt/min
    3. 125 gtt/min
    4. 250 gtt/min

20. A client is admitted to the hospital with a diagnosis of adrenal insufficiency. In preparing to complete the admission history, the nurse anticipates that the client will have experienced:
    1. Decreased muscle tone
    2. Hypertension
    3. Diarrhea
    4. Fever

21. In reviewing the results of the client's blood work, the nurse recognizes that the unexpected value that should be reported to the physician is:
    1. Calcium, 3.9 mEq/L
    2. Sodium, 140 mEq/L
    3. Potassium, 3.5 mEq/L
    4. Magnesium, 2.1 mEq/L

22. The nurse anticipates that the client with a fluid volume excess will manifest a(n):
    1. Increased urine specific gravity
    2. Decreased body weight
    3. Increased blood pressure
    4. Decreased pulse strength

23. The nurse recognizes that the client, based on the imbalance that is present, will require fluid replacement with isotonic solution. One of the isotonic solutions that may be ordered by the physician is:
    1. 0.45% saline
    2. Lactated Ringer's
    3. 5% dextrose in normal saline
    4. 5% dextrose in lactated Ringer's

24. A client has severe anemia and will be receiving blood transfusions. The nurse prepares and begins the infusion. Ten minutes after the infusion has begun, tachycardia, chills, and low back pain develop. After stopping the transfusion, the nurse should:
    1. Administer an antipyretic
    2. Begin an infusion of epinephrine
    3. Run normal saline through the blood tubing
    4. Obtain and send a urine specimen to the laboratory

Chapter 41   Sleep

1. The physiology of sleep is complex. Which of the following is the most appropriate statement in regard to this process?
    1. Ultradian rhythms occur in a cycle longer than 24 hours.
    2. Nonrapid eye movement (NREM) refers to the cycle that most clients experience when in a high-stimulus environment.
    3. The reticular activating system is partly responsible for the level of consciousness of a person.
    4. The bulbar synchronizing region causes the rapid eye movement (REM) sleep in most normal adults.

2. The nurse is alert to clients who may be predisposed to obstructive sleep apnea, including those individuals with:
    1. Heart disease
    2. Respiratory infections
    3. Nasal polyps
    4. Obesity

3. When a client is deprived of sleep, the nurse might assess such symptoms as:
    1. Elevated blood pressure and confusion
    2. Confusion and irritability
    3. Inappropriateness and rapid respirations
    4. Decreased temperature and talkativeness

4. The parents of a newborn wonder when she should start to sleep through the night. The nurse's response should be that in infants, a nighttime pattern of sleep usually develops by:
    1. 1 month
    2. 2 months
    3. 3 months
    4. 6 months

5. The mother of a 2-year-old tells the nurse that the child has started crying and resisting going to sleep at the scheduled bedtime. The nurse should advise the parent to:
    1. Offer the child a bedtime snack
    2. Eliminate one of the naps during the day
    3. Allow the child to sleep longer in the mornings
    4. Maintain consistency in the same bedtime ritual

6. An 11-year-old child in middle school is currently experiencing sleep-related fatigue during classes. Which of the following is the most appropriate response by the school nurse when counseling the child's parents regarding this assessment?
    1. "What are the child's usual sleep patterns?"
    2. "Establish bedtimes for the child and withhold his allowance whenever those times are not adhered to."
    3. "We need to explore other health-related problems, as sleep problems are not likely the cause of his fatigue."
    4. "The bulbar synchronizing region of the child's central nervous system is causing these insomniac problems."

7. In describing the sleep patterns of older adults, the nurse recognizes that they:
   a. Are more difficult to arouse
   b. Require more sleep than middle-aged adults
   c. Take less time to fall asleep
   d. Have a decline in stage 4 sleep

8. For a client who is currently taking a diuretic, the nurse should inform the client that he or she may experience:
   1. Nocturia
   2. Nightmares
   3. Increased daytime sleepiness
   4. Reduced REM sleep

9. As a result of recent studies regarding infant safety during sleep, the nurse instructs the parents to:
   1. Provide a stuffed toy for comfort
   2. Cover the infant loosely with a blanket
   3. Place the infant on its back
   4. Use small pillows in the crib

10. A 74-year-old client has been having sleeping difficulties. To have a better idea of the client's problem the nurse should respond:
    1. "What do you do just prior to going to bed?"
    2. "Let's make sure that your bedroom is completely darkened at night."
    3. "Why don't you try napping more during the daytime?"
    4. "You should always eat something just before bedtime."

11. Which of the following information provided by the client's bed partner is most associated with sleep apnea?
    1. Restlessness
    2. Talking during sleep
    3. Somnambulism
    4. Excessive snoring

12. In teaching methods to promote positive sleep habits at home, the nurse instructs the client to:
    1. Use the bedroom only for sleep or sexual activity
    2. Eat a large meal 1 to 2 hours before bedtime
    3. Exercise vigorously before bedtime
    4. Stay in bed if sleep does not come after ½ hour

13. The nurse is discussing sleep habits with the client in the sleep-assessment clinic. Of the following activities performed before sleeping, the nurse is alert to the one that may be interfering with the client's sleep, which is:
    1. Listening to classical music
    2. Finishing office work
    3. Reading novels
    4. Drinking warm milk

14. It is determined that the client will need pharmacologic treatment to assist with his sleep patterns. The nurse anticipates that treatment with an anxiety-reducing, relaxation-promoting medication will include the use of:
    1. Barbiturates
    2. Amphetamines
    3. Benzodiazepines
    4. Tricyclic antidepressants

15. The nurse is completing an assessment on the client's sleep patterns. A specific question that the nurse should ask to determine the potential presence of sleep apnea is:
    1. "How easily do you fall asleep?"
    2. "Do you have vivid, life-like dreams?"
    3. "Do you ever experience loss of muscle control or falling?"
    4. "Do you snore loudly or experience headaches?"

16. Older adults at the community center are having a discussion on health issues, led by a nurse volunteer. One of the participants asks the nurse what to do about not being able to sleep well at night. The nurse informs the participants that sleep in the evening may be enhanced by:
    1. Drinking an alcoholic beverage before bedtime
    2. Using an over-the-counter sleeping agent
    3. Eliminating naps during the day
    4. Going to bed at a consistent time even if not feeling sleepy

Chapter 42   Comfort

1. Which one of the following nursing interventions for a client in pain is based on the gate-control theory?
   1. Giving the client a back massage
   2. Changing the client's position in bed
   3. Giving the client a pain medication
   4. Limiting the number of visitors

2. The client is receiving an epidural opioid infusion for pain relief. A priority nursing intervention when caring for this client is to:
   1. Use aseptic technique
   2. Label the port as an epidural catheter
   3. Monitor vitals signs every 15 minutes
   4. Avoid supplemental doses of sedatives

3. The client tells the nurse about a burning sensation in the epigastric area. The nurse should describe this type of pain as:
   1. Referred
   2. Radiating
   3. Deep visceral
   4. Superficial or cutaneous

4. The nurse must frequently assess a client experiencing pain. When assessing the intensity of the pain, the nurse should:
   1. Ask about what precipitates the pain
   2. Question the client about the location of the pain
   3. Offer the client a pain scale to objectify the information
   4. Use open-ended questions to find out about the sensation

5. The nurse on a postoperative care unit is assessing the quality of the client's pain. To obtain this specific information about the pain experience from the client, the nurse should ask:
   1. "What does your discomfort feel like?"
   2. "What activities make the pain worse?"
   3. "How much does it hurt on a scale of 1 to 10?"
   4. "How much discomfort are you able to tolerate?"

6. The client will be going home on medication administered through a PCA (patient-controlled analgesia) system. To assist the family members with an understanding of how this therapy works, the nurse explains that the client:
   1. Has control over the frequency of the IV analgesia
   2. Can choose the dosage of the drug received
   3. May request the type of medication received
   4. Controls the route for administering the medication

7. An older client with mild musculoskeletal pain is being seen by the primary care provider. The nurse anticipates that treatment of this client's level of discomfort will include:
   1. Fentanyl
   2. Diazepam
   3. Acetaminophen
   4. Meperidine hydrochloride

8. The nurse tells the client that the urinary catheter insertion may feel uncomfortable. This is most accurately an example of:
   1. Distraction
   2. Reducing pain perception
   3. Anticipatory response
   4. Self-care maintenance

9. The nurse is working on a postoperative care unit in the medical center. Of the following clients, the nurse determines that the individual who is best suited for PCA management is the client who:
   1. Has psychogenic discomfort
   2. Is recovering after a total hip replacement
   3. Experiences renal dysfunction
   4. Recently experienced a cerebrovascular accident (stroke)

10. A client with chronic back pain has an order for a transcutaneous electrical nerve stimulation (TENS) unit for pain control. The nurse should instruct the client to:
    1. Keep the unit on high
    2. Use the unit when pain is perceived
    3. Remove the electrodes at bedtime
    4. Use the therapy without medications

11. A terminally ill client with liver cancer is experiencing great discomfort. A realistic goal in caring for the client is to:
    1. Increasingly administer narcotics to oversedate the client and thereby decrease the pain
    2. Continue to change the analgesics to find the right narcotic that completely alleviates the pain
    3. Adapt the analgesics as the nursing assessment reveals the need for specific medications
    4. Withhold analgesics, as they are not being effective in relieving discomfort

12. A client is having severe, continuous discomfort from kidney stones. Based on the client's experience, the nurse anticipates which of the following findings in the client's assessment?
    1. Tachycardia
    2. Diaphoresis
    3. Pupil dilation
    4. Nausea and vomiting

13. Nurses working with clients in pain need to recognize and avoid common misconceptions and myths about pain. In regard to the pain experience, which of the following is correct?
    1. The client is the best authority on the pain experience.
    2. Chronic pain is mostly psychological in nature.
    3. Regular use of analgesics leads to drug addiction.
    4. The amount of tissue damage is accurately reflected in the degree of pain perceived.

14. A nonpharmacologic approach that the nurse may implement for clients experiencing pain that focuses on promoting pleasurable and meaningful stimuli is:
    1. Acupressure
    2. Distraction
    3. Biofeedback
    4. Hypnosis

15. In caring for the client who is receiving epidural analgesia, an appropriate nursing intervention is to:
    1. Change the tubing every 48 to 72 hours
    2. Change the dressing every shift
    3. Secure the catheter to the outside skin
    4. Use a bulky occlusive dressing over the site

16. The client is experiencing breakthrough pain while taking opioids. An order is written for the client to receive a transmucosal fentanyl "unit." In teaching about this medication, the nurse recognizes that additional instruction is required if the client says that he will:
    1. Swab the "unit" over the cheeks
    2. Chew the "unit" after administration
    3. Take no more than 2 "units" per episode of discomfort
    4. Allow the "unit" to dissolve slowly in the mouth over a period of 15 minutes or more

17. The nurse consults with the primary physician of a client who is experiencing continuous, severe pain. In planning for the client's treatment, the nurse is aware of the principles of pain management and that it is appropriate to expect treatment to include:
    1. Focusing on intramuscular administration of analgesics
    2. Waiting for pain to become more intense before administering opioids
    3. Administering opioid with nonopioid analgesics for severe pain
    4. Administering large doses of opioids initially to clients who have not taken the medications before

18. On entering the room, the nurse discovers that the client is experiencing acute pain. An expected assessment finding for this client is:
    1. Bradycardia
    2. Bradypnea
    3. Diaphoresis
    4. Decreased muscle tension

19. The client is unable to rest even after medication. The nurse decides to give the client a backrub. Which of the following strokes should the nurse use when finishing the backrub?
    1. Long firm strokes down the back
    2. Light strokes while moving up the back in a circular motion
    3. Kneeding movements toward the sacrum
    4. Circular motion upward from buttocks to shoulders

Chapter 43   Nutrition

1. While doing a nutritional assessment of a low-income family, the community health nurse determines that the family's diet is inadequate in protein content. The nurse suggests which of the following foods to increase protein content with little increase in food expenditure?
    1. Oranges and potatoes
    2. Potatoes and rice
    3. Rice and macaroni
    4. Peas and beans

2. A client is suspected of having a fat-soluble vitamin deficiency. To assist the client with this deficiency, the nurse informs the client:
    1. "More exposure to sunlight and drinking milk could solve your nutritional problem."
    2. "Eating more pork, fish, eggs, and poultry will increase your vitamin B complex intake."
    3. "Increasing your protein intake will increase your negative nitrogen imbalance."
    4. "Decreasing your triglyceride levels by eating less saturated fats would be a good health intervention for you."

3. The client is diagnosed with malabsorption syndrome (celiac disease). In teaching about the gluten-free diet, the nurse informs the client to avoid:
    1. Citrus fruits
    2. Vegetables
    3. Red meats
    4. Wheat products

4. The school nurse suspects that a junior high student may have anorexia nervosa. This eating disorder is characterized by:
    1. A lack of control over eating patterns
    2. Self-imposed starvation
    3. Binge/purge cycles
    4. Excessive exercise

5. A client is pregnant for the third time. In regard to her nutritional status, she should:
   1. Limit her weight gain to a maximum of about 25 pounds
   2. Approximately double her protein intake
   3. Increase her vitamin A and milk product consumption
   4. Increase her intake of folic acid

6. The client has had throat surgery and is able to have oral intake. The nurse should offer the client:
   1. Chicken noodle soup
   2. Ginger ale
   3. Oatmeal
   4. Hot tea with lemon

7. The nurse is discussing dietary intake with a client who is human immunodeficiency virus (HIV) positive. The nurse informs the client that the diet will include a:
   1. Restriction of potassium, phosphate, and sodium
   2. Reduction in carbohydrate intake
   3. Decreased protein and increased folic acid intake
   4. Reduction in fat, with smaller, more frequent meals

8. When introducing a feeding to a client with an indwelling gavage tube for enteral nutrition, the nurse should first:
   1. Irrigate the tube with normal saline solution
   2. Check to see that the tube is properly placed
   3. Place the client in a supine position
   4. Introduce some water before giving the liquid nourishment

9. The nurse is caring for a client who is receiving parenteral nutrition (PN). An appropriate intervention related to this therapy is for the nurse to:
   1. Begin the infusion rates at 100 to 150 ml per hour
   2. Maintain a consistent infusion rate
   3. Change the infusion tubing once a week
   4. Monitor protein levels daily

10. A client needs a small-bore nasogastric tube inserted for enteral nutrition (EN). Before the insertion, the nurse correctly states to the client:
    1. "The tube will feel uncomfortable and may make you gag at times when I am inserting it."
    2. "We will mark this tube from the end of your nose to your umbilicus to obtain the right length for insertion."
    3. "Please hold your breath when I insert this small tube through your nose down into your stomach."
    4. "Please tilt your head back after the tube passes the nasopharynx."

11. A client is seen in the outpatient clinic for follow-up of a nutritional deficiency. In planning for the client's dietary intake, the nurse includes a complete protein, such as:
    1. Eggs
    2. Oats
    3. Lentils
    4. Peanuts

12. According to the Food Guide, vegetables should be included in the average adult's diet as:
    1. 1 to 3 servings per day
    2. 2 to 4 servings per day
    3. 3 to 5 servings per day
    4. 6 to 11 servings per day

13. The parent of an 8-year-old asks the nurse about any special nutritional needs for children in this age group. The nurse identifies that children during this period need to:
    1. Increase their intake of B vitamins
    2. Significantly increase iron intake
    3. Maintain a sufficient intake of protein, and vitamins A and C
    4. Increase carbohydrates to meet increased energy needs

14. The nurse who is assisting the client in meal selection realizes that clients who practice Islam or Judaism share an avoidance of:
    1. Alcohol
    2. Shellfish
    3. Caffeine
    4. Pork products

15. After a surgical procedure, the client is advanced to a full liquid diet. The nurse is able to recommend which one of the following foods for this client?
    1. Custard
    2. Pureed meats
    3. Soft fresh fruit
    4. Canned soup

16. A client has an enteral tube in place and is receiving tube feedings. While the nurse is administering the feeding, the client begins to experience abdominal cramping and nausea. The nurse should:
    1. Cool the formula
    2. Remove the tube
    3. Use a more concentrated formula
    4. Decrease the administration rate

17. A client is diagnosed with a peptic ulcer and has come to the primary physician for a follow-up visit. The client asks the nurse what foods are safe to add to his diet. An appropriate response by the nurse is to inform the client that the following may be added to the diet:
    1. Citrus juices
    2. Green vegetables
    3. Frequent glasses of milk
    4. Unlimited decaffeinated coffee

18. The nurse is speaking with parents of a child at a day-care center. The parents ask the nurse about the nutritional needs of their toddler. An appropriate finger food that is identified by the nurse is:
    1. Nuts
    2. Popcorn
    3. Cheerios
    4. Hot dogs

19. A school nurse in a high school is reviewing the nutritional needs of adolescents. The nurse is aware that in this age group:
    1. Girls require less protein
    2. Boys require additional iron
    3. Vitamin B needs are decreased
    4. Energy and caloric needs are decreased

20. The client is assessed by the nurse as having a high risk for aspiration. The nursing diagnosis identified for the client is *Self-care deficit, feeding related to unilateral weakness.* An appropriate technique for the nurse to use when assisting the client with feeding is to:
    1. Place food to the unaffected side of the mouth
    2. Place the client in semi-Fowler's position
    3. Have the client use a straw
    4. Use thinner liquids

21. A nasogastric tube is inserted for the client to receive intermittent tube feedings. An initial chest radiograph is done to confirm placement of the tube in the stomach. After the radiographic confirmation, the most reliable method of checking for tube placement is for the nurse to:
    1. Place the end of the tube in water and observing for bubbling
    2. Auscultate while introducing air into the tube
    3. Measure the pH of the secretions aspirated
    4. Ask the client to speak

22. For the client who is receiving parenteral nutrition via a central venous catheter, the nurse recognizes that a priority is to:
    1. Use sterile technique during the administration of the feedings
    2. Maintain the initial infusion rate at no more than 40 to 60 ml per hour
    3. Complete the administration of the feeding within 12 hours
    4. Have radiographic confirmation of the placement of the catheter

23. A client has been receiving tube feedings and is tolerating them very well. The physician determines that the rate of the intermittent tube feedings may be advanced. The nurse prepares to:
    1. Increase the feedings by 50 ml per day
    2. Start an isotonic formula at ½ strength
    3. Infuse a bolus feeding over a 5- to 10-minute period
    4. Begin feedings with 250 to 500 ml at each interval

24. The nurse is aware that some medications alter the client's taste and may influence the dietary intake. In reviewing the medications taken by the clients on the unit, the nurse will consult with the nutritionist to develop a palatable meal plan for the client taking:
    1. Ampicillin
    2. Morphine
    3. Furosemide
    4. Acetaminophen

25. Food safety is a concern of a group of adults attending the community health clinic. The participants identify to the nurse that they have seen a lot of reports on television about *Escherichia coli* and how dangerous it can be. When asked where the bacteria come from, the nurse responds that a potential source of *E. coli* is:
    1. Sausage
    2. Soft cheeses
    3. Milk products
    4. Ground beef

Chapter 44   Urinary Elimination

1. An assessment is completed by the nurse, and a nursing diagnosis for the oriented adult female client is identified as *Stress incontinence related to decreased pelvic muscle tone*. An appropriate nursing intervention based on this diagnosis is to:
   1. Apply adult diapers
   2. Catheterize the client
   3. Administer urecholine
   4. Teach Kegel exercises

2. A client in the hospital has an indwelling urinary catheter, and the nurse is instructing the nursing assistant in the appropriate care to provide. The nurse teaches the assistant to:
   1. Empty the drainage bag at least q8h
   2. Cleanse up the length of the catheter to the perineum
   3. Use clean technique to obtain a specimen for culture and sensitivity
   4. Place the drainage bag on the client's lap while transporting the client to testing

3. The nurse suspects that the client has a bladder infection based on the client exhibiting an early sign or symptom such as:
   1. Chills
   2. Hematuria
   3. Flank pain
   4. Incontinence

4. The client has an indwelling catheter. The nurse should obtain a sterile urine specimen by:
   1. Disconnecting the catheter from the drainage tubing
   2. Withdrawing urine from a urinometer
   3. Opening the drainage bag and removing urine
   4. Using a needle to withdraw urine from the catheter port

5. Immediately after an intravenous pyelogram (IVP), the nurse should observe the client for which of the following?
   1. Infection in the urinary bladder
   2. An allergic reaction to the contrast material
   3. Urinary suppression caused by injury to kidney tissues
   4. Incontinence as a result of paralysis of the urinary sphincter

6. A client with an excessive alcohol intake has a reduced amount of antidiuretic hormone (ADH). The nurse anticipates the client will exhibit:
   1. Hematuria
   2. An increased blood pressure.
   3. Dry mucous membranes
   4. A low serum sodium level

7. A client is going to have a cystoscopy. Which of the following reflects the correct information that should be taught before the procedure?
   1. "Are you allergic to iodine?"
   2. "There will be no need to have a special consent form."
   3. "You will need to have fluids restricted the evening before the cystoscopy."
   4. "You will probably be given sedatives before the procedure."

8. A postpartum client has been unable to void since her delivery of her baby this morning. Which of the following nursing measures would be beneficial for the client initially?
   1. Increase fluid intake to 3500 ml
   2. Insert indwelling Foley catheter
   3. Rinse the perineum with warm water
   4. Apply firm pressure over the bladder

9. The nurse is visiting the client who has a nursing diagnosis of *Alteration in urinary elimination, retention*. On assessment, the nurse anticipates that this client will exhibit:
   1. Severe flank pain and hematuria
   2. Pain and burning on urination
   3. A loss of the urge to void
   4. A feeling of pressure and voiding of small amounts

10. The unit manager is evaluating the care of a new nursing staff member. Which of the following is an appropriate technique for the nurse to implement to obtain a clean-voided urine specimen?
    1. Apply sterile gloves for the procedure.
    2. Restrict fluids before the specimen collection.
    3. Place the specimen in a clean urinalysis container.
    4. Collect the specimen after the initial stream of urine has passed.

11. The nurse is aware that clients with chronic alterations in kidney function have insufficient amounts of:
    1. Vitamin A
    2. Vitamin D
    3. Vitamin E
    4. Vitamin K

12. In an assessment of a client with reflex incontinence, the nurse expects to find that the client has:
    1. A constant dribbling of urine
    2. An uncontrollable loss of urine when coughing or sneezing
    3. No urge to void and an unawareness of bladder filling
    4. An immediate urge to void but not enough time to reach the bathroom

13. In determining the client's urinary status, the nurse anticipates that the urinary output for an average adult should be:
    1. 800 to 1000 ml per day
    2. 1000 to 1200 ml per day
    3. 1500 to 1700 ml per day
    4. 2000 to 2300 ml per day

14. A timed urine specimen collection is ordered. The test will need to be restarted if the following occurs:
    1. The client voids in the toilet
    2. The urine specimen is kept cold
    3. The first voided urine is discarded
    4. The preservative is placed in the collection container

15. The nurse is working with a client who has a urinary diversion. Included in the plan of care for this client is instruction that:
    1. Special clothing will need to be ordered to fit around the diversion
    2. A stomal bag will need to be worn only at night
    3. A reduction in physical activity will be planned
    4. Special skin care is a priority

16. The nursing instructor is evaluating the student during the catheterization of a female client. The instructor determines that the student has implemented appropriate technique when observed:
    1. Keeping both hands sterile throughout the procedure
    2. Reinserting the catheter if it was misplaced initially in the vagina
    3. Inflating the balloon to test it before catheter insertion
    4. Advancing the catheter 7 to 8 inches

17. A client is receiving closed catheter irrigation. During the shift, 950 ml of normal saline irrigant is instilled, and a total of 1725 ml is found in the drainage bag. The client's urinary output is calculated by the nurse to be:
    1. 775 ml
    2. 950 ml
    3. 1725 ml
    4. 2675 ml

18. A bladder-retraining program for a client in an extended care facility should include:
    1. Providing negative reinforcement when the client is incontinent
    2. Having the client wear adult diapers as a preventive measure
    3. Putting the client on a q2h toilet schedule during the day
    4. Promoting the intake of caffeine to stimulate voiding

19. A 3-year-old child is visiting the pediatric clinic. The nurse suspects that the child has a urinary tract infection. An appropriate method for the nurse to implement to obtain a urine specimen from the child is to:
    1. Use an indwelling catheter
    2. Offer fluids 30 minutes in advance
    3. Apply pressure over the urinary bladder
    4. Place a diaper on the child and squeeze out the specimen

20. A sample is obtained from the client for a routine urinalysis. On reviewing the results of the test, the nurse notes that an expected finding of the urinalysis is:
    1. pH, 8.0
    2. Specific gravity, 1.018
    3. Protein amounts to 12 mg per 100 ml
    4. White blood cell count of five to eight per low-power field casts

21. The client is experiencing urinary retention, and the physician is contacted. The nurse anticipates that a medication that will be ordered to promote emptying of the bladder is:
    1. Oxybutynin chloride (Ditropan)
    2. Bethanechol (Urecholine)
    3. Propantheline (Pro-banthine)
    4. Nystatin (Mycostatin)

22. An order is written for the client's indwelling urinary catheterization to be discontinued. While observing the new staff nurse provide care to this client and implement the prescriber's order, the unit manager determines that further instruction is required for the new nurse in catheter removal if he is observed:
    1. Draping the female client between the thighs
    2. Obtaining a specimen before removal
    3. Cutting the catheter to deflate the balloon
    4. Checking the client's output for 24 hours after removal

23. A condom catheter is to be used for an adult male client in the extended care facility. In the application of the condom catheter, the nurse uses appropriate technique when:
    1. Using sterile gloves
    2. Wrapping the adhesive tape securely around the base of the penis
    3. Leaving a 1- to 2-inch space between the tip of the penis and the end of the catheter
    4. Taping the tubing tightly to the thigh and attaching the drainage bag to the bed frame

24. Urinary elimination may be altered with different pathophysiologic conditions. For the client with diabetes mellitus, the nurse anticipates that an initial urinary sign or symptom will be:
    1. Urgency
    2. Dysuria
    3. Hematuria
    4. Polyuria

Chapter 45   Bowel Elimination

1. The nurse recognizes that changes in elimination occur with the aging process. An expected change in bowel elimination is which of the following:
   1. Absorptive processes are increased in the intestinal mucosa.
   2. Esophageal emptying time is increased.
   3. Changes in nerve innervation and sensation cause diarrhea.
   4. Mastication processes are less efficient.

2. A 6-month-old infant has severe diarrhea. The major problem associated with severe diarrhea is:
   1. Pain in the abdominal area
   2. Electrolyte and fluid loss
   3. Presence of excessive flatus
   4. Irritation of the perineal and rectal area

3. The client is seen in the gastroenterology clinic after having experienced changes in his bowel elimination. A colonoscopy is ordered, and the client has questions about the examination. Before the colonoscopy, the nurse teaches the client that:
   1. No special preparation is required
   2. Light sedation is normally used
   3. No metallic objects are allowed
   4. Swallowing of an opaque liquid is required

4. A client is to have a stool test for occult blood. The nurse is instructing the nursing assistant in the correct procedure for the test. The nursing assistant is correctly informed that:
   1. Sterile technique is used for collection
   2. Stool should be collected over a 3-day period
   3. The specimen should be kept warm
   4. A 1-inch sample of formed stool is needed

5. A client has just had intestinal surgery with the creation of a colostomy. For the first few weeks, the nutritional therapy for this client will include:
   1. Vegetables
   2. Fresh fruit
   3. Whole-grain breads
   4. Poached eggs and rice

6. The client has been admitted to an acute care unit with a diagnosis of biliary disease. The nurse suspects that the feces will appear:
   1. Bloody
   2. Pus filled
   3. Black and tarry
   4. White or clay colored

7. The client asks the nurse recommend bulk-forming foods that may be included in the diet. Which of the following should be recommended by the nurse?
   1. Whole grains
   2. Fruit juice
   3. Rare meats
   4. Milk products

8. The client is taking medications to promote defecation. Which of the following instructions should be included by the nurse in the teaching plan for this client?
   1. Increased laxative use often causes hyperkalemia.
   2. Salt tablets should be taken to increase the solute concentration of the extracellular fluid.
   3. Emollient solutions may increase the amount of water secreted into the bowel.
   4. Bulk-forming additives may turn the urine pink.

9. While undergoing a soapsuds enema, the client complains of abdominal cramping. The nurse should:
   1. Immediately stop the infusion
   2. Lower the height of the enema container
   3. Advance the enema tubing 2 to 3 inches
   4. Clamp the tubing

10. The nurse is caring for clients on a postoperative unit in the medical center. The nurse is alert to the possibility that for 24 to 48 hours of the postoperative period, clients may experience the following as a result of the anesthetic used during the surgery:
    1. Colitis
    2. Stomatitis
    3. Paralytic ileus
    4. Gastrocolic reflex

11. For clients with hypocalcemia, the nurse should implement measures to prevent:
    1. Gastric upset
    2. Malabsorption
    3. Constipation
    4. Fluid secretion

12. The client is to receive a sodium polystyrene sulfonate (Kayexelate) enema. The nurse recognizes that this is used to:
    1. Prevent further constipation
    2. Remove excess potassium from the system
    3. Reduce bacteria in the colon before diagnostic testing
    4. Provide direct antidiarrheal medication to the intestine

13. The appropriate amount of fluid to prepare for an enema to be given to an average size school-age child is:
    1. 150 to 250 ml
    2. 250 to 350 ml
    3. 300 to 500 ml
    4. 500 to 750 ml

14. The nurse is instructing the client in stomal care for an incontinent ostomy. The nurse evaluates achievement of learning goals if the client uses:
    1. Triamcinolone acetamide (Kenalog) spray for a yeast infection
    2. Peroxide to toughen the periostomal skin
    3. A commercial deodorant around the stoma
    4. Alcohol to cleanse the stoma

15. An appropriate measure for the nurse to implement for the client with a nasogastric tube in place is to:
    1. Tape the tube up and around the ear on the side of insertion
    2. Secure the tubing to the bed by the client's head
    3. Mark the tube where it exits the nose
    4. Change the tubing daily

16. The nurse instructs the client that, before the fecal occult blood test (FOBT), she may eat:
    1. Whole wheat bread
    2. A lean, T-bone steak
    3. Veal
    4. Salmon

UNIT 8 CLIENTS WITH SPECIAL NEEDS

Chapter 46 Mobility and Immobility

1. A client has been on prolonged bed rest, and the nurse is observing for signs associated with immobility. In assessment of the client, the nurse is alert to a(n):
   1. Increased blood pressure
   2. Decreased heart rate
   3. Increased urinary output
   4. Decreased peristalsis

2. A 61-year-old client recently had left-sided paralysis from a cerebrovascular accident (stroke). In planning care for this client, the nurse implements which one of the following as an appropriate intervention?
   1. Encourage an even gait when walking in place.
   2. Assess the extremities for unilateral swelling and muscle atrophy.
   3. Encourage holding the breath frequently to hyperinflate his lungs.
   4. Teach the use of a two-point crutch technique for ambulation.

3. Two nurses are standing on opposite sides of the bed to move the client up in bed with a draw sheet. Where should the nurses be standing in relation to the client's body as they prepare for the move?
   1. Even with the thorax
   2. Even with the shoulders
   3. Even with the hips
   4. Even with the knees

4. A client is leaving for surgery, and because of preoperative sedation, needs complete assistance to transfer from the bed to the stretcher. Which of the following should the nurse do first?
   1. Elevate the head of the bed
   2. Explain the procedure to the client
   3. Place the client in the prone position
   4. Assess the situation for any potentially unsafe complications

5. A client has sequential compression stockings in place. The nurse evaluates that they are implemented appropriately by the new staff nurse when the:
   1. Initial measurement is made around the client's calves
   2. Intermittent pressure is set at 40 mm Hg
   3. Stockings are wrapped directly over the leg from ankle to knee
   4. Stockings are removed every hour during application

6. The nurse assesses that the client has torticollis, and that this may adversely influence the client's mobility. This individual has a(n):
   1. Exaggeration of the lumbar spine curvature
   2. Increased convexity of the thoracic spine
   3. Abnormal anteroposterior and lateral curvature of the spine
   4. Contracture of the sternocleidomastoid muscle with a head incline

7. An immobilized client is suspected as having atelectasis. This is assessed by the nurse, on auscultation, as:
   1. Harsh crackles
   2. Wheezing on inspiration
   3. Diminished breath sounds
   4. Bronchovesicular whooshing

8. The best approach for the nurse to use to assess the presence of thrombosis in an immobilized client is to:
   1. Measure the calf and thigh diameters
   2. Attempt to elicit Homan's sign
   3. Palpate the temperature of the feet
   4. Observe for a loss of hair and skin turgor in the lower legs

9. A client is getting up for the first time after a period of bed rest. The nurse should first:
   1. Assess respiratory function
   2. Obtain a baseline blood pressure
   3. Assist the client to sit at the edge of the bed
   4. Ask the client if he or she feels light-headed

10. To promote respiratory function in the immobilized client, the nurse should:
    1. Change the client's position q4-8h
    2. Encourage deep breathing and coughing every hour
    3. Use oxygen and nebulizer treatments regularly
    4. Suction the client every hour

11. Antiemboli stockings (TEDs) are ordered for the client on bed rest after surgery. The nurse explains to the client that the primary purpose for the elastic stockings is to:
    1. Keep the skin warm and dry
    2. Prevent abnormal joint flexion
    3. Apply external pressure
    4. Prevent bleeding

12. To provide for the psychosocial needs of an immobilized client, an appropriate statement by the nurse is:
    1. "The staff will limit your visitors so that you will not be bothered."
    2. "A roommate can be a real bother. You'd probably rather have a private room."
    3. "Let's discuss the routine to see if there are any changes we can make."
    4. "I think you should have your hair done and put on some make-up."

13. To reduce the chance of external hip rotation in a client on prolonged bed rest, the nurse should implement the use of a:
    1. Footboard
    2. Trochanter roll
    3. Trapeze bar
    4. Bed board

14. To reduce the chance of plantar flexion (foot drop) in a client on prolonged bed rest, the nurse should implement the use of:
    1. Trapeze bars
    2. High-top sneakers
    3. Trochanter rolls
    4. 30-degree lateral positioning

15. A client is admitted to the medical unit following a cerebrovascular accident (CVA). There is evidence of left-sided hemiparesis and the nurse will be following up on range of motion and other exercises performed in physical therapy. The nurse correctly teaches the client and family members which one of the following principles of range-of-motion exercises?
    1. Flex the joint to the point of discomfort
    2. Work from proximal to distal joints
    3. Move the joints quickly
    4. Provide support for distal joints

Chapter 47 Skin Integrity and Wound Care

1. The nurse determines that the client's wound may be infected. To perform an aerobic wound culture, the nurse should:
   1. Collect the superficial drainage
   2. Collect the culture before cleansing the wound
   3. Obtain a culturette tube and use sterile technique
   4. Use the same technique as for collecting an anaerobic culture

2. Pressure ulcers form primarily as a result of:
   1. Nitrogen buildup in the underlying tissues
   2. Prolonged illness or disease
   3. Tissue ischemia
   4. Poor nutrition

3. The nurse notes that a client's skin is reddened, with a small abrasion and serous fluid present. The nurse should classify this stage of ulcer formation as:
   1. Stage 1
   2. Stage 2
   3. Stage 3
   4. Stage 4

4. The client has rheumatoid arthritis, is prone to skin breakdown, and is also somewhat immobile because of arthritic discomfort. Which of the following is the best intervention for the client's skin integrity?
   1. Having the client sit up in a chair for 4-hour intervals.
   2. Keeping the head of the bed in a high Fowler's position to increase circulation.
   3. Keeping a written schedule of turning and positioning.
   4. Encouraging the client to perform pelvic muscle training exercises several times a day.

5. On changing the client's dressing, the nurse notes that the wound appears to be granulating. An appropriate noncytoxic cleansing agent selected by the nurse is:
   1. Sterile saline
   2. Hydrogen peroxide
   3. Povidone-iodine (Betadine)
   4. Sodium hypochlorite (Dakin's solution)

6. A client requires wound debridement. The nurse is aware that which one of the following statements is correct regarding this procedure?
   1. It provides a clean base for healing.
   2. Autolytic treatment requires irrigation.
   3. Mechanical methods involve direct surgical removal of the eschar layer of the wound.
   4. Enzymatic debridement may be implemented independently by the nurse whenever it is required.

7. The nurse prepares to irrigate the client's wound. The primary reason for this procedure is to:
   1. Decrease scar formation
   2. Remove debris from the wound
   3. Improve circulation from the wound
   4. Decrease irritation from wound drainage

8. When turning a client, the nurse notices a reddened area on the coccyx. What skin care interventions should the nurse use on this area?
   1. Clean the area with mild soap, dry, and add a protective moisturizer.
   2. Apply a dilute hydrogen peroxide and water mixture, and use a heat lamp on the area.
   3. Soak the area in normal saline solution.
   4. Wash the area with an astringent, and paint it with povidone-iodine (Betadine).

9. A client with a large abdominal wound requires a dressing change every 4 hours. The client will be discharged to the home setting where the dressing care will be continued. Which of the following is true concerning this client's wound-healing process?
   1. An antiseptic agent is best followed with a rinse of sterile saline solution.
   2. A heat lamp should be used every 2 hours to rid the wound area of contaminants.
   3. Sterile technique should be emphasized to the client and family.
   4. A dressing covering will allow the wound area to remain moist.

10. On inspection of the client's wound, the nurse notes that it appears infected and has a large amount of exudate. An appropriate dressing for the nurse to select based on the wound assessment is:
   1. Foam
   2. Hydrogel
   3. Hydrocolloid
   4. Transparent film

11. A client has a healing abdominal wound. The wound has minimal exudate and collagen formation. The wound is identified by the nurse as being in which phase of healing?
   1. Primary intention
   2. Inflammatory phase
   3. Proliferative phase
   4. Secondary intention

12. A client comes to the emergi-center after an injury. The nurse implements appropriate first aid for the client when:
   1. Removing any penetrating objects
   2. Elevating an affected part that is bleeding
   3. Vigorously cleaning areas of abrasion or laceration
   4. Keeping any puncture wounds from bleeding

13. The nurse is concerned that the client's midsternal wound is at risk for dehiscence. Which of the following is the best intervention to prevent this complication?
   1. Administering antibiotics to prevent infection.
   2. Using appropriate sterile technique when changing the dressing.
   3. Keeping sterile towels and extra dressing supplies near the client's bed.
   4. Placing a pillow over the incision site when the client is deep breathing or coughing.

14. After a head injury, the client has th drainage coming from the left ear. The nur describes this drainage as:
   1. Serous
   2. Purulent
   3. Cerebrospinal fluid
   4. Serosanguinous

15. Which nursing entry is most complete describing a client's wound?
   1. Wound appears to be healing we Dressing dry and intact.
   2. Wound well approximated with minim drainage.
   3. Drainage size of quarter; wound pin 4×4's applied.
   4. Incisional edges approximated witho redness or drainage, two 4×4's applied.

16. The nurse recognizes that skin integrity ca be compromised by being exposed to bo fluids. The greatest risk exists for the clie who has exposure to:
   1. Urine
   2. Purulent exudates
   3. Pancreatic fluids
   4. Serosanguinous drainage

17. The client is scheduled for a dressing chang When removing the adhesive tape used secure the dressing, the nurse should lift th edge and hold the tape:
   1. At a 45-degree angle to the skin surfa while pulling away from the wound
   2. At a right angle to the skin surface whi pulling toward the wound
   3. At a right angle to the skin surface whi pulling away from the wound
   4. Parallel to the skin surface while pullir toward the wound

18. When cleaning a wound, the nurse should
   1. Go over the wound twice and discard th swab
   2. Move from the outer region of the wour toward the center
   3. Start at the drainage site and move ou ward with circular motions
   4. Use an antiseptic solution followed by normal saline rinse

9. The client has a large, deep wound on the sacral region. The nurse correctly packs the wound by:
   1. Filling two thirds of the wound cavity
   2. Leaving saline-soaked folded gauze squares in place
   3. Putting the dressing in very tightly
   4. Extending only to the upper edge of the wound

0. The nurse is aware that application of cold is indicated for the client with:
   1. Menstrual cramping
   2. An infected wound
   3. A fractured ankle
   4. Degenerative joint disease

1. The client has a stage IV ulcer. In accordance with the Agency for Health Care Policy and Research (AHCPR), the nurse recommends that the client should have a:
   1. Foam mattress
   2. Air-fluidized bed
   3. Rotokinetic bed
   4. Static support surface

2. The nurse uses the Norton Scale in the extended care facility to determine the client's risk for pressure ulcer development. Which one of the following scores, based on this scale, places the client at the highest level of risk?
   1. 6
   2. 8
   3. 15
   4. 19

3. The client requires support, and an abdominal binder is ordered. The nurse correctly implements the use of a binder by:
   1. Using it as a replacement for underlying dressings
   2. Keeping it loose for client comfort
   3. Having the client sit or stand when it is applied
   4. Making sure the client has adequate ventilatory capacity

24. The client is brought into the emergency department with a knife wound. The nurse correctly documents the client's wound as a(n):
   1. Contusion wound
   2. Clean wound
   3. Acute wound
   4. Intentional wound

25. The nurse is planning a program on wound healing and includes information that smoking influences healing by:
   1. Suppressing protein synthesis
   2. Creating increased tissue fragility
   3. Depressing bone marrow function
   4. Reducing functional hemoglobin in the blood

26. To reduce pressure points that may lead to pressure ulcers, the nurse should:
   1. Position the client directly on the trochanter when side-lying
   2. Use a donut device for the client when sitting up
   3. Elevate the head of the bed as little as possible
   4. Massage over the bony prominences

27. The client is experiencing low back pain and is to have an aquathermia pad applied. The nurse recognizes that safe application of heat to a client's injury includes:
   1. Providing a timer for the client
   2. Allowing the client to adjust the temperature for comfort
   3. Placing the pad directly onto the area requiring treatment
   4. Using the highest temperature that is tolerated by the client

28. In reviewing the client's nutritional intake, the nurse wants to recommend intake of foods that will specifically promote collagen synthesis and capillary wall integrity. The nurse suggests to the client to eat:
   1. Fish
   2. Eggs
   3. Liver
   4. Citrus fruits

29. A client on the medical unit is taking steroids and also has a wound from a minor injury. To promote wound healing for this client, the nurse recommends that the following be specifically added:
   1. Iron
   2. Folic acid
   3. Vitamin A
   4. B complex vitamins

Chapter 48   Sensory Alterations

1. During a community screening, the nurse informs a 50-year-old African-American client about the frequency of eye examinations. It is recommended that individuals in this age group have eye examinations:
   1. Every 3 to 4 months
   2. Every 6 months
   3. Every 1 to 2 years
   4. Every 4 years

2. With advancing age, which of the following normal physiological changes in sensory function occurs?
   1. Decreased sensitivity to glare
   2. Increased number of taste buds
   3. Difficulty discriminating vowel sounds
   4. Decreased sensitivity to pain

3. The nurse teaches a client that prolonged use of the antibiotic streptomycin may result in:
   1. Damage to the auditory nerve
   2. Alteration in perception
   3. Optic irritation
   4. Loss of taste

4. Which of the following occupations poses the least risk for sensory alterations?
   1. Waiter
   2. Welder
   3. Computer programmer
   4. Construction worker

5. The nurse is working with a client with moderate hearing impairment. To promote communication with this client, the nurse should:
   1. Use a louder tone of voice than normal
   2. Use visual aids such as the hands and eyes when speaking
   3. Approach a client quietly from behind before speaking
   4. Select a public area to have a conversation

6. The client has hyperesthesia apparently associated with a neurologic trauma. Which of the following is an appropriate nursing intervention in regard to the client's sense of touch?
   1. Reminding the client of the need to have frequent tactile contact
   2. Keeping the client loosely covered with sheets and blankets
   3. Allowing the client to lie motionless
   4. Using touch as a form of therapy

7. The client has experienced a cerebrovascular accident (stroke) with resultant expressive aphasia. The nurse promotes communication with this client by:
   1. Speaking very loudly and slowly
   2. Speaking to the client on the unaffected side
   3. Using a picture chart for the client's responses
   4. Using hand gestures to convey information to the client

8. The client was working in the kitchen and was splashed in the face with a caustic cleaning agent. His eyes were affected, and he was brought to the hospital for treatment. After cleansing and evaluation, his eyes were bandaged. When assisting this client who has temporary visual loss to eat, the nurse should:
   1. Feed the client the entire meal
   2. Allow the client to experiment with food
   3. Orient the client to the location of the foods on the plate
   4. Encourage the family to feed the client

394   Test Bank

9. The nurse completes a safety assessment during a home visit to an older adult client. Of the following observations made by the nurse, the one that is of greatest concern for this client who has evidence of sensory impairment is:
   1. Low-pile carpeting throughout the home
   2. A handrail on the stairs that extends the full length
   3. Higher wattage iridescent lighting in all the rooms
   4. The gray/black settings on the stove handles

10. A client is legally blind in both eyes. Which of the following is the most appropriate statement for the nurse to make to the client regarding providing the client with assistance?
    1. "I will walk in front of you, and you can hold onto my belt."
    2. "I know that you must need me to be your sighted guide to get around in this facility."
    3. "I will warn you of upcoming curbs or stairs."
    4. "I will get you a wheelchair so that I can move you around safely."

11. A 79-year-old client drives his car in the local areas near his home. The most appropriate driving tip for the nurse to give this client is:
    1. "Go very, very slowly so you will have some chance of reacting."
    2. "Take your time on long road trips when you are by yourself. "
    3. "Remember to keep your car maintained with regular checkups."
    4. "To avoid sun glare, you should drive at night."

12. An older adult client in a nursing home has visual and hearing losses. The nurse is alert to which of the following signs that represents the effects of sensory deprivation?
    1. Diminished anxiety
    2. Improved task completion
    3. Altered spatial perception
    4. Decreased need for physical stimulation

13. During a home safety assessment, the nurse identifies that a number of hazards. Of the following hazards that are noted by the nurse, which one represents the greatest risk for this client with diabetic peripheral neuropathy?
    1. Improper water heater settings
    2. Absence of smoke detectors
    3. Cluttered walkways
    4. Lack of bathroom grab bars

14. The nurse in the pediatric clinic is checking the basic visual acuity of a 4-year-old child. The nurse should have the child:
    1. Use the standard Snellen chart
    2. Read a few lines from children's book
    3. Follow the peripheral movement of an object
    4. Identify crayon colors

15. For a client with receptive aphasia, which one of the following nursing interventions is the most effective?
    1. Providing the client with a letter chart to use to answer complex questions
    2. Using a system of simple gestures and repeated behaviors to communicate
    3. Offering the client a notepad to write questions and concerns
    4. Obtaining a referral for a speech therapist

16. The nurse recommends follow-up auditory testing for a child who was exposed in utero to:
    1. Excessive oxygen
    2. Diabetes
    3. Respiratory infection
    4. Rubella

17. The family of an older client asks the nurse how the stairways and hallways in the home may be enhanced to promote safety. In addition to extra lighting, the nurse recommends the use of paint and decorations that are:
    1. Red and yellow
    2. Black and white
    3. Brown and green
    4. Blue and purple

18. The nurse is working with older adult clients in an extended care facility. To enhance the clients' gustatory sense, the nurse should:
    1. Mix foods together
    2. Assist with oral hygiene
    3. Provide foods of similar texture and consistency
    4. Make sure foods are extremely spicy

19. A home safety measure specific for a client with diminished olfaction is the use of:
    1. Smoke detectors on all levels
    2. Extra lighting in hallways
    3. Amplified telephone receivers
    4. Mild water heater temperatures

20. The nurse has completed the admission assessment for a client admitted to the hospital's subacute care unit. Of the following nursing diagnoses identified by the nurse, the one that takes the highest priority is:
    1. *Social isolation*
    2. *Injury, risk for*
    3. *Adjustment, impaired*
    4. *Communication, impaired verbal*

21. While participating in a community auditory screening, the nurse is alert to the population that has the greatest prevalence of problems. The nurse is aware that hearing impairment is more common for:
    1. Caucasians
    2. Asian-Americans
    3. African-Americans
    4. Native Americans

22. The nurse is visiting the day-care center for routine assessment of the children. After spending time with the children in one of the playrooms, the nurse suspects that a child has a visual deficit as a result of observing:
    1. Poor balance and gait
    2. An increase in weight
    3. Sitting and rocking back and forth
    4. A failure to respond when touched

Chapter 49 Care of Surgical Clients

1. A 43-year-old client is scheduled to have gastrectomy. Which of the following is major preoperative concern?
    1. The client's brother had a tonsillectom at age 11 years
    2. The client smokes a pack of cigarettes day
    3. The presence of an intravenous (IV) inf sion
    4. A history of employment as a comput programmer

2. An appendectomy is appropriately docu mented by the nurse as:
    1. Diagnostic surgery
    2. Palliative surgery
    3. Ablative surgery
    4. Reconstructive surgery

3. An obese client is admitted for abdomin surgery. The nurse recognizes that this clien is more susceptible to the postoperativ complication of:
    1. Anemia
    2. Seizures
    3. Protein loss
    4. Dehiscence

4. The nurse is working in a postoperative ca unit in an ambulatory surgery center. Of th following clients that have come to have su gery, the client at the greatest risk durin surgery is a:
    1. 78-year-old taking an analgesic agent
    2. 43-year-old taking an antihypertensi agent
    3. 27-year-old taking an anticoagulant agen
    4. 10-year-old taking an antibiotic agent

5. A 92-year-old client is scheduled for a colectomy. Which normal physiologic change that accompanies the aging process increases this client's risk for surgery?
   1. An increased tactile sensation
   2. An increased metabolic rate
   3. A relaxation of arterial walls
   4. Reduced glomerular filtration

6. The nurse is completing the preoperative checklist for an adult female client is who is scheduled for an operative procedure later in the morning. Which of the following preoperative assessment findings for this client indicates a need to contact the surgeon?
   1. Hgb, 14 g/100 ml
   2. BUN, 15 mg/100 ml
   3. Platelets, 300,000/mm^3
   4. Serum creatinine, 3.2 mg/100 ml

7. The nurse is evaluating the following: *"Client describes surgical procedures and postoperative treatment"* and determines that the client has not achieved this outcome. The nurse should:
   1. Obtain the consent, as this is expected with preoperative anxiety
   2. Teach the client all about the procedure
   3. Ask the unit manager to assist with a teaching plan
   4. Inform the surgeon so that information can be provided

8. Which of the following statements most accurately reflects nursing accountability in the intraoperative phase?
   1. "I would like to see the client have a regional anesthetic rather than a general anesthetic."
   2. "A sponge seems to be missing, so a recount should be done of all the sponges that have been removed."
   3. "Did the client receive the medications and sign the consent?"
   4. "The client looks to be reactive and stable."

9. The client will have an incision in the lower left abdomen. Which of the following measures by the nurse will help decrease discomfort in the incisional area when the client coughs postoperatively?
   1. Applying a splint directly over the lower abdomen
   2. Keeping the client flat with her feet flexed
   3. Turning the client onto the right side
   4. Applying pressure above and below the incision

10. The nurse is evaluating the client in the hospital's postanesthesia care unit (PACU) and determines that the Aldrete score is 8. Based on this assessment, the nurse anticipates that the client will:
    1. Be sent to the intensive care unit
    2. Be discharged back to his room on the nursing unit
    3. Remain in the PACU until the score improves
    4. Return to the operating room for surgical evaluation

11. A client is in the PACU recovering from a vagotomy and pyloroplasty. Which of the following is a normal expectation of the client in this stage of recovery?
    1. Returned normal bowel sounds on auscultation
    2. Pain that is relieved with noninvasive comfort measures
    3. Voluntary bladder control and function
    4. A subdued level of consciousness and neurologic function

12. The client is scheduled for abdominal surgery and has just received the preoperative medications. The nurse should:
    1. Keep the client quiet
    2. Obtain the consent
    3. Prepare the skin at the surgical site
    4. Place the side rails up on the bed or stretcher

13. The nurse is completing the preoperative checklist for an adult client who is scheduled for an operative procedure later in the morning. Which of the following preoperative assessment findings for this client indicates a need to contact the anesthesiologist?
    1. Temperature, 100° F
    2. Pulse, 90
    3. Respirations, 20
    4. Blood pressure, 130/74

14. In the postoperative period, the nurse recognizes that an early sign of malignant hyperthermia is:
    1. Fever
    2. Tachycardia
    3. Muscle relaxation
    4. Skin pallor

15. The client tells the nurse, "Blowing into this tube thing (incentive spirometer) is a ridiculous waste of time." The nurse explains that the specific purpose of the therapy is to:
    1. Directly remove excess secretions from the lungs
    2. Increase pulmonary circulation
    3. Promote lung expansion
    4. Stimulate the cough reflex

16. The female client is on the surgical unit and being readied for abdominal surgery with general anesthesia early in the afternoon. In preparing this client for surgery, the nurse should:
    1. Leave all of her jewelry intact
    2. Provide her with sips of water for a dry mouth
    3. Remove her make-up and nail polish
    4. Remove her hearing aid before transport to the operating room

17. The client asks the nurse the purpose of having medications [meperidine (Demerol) and hydroxyzine (Vistaril)] given before surgery. The nurse should inform the client that these particular medications:
    1. Reduce preoperative fear
    2. Promote emptying of the stomach
    3. Reduce body secretions
    4. Ease the induction of the anesthesia

18. A client who receives general or regional anesthesia in an ambulatory surgery center:
    1. Has to meet identified criteria to be discharged home
    2. Will remain in the phase I recovery area longer than a hospitalized client
    3. Is allowed to ambulate as soon as being admitted to the recovery area
    4. Is immediately given liberal amounts of fluid to promote the excretion of the anesthesia

19. After abdominal surgery, the nurse suspects that the client may be having internal bleeding. Which of the following findings is indicative of this complication?
    1. Increased blood pressure
    2. Incisional pain
    3. Abdominal distention
    4. Increased urinary output

20. After discharge from the PACU, the client returned to the surgical nursing unit at 10:00 AM. It is now 11:30 AM, and the client is not experiencing any complications or difficulties. The nurse will plan to measure the client's vital signs:
    1. Every 15 minutes
    2. Every 30 minutes
    3. Every 1 hour
    4. Every 4 hours

21. The client had surgery in the morning that involved the right femoral artery. To assess the client's circulation status to the right leg, the nurse will make sure to check the pulse at the:
    1. Radial artery
    2. Ulnar artery
    3. Brachial artery
    4. Dorsalis pedis artery

22. On admission to the PACU, the client who has no orthopedic or neurologic restrictions is positioned with the:
    1. Bed flat and the client's arms to the sides
    2. Client's neck flexed and body positioned laterally
    3. Head of the bed slightly elevated with the client's head to the side
    4. Client's arms crossed over the chest and the bed in high Fowler's position

23. A client who is scheduled for surgery is found to have thrombocytopenia. A specific postoperative concern for the nurse for this client is:
    1. Hemorrhage
    2. Wound infection
    3. Fluid imbalance
    4. Respiratory depression

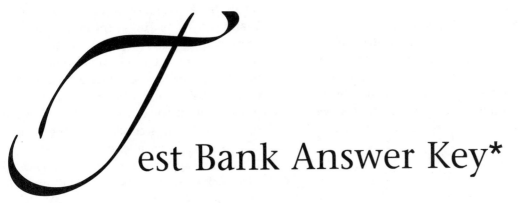

_T_est Bank Answer Key*

_C_hapter 1

1. 1, p. 3
Rationale:
1. Florence Nightingale believed the role of the nurse was to put the client's body in the best state to remain free of disease or to recover from disease.
2. Although Florence Nightingale may have addressed meeting the psychological needs of her patients, it is not the focus of her theory. The goal of Nightingale's theory is to facilitate "the body's reparative processes" by manipulating the client's environment.
3. Florence Nightingale thought the human body had reparative properties of its own if it were just cared for in a way to recover from disease. Her theory did not focus on achieving a maximal level of wellness.
4. Florence Nightingale believed the nurse was in charge of another's health. Although she interacted with her patients by reading to them, her theory of nursing care did not focus on interpersonal interactions.

Donald Venes, ed: *Taber's cyclopedic medical dictionary*, ed. 19, F.A. Davis Publishers, Philadelpha, 1997.
*Question number is followed by the correct answer and page reference in text.

2. 4, p. 22
Rationale:
4. The National League for Nursing (NLN) is the professional nursing organization concerned with nursing education. The NLN provides accreditation to nursing programs that seek and meet the NLN accreditation requirements.
1. The American Nurses Association (ANA) is concerned with the nursing profession and issues affecting health care, including standards of care.
2. The International Council of Nurses (ICN) is concerned about issues of health care and the nursing profession, including the provision of an international power base for nurses.
3. The Congress of Nursing Practice is the part of the ANA concerned with the legal aspects of nursing practice, public recognition of the importance of nursing, and how trends in health care affect nursing practice.

3. 3, p. 17
Rationale:
3. A master's degree is nursing is required to become a nurse practitioner.

1. Diploma programs in nursing require 3 years of education, after which the graduate may become a registered nurse, but not a nurse practitioner.
2. The baccalaureate degree program generally requires 4 years of study in a college or university, after which the graduate may become a registered nurse, not a nurse practitioner.
4. Doctoral programs focus on the application of research findings to clinical practice. The doctoral degree is beyond the master's degree.

4. 1, p. 22
Rationale:
1. The ANA hires lobbyists at the state and federal level to promote the advancement of health care and the economic and general welfare of nurses.
2. State boards of nursing focus primarily on licensure of nurses within their own state.
3. The National Student Nurses Association focuses on issues of importance for nursing students.
4. The American Hospital Association does not focus on nurses' economic issues and the advancement of the role of nurses.

5. 3, p. 18
Rationale:
3. Although most states have similar practice acts, each individual state has its own Nurse Practice Act that regulates the licensure and practice of nursing within that state. Knowledge of the Nurse Practice Act is necessary to provide safe and legal nursing care.
1. Standards of nursing practice are specific not to a city, but rather to the profession itself.
2. Although the clinical ladder of mobility may be of interest in regard to professional advancement, it is not the most important factor when practicing nursing in another state. Knowledge of the Nurse Practice Act to provide safe and legal nursing care is of higher importance.
4. Regardless of where a nurse practices, the nurse should strive to remain current in nursing skills, knowledge, and theory through continuing education offerings.

6. 1, p. 19
Rationale:
1. The nurse, in caring for this client, will coordinate the activities of other members of the health care team. This client may require the assistance of a nursing assistant to provide personal care until the client is less fatigued. A nutritionist may be necessary for diet evaluation, planning, and teaching. A nurse may provide education on the dialysis therapy and perform the skill necessary until the client is able to do so independently.
2. The nurse may include patient teaching in the client's care, but more is required to meet the needs of this client.
3. The nurse is not performing in the role of counselor.
4. Clear communication will be necessary for the client to understand self-care measures regarding dialysis. The role of communicator does not, however, entirely meet the client's physical needs at this time.

7. 1, p. 20
Rationale:
1. Most nurses provide direct client care in the hospital setting.
2. Although opportunities for providing patient care in the client's home are increasing, the majority of nurses are not employed in this setting.
3. Significantly fewer nurses work in an ambulatory care setting.
4. The majority of nurses do not work in nursing homes or extended care settings.

8. 3, p. 14, 19
Rationale:
3. An occupational therapist is one who provides assessment and intervention to ameliorate physical and psychological deficits that interfere with the performance of activities and tasks of living, including one's employment.
1. A respiratory therapist provides treatment to preserve or improve pulmonary function.
2. A physician's assistant performs tasks usually done by physicians and works under the direction of a supervising physician.

4. A physical therapist is responsible for the patient's movement system. A physical therapist may use exercises as an intervention to improve a client's mobility.

9. 4, p. 4
Rationale:
4. In 1923, the Goldmark Report identified the need for increased financial support to university-based schools of nursing.
1. In 1975, the NLN required theory-based curriculum for accreditation.
2. The Brown Report of 1948 concluded that all nursing education programs should be affiliated with universities and should have their own budgets.
3. The National Commission on Nursing and Nursing Education Report of 1965 recommended that nursing roles and responsibilities be clarified in relation to other health care professionals.

10. 4, pp. 4 to 5
Rationale:
4. In 1893, Lillian Wald and Harriet Brewster opened the Henry Street Settlement, which was the first community health service for the poor.
1. In 1894, Isabel Hampton Robb was the first superintendent of the Johns Hopkins Training School in Baltimore, Maryland.
2. Isabel Hampton Robb was one of the original founders of the *American Journal of Nursing*.
3. The first nurses training school in Canada was founded in 1874: St. Catherine's, Ontario.

11. 1, p. 18
Rationale:
1. Set minimum practice requirements are based on the certification the nurse is seeking. After passing the initial examination, the nurse maintains certification by ongoing continuing education and clinical or administrative practice.
2. A specialized examination is given according to the specific area of nursing practice in which certification is being sought.
3. A master's degree in nursing is not required for certification in a specialty area.

4. Individual states do not grant certification by request. Certification in a specialty area requires passing the examination for certification in that area and meeting minimal practice requirements.

12. 1, pp. 10, 19
Rationale:
1. As a client advocate, the nurse protects the client's human and legal rights and provides assistance in asserting those rights if the need arises. Performing in the role of patient advocate fulfills a measurement criterion for the professional performance standard of ethics.
2. Participating in data collection is a measurement criterion for the professional performance standard of quality of practice.
3. Consulting with health care providers is a measurement criterion for the professional performance standard of collaboration.
4. The nurse who seeks experiences to maintain clinical skills is fulfilling a measurement criterion for the professional performance standard of education.

13. 1, p. 3
Rationale:
1. The Civil War stimulated the growth of nursing in the United States. Nurses were in demand to tend to the soldiers of the battlefield.
2. Throughout history, nurses and their professional organizations have lobbied for health care legislation to meet the needs of clients. However, legislation was not responsible for the growth of nursing in the 19th century.
3. Although Florence Nightingale had great impact on the practice of nursing, she was not the cause for the growth of nursing in the United States during the 19th century.
4. The women's movement has encouraged nurses to seek greater autonomy and responsibility in providing care and has caused female clients to seek more control of their health and lives. The women's movement was not responsible for the growth of nursing in the 19th century.

14. 2, p. 17
Rationale:

2. An in-service education program is instruction or training provided by a health care agency or institution for its employees.
1. A workshop at a nursing convention is an example of a continuing education program.
3. Credit courses at a college are examples of continuing education that could possibly be applied toward furthering one's degree.
4. Noncredit courses offered via the Internet are examples of a continuing education program.

15. 4, p. 5
Rationale:

4. In recent decades, a higher incidence has been found of chronic, long-term illness.
1. With shortened hospital stays, client acuity has increased, not decreased.
2. Hospitals stays have decreased, not increased. Lengths of stay have shortened with a trend toward home care, health promotion, and illness prevention.
3. With increased public awareness and increasing health care costs, greater emphasis has been placed on health promotion and illness prevention.

16. 4, p. 6
Rationale:

4. The nurse may educate the client in such areas as exercise, nutrition, and healthy lifestyles to assist the client in health promotion and illness prevention.
1. By administering medication, the nurse is assisting to restore a person to health or maintain one's health.
2. A nurse who treats a foot ulcer is assisting a client to restore health, rather than promoting healthy behaviors.
3. Obtaining an operative consent pertains to legal aspects of care and is not considered a ealth promotion activity.

Chapter 2

1. 1, p. 28
Rationale:

1. During most of the 20th century, little restriction was placed on the prescription of care and treatment of clients. As a result, health care costs grew out of control.
2. The increase in members within the work force is not responsible for the dramatic increase in health care costs.
3. There is an increased incidence of chronic disease in the United States, and hospitalized clients are more acutely ill. Neither condition accounts for the dramatic increase in health care costs from 1965 to 1985.
4. After the "baby boom," the birth rate proportionately declined from 1965 to 1985.

2. 1, p. 28
Rationale:

1. As a means to reduce health care costs, in 1983, Congress established the prospective payment system in which hospitals are reimbursed a set dollar amount for each diagnosis-related group, regardless of the length of stay or use of services in the hospital.
2. Federal guidelines for treatment have not been used to reduce the cost of health care. Rather, the focus has been on financial reimbursement.
3. State limits on health care fees have not been used nationwide to reduce health care costs.
4. Court review of insurance coverage has not been a primary intervention to reduce health care costs.

3. 1, p. 29
Rationale:

1. Nursing typically makes up a large percentage of a health care institution's labor budget. To save money, an organization may hire fewer nurses and instead hire less-educated technical staff, placing greater responsibility on the nurse.
2. Nurses do not necessarily achieve higher salary levels than do other health care professionals.

. The impact of cost control on nurses is not because nurses provide client care without direct reimbursement from the client.
. Nurses do not deliver the least cost-effective care. Many negative, and costly, outcomes may be avoided when patients are under the direct care of a registered nurse.

. 3, p. 31
ationale:
. Examples of health promotion activities include exercise classes, prenatal care, well-baby care, nutrition counseling, and family planning.
. An immunization clinic is an example of an illness prevention service.
. A diabetic support group may be an example of a rehabilitation service to adapt to a change in lifestyle.
.. A smoking-cessation clinic may be a part of rehabilitation or offered as an illness prevention service.

. 3, pp. 30, 34, 35
Rationale:
. A state-owned psychiatric hospital is an example of the secondary level of care in which clients with signs and symptoms of disease are diagnosed and treated.
.. A home health agency is an example of either restorative or continuing care, depending on the client's condition.
.. Hospice care is an example of continuing care.
.. A nursing home is an example of continuing care.

. 4, p. 32
Rationale:
.. Exposure to environmental hazards within the workplace, such as noise exposure, is one aspect of occupational safety and health.
.. Motorcycle helmets do not fit within the occupational safety and health category.
.. Firearms do not fit within the occupational safety and health category.
.. Swimming lessons do not fit within the occupational safety and health category.

7. 1, p. 29
Rationale:
1. A preferred provider organization (PPO) is characterized by a contractual agreement between a set of providers (e.g., hospitals, physicians, or clinics) and a purchaser (i.e., the corporation's insurance plan). Comprehensive health services are provided at a discount to the companies under contract. Enrollees are limited to a list of "preferred" hospitals, physicians, and providers. An enrollee pays more out-of-pocket expenses for using a provider not on the list.
2. A Medicare health maintenance organization (HMO) is the same as a managed care organization (all care provided by a primary care physician) but designed to cover costs of senior citizens.
3. Private insurance is the traditional fee-for-service plan in which payment is computed after services are provided, based on the number of services used.
4. In third party payment, an entity (other than the patient or health care provider) reimburses health care expenses. Third party payers include insurance companies, governmental agencies, and employers.

8. 3, p. 29
Rationale:
3. Medicaid is a federally funded, state-operated program of medical assistance to people with low incomes. Individual states determine eligibility and benefits.
1. This option describes Medicare.
2. This option describes Medicare Part A.
4. This option does not describe Medicaid.

9. 2, p. 42
Rationale:
2. Health care providers are defining and measuring quality in terms of outcomes. An outcome is a measure of what actually does or does not happen as a result of a process of care.
1. The focus in quality care management is on the outcome, not the process.

3. Quality care management is not used exclusively in the acute care setting. It may be used in various health care settings.
4. Because quality care management is based on achieving outcomes, it does not allow a high degree of flexibility for the nurse in delivering care.

10. 2, p. 34
Rationale:
2. With the case management model of care, the case manager coordinates the efforts of all disciplines to achieve the most efficient and appropriate plan of care. Continuity of care is of primary importance.
1. Case management is not entirely based on the level of care required.
3. The physician may or may not be the coordinator of client care. The case manager typically is a nurse or social worker.
4. If the efforts of all disciplines are well managed, repetition or delays may be avoided, with a resultant shortened hospital stay. Therefore this focus of care may not be more expensive.

11. 2, p. 28
Rationale:
2. Inpatient hospital services for Medicare clients are reimbursed a set amount for each diagnosis-related group (DRG), regardless of the client's length of stay or use of services in the hospital.
1. Capitation is the payment mechanism in which providers receive a fixed amount per enrollee of a health care plan.
3. Medicare is based not on fixed payments, but rather on a set dollar amount according to the DRG.
4. The payment mechanism that Medicare uses is not direct contracting.

12. 2, p. 32
Rationale:
2. Nurse-managed clinics focus on health promotion and health education, disease prevention, chronic disease management, and support for self-care and caregivers.

1. Same-day surgery is not offered in a nurse managed clinic.
3. Psychiatric therapy is not offered in a nurse managed clinic.
4. Physical therapy is not typically offered in a nurse-managed clinic.

13. 4, p. 35
Rationale:
4. A home health care agency provides health services to individuals and families in their home to promote, maintain, or restore health or to maximize the level of independence while minimizing the effects of disability and illness.
1. Assisted living is a long-term care setting in which clients need some assistance with activities of daily living, but otherwise remain independent.
2. An ambulatory health center is not the best referral for restorative care.
3. A sub–acute care unit is not the best referral for restorative care.

14. 3, p. 38
Rationale:
3. This option describes assisted living. A group of residents live together, each resident having his or her own room, yet sharing dining and social activity areas.
1. Respite care is a service that provides short-term relief for persons providing home care to the ill or disabled.
2. Rehabilitative care includes physical, occupational, and speech therapy and social services to help restore a person to the fullest ability.
4. An extended care facility provides intermediate medical, nursing, or custodial care for clients recovering from acute or chronic illness or disabilities.

15. 4, p. 34
Rationale:
4. Discharge planning should begin at the time of admission to the hospital, by using the strengths and resources of the client, providing resources to meet the client's limitations, and focusing on improving the client's long-term outcomes.

1. The client's diagnosis does not have to be established before discharge planning can begin.
2. Discharge planning should include preparation for long-term needs of the client.
3. Acute care therapies may affect a client's discharge and should be a part of the plan from the beginning.

16. 4, p. 29
Rationale:
4. In a managed care organization (MCO), a primary care physician provides all care, and the focus is on health maintenance and primary care.
1. In an MCO, referral by the primary care physician is necessary for access to specialists and for hospitalization.
2. An MCO does not necessarily provide reimbursement for all health services requested.
3. An MCO does not offer additional coverage for illness-oriented care. The focus is on health maintenance and primary care.

17. 3, p. 30
Rationale:
3. Administering a bronchodilating medication is an example of secondary care (acute care).
1. Well-baby care is an example of preventive care.
2. A blood pressure screening is an example of illness prevention in the level of preventive care.
4. Rehabilitation is an example of the restorative level of care.

Chapter 3

1. 4, pp. 48, 49
Rationale:
4. Community health nursing strives to safeguard and improve the health of populations in the community as well as providing direct care services to subpopulations within a community.

1. Nurses who become expert in community health practice may have advanced nursing degrees, yet the baccalaureate-prepared generalist also can become quite competent in formulating and applying population-focused assessments and interventions.
2. Public health nursing focuses on the needs of populations. Community health nursing has a broader focus, with an emphasis on the health of a community. The community health nurse merges public health knowledge with nursing theory. The community health nurse considers the needs of populations and is prepared to provide direct care services to subpopulations within a community.
3. Public health nursing is concerned with trends and patterns influencing the incidence of disease within populations. A community health nurse may be involved in direct client care for disease within a community.

2. 3, p. 55
Rationale:
3. With the goal of helping clients assume responsibility for their own health care, the community health nurse must assess a client's learning needs and readiness to learn within the context of the individual, the systems the individual interacts with, and the resources available for support. Asking the client about what foods he or she should eat may help the nurse assess the client's level of knowledge regarding nutrition, as well as the client's food preferences. It also enables the client to become a participant in his or her care.
1. Telling the client what foods to buy does not encourage the client to assume responsibility for managing health care.
2. The nurse should first assess the resources available, and then encourage the client to do his or her own shopping.
4. Providing information on food sources and stores with reasonable pricing may be appropriate after the nurse has determined what information the client requires to meet nutritional needs.

3. 4, pp. 52, 53
Rationale:
4. A client with substance abuse has health and socioeconomic problems. Frequently these clients may avoid health care for fear of judgmental attitudes by health care providers and concern over being reported to criminal authorities.
1. An abused client in a shelter has sought protection, so currently should be at less risk.
2. Although considered to be a member of a vulnerable population, the older adult who takes medication for a chronic disease such as hypertension is taking measures to maintain health.
3. A schizophrenic client in outpatient therapy is currently at less risk because he or she is receiving treatment.

4. 3, p. 53
Rationale:
3. The goal of tertiary prevention is to preclude further deterioration of physical and mental function in a person who has an existing illness, and to have the client use whatever residual function is available for maximal enjoyment of and participation in life's activities.
1. Primary prevention is aimed at general health promotion.
2. Secondary prevention is aimed at early recognition and treatment of disease.
4. Health promotion is aimed at reducing the incidence of disease and its impact on people.

5. 4, p. 56
Rationale:
4. This response demonstrates the nurse acting as client advocate by identifying and assisting the client in contacting the appropriate agency for information and resources to meet the client's needs.
1. This response points out the difference in cost for dialysis in the home versus that in the hospital, but does not meet the client's need to reduce the expenses of his therapy. The nurse is not demonstrating patient advocacy.

2. Asking the client whether he has considered renal transplantation does not demonstrate client advocacy.
3. Telling the client that this is the best treatment for him does not address his financial concerns. The nurse is not demonstrating patient advocacy with this response.

6. 4, p. 57
Rationale:
4. When assessing the structure or locale of a community, the nurse should travel around the neighborhood or community and observe its design, the location of services, such as water and sanitation, and the locations where residents congregate.
1. Collecting demographic data on age distribution would be an assessment of the community's population.
2. Visiting neighborhood schools to review health records is an example of assessing a social system within a community.
3. Interviewing clients to determine cultural makeup of subgroups is an example of assessing the population within a community.

7. 2, p. 56
Rationale:
2. As a change agent, the nurse seeks to implement new and more effective approaches to problems. The nurse creates change by working with and empowering individuals and their families to solve problems or to become instrumental in changing aspects affecting their health care.
1. Telling community members how to manage their health care needs may meet resistance. It does not enable clients and their families to take responsibility for their health care.
3. Making decisions for clients does not enable individuals to assume responsibility for their health care decisions.
4. The community-based nurse acting as a change agent may be an excellent resource for health information to members of the community. Ultimately, however, the community members will take an active role to create change for themselves and will assume responsibility for their health care decisions.

408   Test Bank Answer Key

8. 3, p. 56
Rationale:

3. Directing clients to appropriate resources and to improve continuity of care requires the nurse to know those resources well. A physical therapist is responsible for the patient's movement system and is likely to be needed after hip-replacement surgery.

1. A social worker may or may not be necessary.
2. A dietician may or may not be necessary.
4. A respiratory therapist would not be necessary unless the client experienced a respiratory complication or had a pre-existing respiratory condition.

9. 3, p. 47
Rationale:

3. Because hospital stays are being shortened to control health care costs, clients are returning home more acutely ill. This is the largest contributing factor to the increase in the need for and use of home care.

1. Government funding of home care is not the largest contributing factor to the increase in the need for and use of home care.
2. The existence of more single-income families is not the largest contributing factor to the increase in the need for and use of home care.
4. Seven-days-per-week services are available for the elderly in a variety of settings, such as in acute care or long-term care, not just in the home care setting. Being able to provide daily services for the elderly in the home care setting is not the largest contributing factor to the increase in the need for and use of home care.

10. 1, p. 48
Rationale:

1. The overall goals of *Healthy People 2010* are to increase the life expectancy and quality of life and to eliminate health disparities.
2. The initiative of *Healthy People 2010* is to improve the delivery of health care services to the general public. The overall goal did not focus on reducing health care costs.
3. Although MCOs may increase in number, this was not a goal of the *Healthy People 2010* initiative.
4. Establishing the credentials of care providers was not a goal of *Healthy People 2010*.

Chapter 4

1. 4, p. 62
Rationale:

4. A theory is a set of concepts, definitions, relations, and assumptions that project a systematic view of phenomena.
1. Statements that describe concepts or connect concepts are called assumptions.
2. Mental formulations of objects or events are called concepts.
3. Aspects of reality that can be consciously sensed are called phenomena.

2. 2, p. 64
Rationale:

2. Descriptive theories describe phenomena, speculate on why phenomena occur, and describe the consequences of phenomena.
1. Prescriptive theories address nursing interventions and predict the consequence of a specific nursing intervention.
3. Grand theories provide the structural framework for broad, abstract ideas about nursing.
4. Middle-range theories address specific phenomena or concepts and reflect practice.

3. 4, p. 62
Rationale:

4. Environment/situation includes all possible conditions affecting the client and the setting in which health care needs occur, such as the home, school, workplace, or community.
1. Person refers to the recipient of nursing care, including individual clients, families, and the community.
2. Health is the goal of nursing care.
3. Nursing care refers to the "diagnosis and treatment of human responses to actual or potential health problems" (ANA, 1995).

4. 1, p. 68
Rationale:

1. Neuman's framework for practice included nursing actions as primary, secondary, or tertiary levels of prevention in caring for clients holistically. Secondary prevention strengthens internal defenses and resources by establishing priorities and treatment plans for identified symptoms.

2. The goal of Orem's theory is to promote attainment of self-care.
3. Roy's theory focuses on adaptation.
4. In Henderson's theory, nurses help the client to perform 14 basic needs.

5. 4, pp. 65, 69
Rationale:
4. As in Benner and Wrubel's theory, Watson emphasized caring in her theory. Watson's model is designed around the caring process, assisting clients in attaining or maintaining health or in dying peacefully. The key emphasis of her theory is that caring is the moral ideal: mind-body-soul engagement with another.
1. Self-care is central to Orem's theory.
2. The key emphasis of Johnson's theory is that subsystems exist in dynamic stability.
3. The key emphasis of Roy's theory is that stimuli disrupt an adaptive system.

6. 1, p. 64
Rationale:
1. According to systems theory, a system is made up of parts that rely on one another, are interrelated, share a common purpose, and together form a whole. A client's interaction with the environment is an example of an open system. The nurse understands that factors that change the environment also can have an impact on the system.
2. Maslow's hierarchy of human needs is an interdisciplinary theory useful in planning individualized care.
3. Determining a client's attitudes toward health behaviors follows a health-and-wellness theoretical model.
4. Focusing on the response of a client to the process of growth and development is consistent with developmental theories.

7. 3, p. 68
Rationale:
3. The goal of Orem's theory is to help the client perform self-care.
1. The goal of Nightingale's theory is to facilitate "the body's reparative processes" by manipulating the client's environment.

2. The goal of Henderson's theory is to work independently with other health care workers assisting the client to gain independence as quickly as possible.
4. The goal of King's theory is to use communication to help the client reestablish positive adaptation to the environment.

8. 4, p. 67
Rationale:
4. The framework for practice according to Martha Roger's theory is the unitary human continuously changing and coexisting with the environment.
1. Abdellah's nursing theory includes 21 nursing problems within four major client needs in the framework for practice.
2. Nightingale's theory includes manipulation of the client's environment (i.e., appropriate noise, nutrition, hygiene, light, comfort, socialization, and hope) in the framework for practice.
3. Johnson's theory includes seven categories of behavior and behavioral balance in the framework for practice.

9. 3, p. 67
Rationale:
3. Stress reduction is the goal of the systems model of nursing practice according to Neuman's theory.
1. Peplau's theory focuses on the interpersonal process as the maturing force for personality.
2. Orlando's theory focuses on the interpersonal process to alleviate distress.
4. Parse's theory focuses on indivisible beings and the environment co-creating health.

10. 2, pp. 67, 69
Rationale:
2. Leininger states that care is the essence of nursing and the dominant, distinctive, and unifying feature of nursing. Caring also is central to Benner and Wrubel's theory, depicting personal concern as an inherent feature of nursing practice.
1. The theories of Roy and Johnson focus on the client's adaptation to demands.

3. Neuman's theory places emphasis on achieving a maximum level of wellness. Abdellah's theory also addressed the person as a whole.
4. King's theory and Peplau's theory share a similarity with a focus on interpersonal communication.

11. 2, p. 68
Rationale:
2. The goal of nursing, according to Orem, is to increase the client's ability to meet biologic, psychological, developmental, or social needs independently.
1. According to Henderson, nurses help clients to perform 14 basic needs.
3. Abdellah's theory emphasizes the delivery of nursing care for the whole person.
4. Neuman's theory is concerned with the whole person. According to Neuman, the focus of nursing is on the variables affecting the client's response to a stressor.

Chapter 5

1. 2, p. 77
Rationale:
2. An example of an exploratory type of research is to develop or refine a hypothesis about the relations among phenomena.
1. An example of a historical type of research is to establish facts and relations concerning past events.
3. An example of a descriptive type of research is accurately to portray characteristics of persons, situations, or groups and the frequency with which certain events or characteristics occur.
4. An example of an evaluation type of research is to test how well a program, practice, or policy is working.

2. 4, p. 82
Rationale:
4. HIPAA regulations identify how protected health information of potential research subjects is to be managed. The researcher must be able to ensure that the data will be protected and used only by the researcher.

1. HIPAA regulations should not influence the area of cost in nursing research.
2. The focus of HIPAA regulations is not on where a study may be published.
3. HIPAA regulations should not influence the type of study conducted.

3. 2, p. 81
Rationale:
2. Nurses with a baccalaureate degree are prepared to read research critically and use existing standards to determine the readiness of the findings for clinical practice. They also participate in research activities through identification of clinical problems in nursing practice.
1. Nurses with a master's degree assume the role of clinical expert and are able to create a climate in which research-based change can be implemented into practice.
3. Doctorally prepared nurses are prepared to design studies independently including the development of methods of inquiry relevant to nursing.
4. Doctorally prepared nurses are responsible for acquiring funding for research from public and private sources.

4. 4, p. 82
Rationale:
4. As a component of informed consent, research subjects are given full and complete information about the purpose of the study, procedures, data collection, potential harm and benefits, and alternative methods of treatment.
1. In the case of research, institutions have Health Information Portability and Privacy Act (HIPAA) regulations that identify how protected health information of research subjects is to be managed. The nurse researcher who follows HIPAA guidelines is following the principle of protection of subjects.
2. Research aspects such as minimizing the risk to participants, allowing reasonable risk to participants in relation to anticipated benefits, and monitoring the research to ensure the safety of participants follows the ethical standard of freedom from harm.

3. Confidentiality guarantees that any information provided by the subject will not be reported in any manner that identifies the subject and will not be made accessible to people outside the research team. Describing how confidentiality is maintained is a component of informed consent.

5. 2, p. 82
Rationale:
2. Using data obtained before the initiation of the study would be a breach of privacy because the participant has not yet given informed consent for use of those data.
1. Within the consent document, the researcher must outline alternative methods of treatment and alternatives to participation, including the right to withdraw from the study at any given time.
3. One component of informed consent is the inclusion of informing the research subject of the potential harm and benefits. This would include the risks to the subject (including financial risks) and the potential for no benefit.
4. Adhering to verbal and written agreements is central to informed consent and the implementation of ethical research.

6. 4, p. 84
Rationale:
4. The Methods section of a study includes the description of the sample (what or who was studied), type of data collected, and the device or instrument used to measure empirical information.
1. The Introduction section presents the purpose, a summary of literature used to formulate the study, and the hypothesis tested or the research questions posed.
2. The Conclusion consists of the author summarizing implications that can be drawn from the study.
3. The Results section contains a description of the results obtained in the study, including appropriate statistical tests used to analyze the data.

7. 2, p. 80
Rationale:
2. After identifying the problem, the next step in the research process is to review the literature to determine what is known about the problem.
1. After identification of the problem and review of the literature, the researcher will design the study protocol. Selecting the population is a component of this phase of the research process.
3. Identifying the instrument to use for data analysis occurs during the process of designing the study protocol. This step would occur during the study design phase of the research process after problem identification and literature review has taken place.
4. Obtaining necessary approvals is part of conducting the study, which follows the design phase in the research process.

8. 3, p. 77
Rationale:
3. Correlational research explores the interrelations among variables of interest (such as factors affecting client comfort) without any active intervention by the researcher.
1. Historical research is designed to establish facts and relations concerning past events. It would not use prospective groups of clients.
2. In experimental research, the investigator controls the study variable and randomly assigns subjects to different conditions.
4. Evaluation research tests how well a program, practice, or policy is working.

9. 2, p. 77
Rationale:
2. In experimental research, the investigator controls the study variable (use of humor) and randomly assigns subjects to different conditions (those who receive humor as an intervention, and those who do not).

1. The effects of therapeutic touch on a geriatric client with Alzheimer's disease lends itself to the nursing process as a nursing intervention, perhaps to assist a client in meeting a goal of preventing social isolation. To use the experimental research process, other clients would have to be involved (i.e., a group of clients with Alzheimer's disease who receive therapeutic touch, and a group of clients with Alzheimer's disease who do not receive therapeutic touch to determine whether therapeutic touch had any effect).

3. Determining the blood-pressure patterns of a client who recently had a cerebrovascular accident is a part of the assessment phase of the nursing process. No variable is being controlled by the nurse, as would be in an experimental research study.

4. Setting priorities in nursing diagnosis for client care is an example of using the nursing process.

10. 4, p. 76
Rationale:
4. Trying various ways of resolving client's health care needs or evaluating health care products, as in trying different types of colostomy dressings for maximal effect, is an example of the problem-solving strategy for knowledge acquisition.

1. Practicing skills is an example of gaining experience to increase one's knowledge.

2. Information seeking is a strategy used to obtain knowledge from experts in a particular field.

3. Reviewing Maslow's hierarchy in a reference textbook or on the Internet is another example of acquiring knowledge through information seeking.

11. 2, p. 84
Rationale:
2. A description of the clients used is found in the Methods section of the research study.

1. The introductory section presents the purpose of the study, a summary of literature, and the hypotheses tested or questions posed.

3. The Results section contains a description of the results obtained in the study, including appropriate statistical tests used to analyze the data.

4. The Discussion section presents the author's interpretation of the results, including conclusions and implications that can be drawn form the study.

12. 4, p. 84
Rationale:
4. Determination of whether the subjects and environment in the study are similar to the clients for whom the nurse provides care in the particular practice setting is necessary before research can be considered for use in practice.

1. Even though research may indicate that ethical principles were maintained, it does not necessarily mean that it is feasible to apply the findings in practice. For example, cost issues may limit the use of research findings.

2. Although cost may be a consideration in determining the feasibility of applying research findings, it is not the priority consideration for research use. The research findings would first have to be applicable to the practice setting and client population.

3. The number of journals that published the research results of the study should not be the priority consideration in implementation of its findings. To judge the scientific worth of the study, however, it is important to examine the amount of supportive evidence provided by other scientific studies that have obtained similar results.

13. 1, p. 79
Rationale:
1. This question is an example of a predictive type of question because it connects stress reduction with the use of guided imagery.

2. This question does not predict any outcome, but rather focuses on frequency of a response, which could be used in data collection.

3. This question does not predict any type of outcome, but rather explores meaning to gain understanding.

4. This question explores factors that affect a phenomenon. It is not a predictive type of question.

Chapter 6

1. 3, p. 91
Rationale:
3. When formulating a definition of "health," a person should consider the total person, as well as the environment in which the person lives. Health generally implies a state of well-being, which is ultimately defined in terms of the individual.
1. Health is considered to be more than merely the absence of disease.
2. The definition of health has broadened beyond the physiological state to include mental, social, and spiritual well-being.
4. An individual who has the ability to pursue activities of daily living may not define himself or herself as being healthy. Life conditions such as environment, diet, and lifestyle practices may negatively affect one's health long before one is unable to perform activities of daily living.

2. 2, p. 91
Rationale:
2. Two overarching goals for *Healthy People 2010* are (1) to increase quality and years of healthy life, and (2) to eliminate health disparities.
1. Reducing health care costs was not a goal for *Healthy People 2010*.
3. Investigation of substance abuse was not one of the main, overarching goals for *Healthy People 2010*.
4. Determining acceptable morbidity rates was not one of the main, overarching goals for *Healthy People 2010*.

3. 4, p. 96
Rationale:
4. Using a holistic approach involves consideration of all factors that may affect a client's level of well-being in all dimensions, not just physical health. Factors such as diet and exercise can influence one's level of health.
1. Directing the client in exercise does not address the many factors that may affect one's level of health. This response does not facilitate the client's seeing the connection between lifestyle choices and well-being.

2. Directing the client to follow physician's orders, although important, does not describe a holistic approach of nursing care. A holistic approach may include a discussion of diet and exercise and the effect these factors have on blood glucose. The aim is for the client to take responsibility for his or her health and choices that may affect health.
3. Viewing laboratory test results is a part of nursing assessment. To approach the client holistically, the nurse would need also to assess the client's diet and activity level.

4. 1, p. 97
Rationale:
1. Risk factors are anything that increases the vulnerability of an individual or group to an illness or accident. This client is identifying the physical risk factor of genetic predisposition to heart disease.
2. An example of an active strategy would be weight reduction or smoking cessation where the client is actively involved in measures to improve present and future levels of wellness.
3. A negative health behavior is a behavior that may negatively affect one's health. An example of a negative health behavior would be consistently drinking alcohol in excess.
4. Health beliefs are a person's ideas, convictions, and attitudes about health and illness. An example of a health belief would be the client statement, "Heart disease runs in our family. I know I will have heart disease anyway, so why exercise?"

5. 1, p. 100
Rationale:
1. During the contemplation stage, the client is considering a change within the next 6 months. The client may be ambivalent initially, but will more likely accept information as more belief develops in the value of change.
2. During the preparation stage, the client is making small changes in preparation for a change in the next month. At this point, the client believes advantages outweigh disadvantages in behavior change.
3. During the active stage, the client is actively engaged in strategies to change behavior.

414   Test Bank Answer Key

4. During the maintenance stage, the client has sustained change over time.

6. 4, p. 95
Rationale:
4. External variables influencing a person's health beliefs and practices include family practices, cultural background, and socioeconomic factors, such as income. Economic variables may affect a client's level of health by increasing the risk for disease and influencing how or at what point the client enters the health care system. A person's compliance with the treatment to maintain or improve health also is affected by economic status.
1. Religious practices are one way in which people exercise spirituality. Spirituality is considered to be an internal variable.
2. An example of an internal variable that can influence health beliefs and practices of a client includes emotional factors, such as the reaction to heart disease.
3. Educational background is an internal variable that can influence the health beliefs and practices of a client.

7. 2, p. 98
Rationale:
2. The secondary prevention level focuses on early diagnosis and prompt treatment as well as on disability limitations. Adequate treatment for the electrolyte imbalance is sought to prevent further complications.
1. The primary prevention level focuses on health promotion and specific protection measures such as immunizations and personal hygiene.
3. The tertiary prevention level focuses on restoration and rehabilitation.
4. Health promotion is a focus of the primary prevention level.

8. 4, pp. 97, 98
Rationale:
4. Tertiary prevention occurs when a defect or disability is permanent and irreversible. Care of the hospice nurse at this level aims to help the client and the client's family achieve as high a level of functioning as possible, despite the limitations caused by the cancer.

1. Teaching a client how to irrigate a new colostomy would be an example of secondary prevention. If the colostomy is to be permanent, care may later move to the tertiary level of prevention.
2. Providing a class on hygiene for an elementary school class would be an example of the primary level of prevention.
3. Informing a client about available immunizations would be an example of primary prevention.

9. 2, p. 99
Rationale:
2. Excessive sunbathing is a lifestyle risk factor for skin cancer.
1. Obesity is a physiological risk factor.
3. Overcrowded housing is an environmental risk factor.
4. An industrial-based occupation is an environmental risk factor.

10. 3, pp. 91, 92
Rationale:
3. In the Health Belief Model, the nurse focuses on the relation between a person's beliefs and health behaviors. By focusing on the client's perceptions of health, the nurse is better able to understand and predict how a client will comply with health care therapies.
1. Basic human need for survival is a component of Maslow's hierarchy of needs model.
2. The nurse who focuses on the functioning of the individual in all dimensions is following a holistic health model.
4. In the health promotion model, the nurse focuses on the multidimensional nature of clients and their interaction with the environment.

11. 3, p. 103
Rationale:
3. The effects of illness on the client and family have created change in family dynamics. Family dynamics is the process by which the family functions, makes decisions, gives support to individual members, and copes with everyday changes and challenges.

1. Body image is the subjective concept of physical appearance. The client did not express concerns regarding body image.
2. Illness behavior refers to how people monitor their bodies, define and interpret their symptoms, take remedial actions, and use the health care system. The client did not express change in illness behavior.
4. Self-concept is a mental self-image of strengths and weaknesses in all aspects of personality. The client did not express a change in self-concept.

12. 1, pp. 95, 102
Rationale:
1. Emotional factors, such as the client's degree of anxiety, are internal variables that can influence the client's health status.
2. An example of an external variable that can influence the client's health status is the use of family remedies.
3. Socioeconomic factors, such as location and type of occupation, are external variables that can influence the client's health status.
4. Socioeconomic factors, including available health insurance coverage, are examples of external variables that can influence the client's health status.

Chapter 7

1. 1, p. 111
Rationale:
1. Acquiring assistance from a staff member before performing a new procedure demonstrates caring behavior toward a client. If the graduate nurse has the assistance of someone who is skilled in the procedure, the client will be less likely to experience anxiety, and the procedure will likely be completed quicker.
2. Performing new treatments as quickly as possible may convey a message that the nurse does not have time for the client, or does not value the client as a person.
3. Being honest is important, but informing clients of a lack of experience may only increase the client's level of anxiety.

4. Avoiding uncomfortable situations does not demonstrate caring behavior toward the client. In contrast, it demonstrates detachment and a lack of commitment on the part of the nurse.

2. 4, p. 108
Rationale:
4. According to Benner, caring means that persons, events, projects, and things matter to people.
1. According to Leininger, caring is the central, unifying, and dominant domain distinguishing nursing from other health disciplines and is necessary for the health and survival of all individuals.
2. Watson defines caring as a new consciousness and moral idea.
3. Swanson defines caring as a nurturing way of relating to a valued other, toward whom one feels a personal sense of commitment and responsibility.

3. 4, p. 110
Rationale:
4. According to Swanson, enabling is defined as facilitating the other's passage through life transitions (e.g., birth, death) and unfamiliar events (e.g., self-injection of insulin).
1. Staying with the client before surgery would be an example of Swanson's "being with" in the caring process.
2. Performing a catheterization skillfully would be an example of Swanson's "doing for" in the caring process.
3. Assessing the client's health history would be an example of Swanson's "knowing" in the caring process.

4. 1, p. 111
Rationale:
1. According to Riemen, the nurse being physically present with the client provides a perception of caring, which is shared by both female and male clients.

2. Promotion of autonomy was not found to be a perception of caring behavior by female and male clients in Riemen's study. Mayer found promotion of autonomy to be identified as nursing caring behavior as perceived by families of clients with cancer.
3. Mayer found knowledge of injection technique to be perceived as a nursing caring behavior by cancer clients.
4. Speed of treatment completion was not perceived as a nursing caring behavior.

5. 1, p. 111
Rationale:
1. Nurses must focus on building a relationship that allows them to learn what is important to their clients.
2. Gathering assessment data is not the most important aspect of knowing a client in relation to caring. Data gathering does not ensure that the nurse will be able to determine the client's perceptions and unique expectations. Success in knowing a client lies in the relationship that is established.
3. Treating discomforts quickly is not the most important aspect of knowing a client.
4. If a nurse is assuming the emotional needs of a client, then the nurse most likely lacks knowing of the client. It is more important to have a relationship in which the nurse can verify what emotional needs the client is experiencing. Knowing who clients are helps the nurse to select those caring approaches that are most appropriate to the client's needs.

6. 3, pp. 110, 112
Rationale:
3. When the nurse closes the door and covers the client during a bath, the nurse is displaying behaviors that make the client feel valued as a human being. The nurse is attending to the client and is preserving the client's dignity.
1. Keeping family members informed is perceived as a caring behavior by family; however, the nurse must first have the client's permission to do so.

2. Calling the client by his or her first name during an admission interview may not demonstrate caring behavior, because a caring relationship has not yet been established. The nurse would be assuming that it is acceptable to the client to call him or her by first name. The nurse should enter the relationship with respect for the client and avoid making assumptions.
4. Sharing personal information about the client with the roommate would be a breach of confidentiality.

7. 4, p. 112
Rationale:
4. Persons who do not experience care in their lives often find it difficult to act in caring ways. The nurse manager who demonstrates a gentle bath acts as a role model and conveys the value of caring. The staff member also may feel more valued because the nurse manager took the time to be with the staff member individually.
1. Telling the staff member how to give baths is less apt to change behavior. The staff member must see why it is important before he or she is likely to be motivated to change the behavior.
2. Providing the staff member with resources to read does not ensure that the staff member will read them or change the behavior.
3. Asking another staff member to provide special skin care does not address the problem of poor hygienic care by the staff member.

8. 4, p. 108
Rationale:
4. A key element of Leininger's theory is transcultural perspectives. Leininger stresses that even though human caring is a universal phenomenon, the expressions, processes, and patterns of caring vary among cultures.
1. Swanson's theory describes caring as consisting of five categories or processes.
2. Being connected with others is a key element of Benner and Wrubel's theory.
3. A key element in Watson's theory is spiritual dimensions and healing.

Test Bank Answer Key 417

Chapter 8

1. 2, p. 120

Rationale:

2. Ethnicity refers to a shared identity related to social and cultural heritage, such as values, language, geographic space, and racial characteristics. Race refers to biologic attributes.
1. A variant cultural pattern is a unique factor within a cultural group.
3. Subcultures refer to subgroups within a race.
4. Ethnocentrism is the root of biases and prejudices, comprising beliefs and attitudes associating negative permanent characteristics with people who are perceived to be different from the valued group.

2. 3, p. 132

Rationale:

3. Cultural groups consist of units of social organization delineated by kinship, status hierarchy, and appropriate roles for their members. Sensitivity to social organization is the recognition of the client's status and role in the family.
1. Sensitivity to communication patterns would be the recognition of the client's language usage.
2. Culture is the framework used in defining social phenomena, such as when a person is considered to be healthy or in need of intervention. The way an individual defines health and health practices must be understood by the nurse to best meet the needs of the client. Sensitivity to social organization is not met by recognizing the definition of health for an individual.
4. Psychological characteristics and coping mechanisms may be expressed in a variety of ways across cultures. Sensitivity to social organization is not demonstrated by the recognition of psychological characteristics and coping mechanisms of a particular culture.

3. 1, p. 123

Rationale:

1. Traditional Western medicine uses medication administration as a method of treatment.
2. Spiritual advising is not used in traditional Western medicine, but may be seen in the African-American cultural group.
3. Acupuncture is an alternative therapy often used in non-Western cultures such as the Chinese and Southeast Asians.
4. Herbal therapy is an alternative therapy often used in non-Western cultures, but not in traditional Western medicine.

4. 2, p. 132

Rationale:

2. Lactose intolerance is frequently observed among Asians, Africans, and Hispanics.
1. Hypertension is commonly seen in African Americans.
3. Aboriginal Canadians descended from Native North American Indians, and those living on reservations have a higher incidence of tuberculosis.
4. Diabetes mellitus is commonly seen among Utes, Pimas, and Papago Indians.

5. 4, p. 129

Rationale:

4. An appropriate strategy for communicating with clients who are not fluent in English is to incorporate hand gestures and pictures.
1. Speaking in a louder tone of voice will not help the client understand the English language.
2. Responding to the client by his or her first name may demonstrate a lack of respect. The nurse should introduce him or herself and then request the client to introduce him or herself.
3. An interpreter is not necessary for all communication. However, an interpreter must be used for communicating to the client information about his or her medical condition. It is not acceptable for family members to translate health care information, but they can assist with ongoing interaction during the client's care.

6. 4, p. 120
Rationale:
4. An example of an invisible (less observable) component of a culture is having a belief in supernatural influences.
1. Using cotton undergarments for clothing is a visible (easily seen) component of culture.
2. An example of a visible (easily seen) component of culture is the wearing of an amulet or charm.
3. An example of a visible (easily seen) component of culture is using prayer beads or candles.

7. 2, p. 133
Rationale:
2. Because time takes on different meanings from one culture to another, the nurse should maintain a flexible attitude and not become emotionally upset when the client requests procedures to be done at different times. When making appointments and referrals, anticipated barriers to time adherence should be explored and managed with the client.
1. For organizational purposes, nurses should seek clients' input, and together the nurse and client may set a time to do procedures.
3. Although the client's input should be sought, it is not realistic to have the clients set their own times for nursing care activities regardless of the schedule. Some procedures may be required more frequently than the client would set, or the nurse may be unable to meet the needs of several clients on the unit at the same time.
4. Maintaining set times for treatments and informing the client of the schedule does not take into consideration the client's time orientation.

8. 4, p. 119
Rationale:
4. By 2020, the population of Hispanic and Latino populations is predicted to triple.
1. Population projections beyond 2000 show the growth of Hispanics/Latinos, Asian-Americans, and African-Americans outpacing the growth of white, European-descended groups.

2. This is not a true statement. The African-American group is projected to double by 2020.
3. This is not a true statement. By 2020, the population of African-Americans is predicted to double, and that of Asian-Americans and Hispanics/Latinos, to triple.

9. 4, p. 120
Rationale:
4. Acculturation is the process of adapting to and adopting a new culture.
1. Biculturalism occurs when an individual identifies equally with two or more cultures.
2. Assimilation occurs when an individual gives up his or her ethnic identity in favor of the dominant culture.
3. Socialization into one's primary culture as a child is known as enculturation.

10. 3, p. 127
Rationale:
3. Holding back more-potent pain medication for a client who had a minor procedure is an example of a cultural imposition of the nurse on a client.
1. Adaptation of the client's room to accommodate extra family members is not an example of cultural imposition on a client, but rather is meeting the client's need by providing culturally congruent care.
2. Seeking information on gender-congruent care for an Egyptian client is an example of the desire to provide culturally congruent care.
4. Encouraging family to assist with the client's care is not an example of cultural imposition on a client. Western culture tends to follow a pattern of caring that focuses on self-care and self-determination, whereas non-Western cultures typically have care provided by others.

11. 2, p. 123
Rationale:
2. Non-Western cultures rely on family members to provide care.
1. This is unlikely, as non-Western cultures depend on family members.

Test Bank Answer Key   419

3. Self-care is a caring pattern of Western cultures. The client's behavior is more likely a result of her cultural background rather than of a lack of motivation.
4. The client's behavior is not indicative of denial of traditional treatment, but rather it is indicative of her culture.

12. 3, pp. 123, 124
Rationale:
3. Rather than dismissing the practice as dangerous and incompatible with Western medicine, practitioners should investigate further whether the practice needs changing.
1. The nurse may be making a false statement. Consultation and collaboration with herbalists can prevent unwarranted distress for the client and nurse.
2. Asking the client why additional remedies are being used may make the client feel defensive. The nurse must first determine what herbs are being used.
4. Contacting the physician is not the first action to be taken by the nurse. The nurse should initially determine what herbs are being used and their effectiveness.

13. 3, p. 125
Rationale:
3. Modesty is a strong value among Afghan and Arab women.
1. Modesty is not an especially important issue for African-American women.
2. Modesty is not an especially important issue for Native American women.
4. Modesty is not an especially important issue for Filipino women.

14. 1, p. 125
Rationale:
1. Religious beliefs may prohibit the presence of males, including husbands, from the delivery room. This may be observed among devout Muslims, Hindus, and Orthodox Jews.
2. Hispanic men typically do not have religious or cultural beliefs that would prohibit them from the delivery room.

3. Korean men typically do not have religious o cultural beliefs that would prohibit them from the delivery room.
4. Catholic men typically do not have religiou or cultural beliefs that would prohibit then from the delivery room.

15. 4, p. 124
Rationale:
4. The nurse should first determine if it is per missible for the item to remain in place dur ing the procedure.
1. Removing the bracelet may create unneces sary stress for the client.
2. Taping the bracelet in place may be appropri ate after the nurse determines that the item may remain in place during the procedure.
3. Asking the client to remove the item may cre ate unnecessary stress for the client.

16. 4, p. 127
Rationale:
4. Some Buddhists may refuse to move the dead body after death because of their belief tha the spirit of the dead takes some time to leave the body. They define death as the absence o consciousness and loss of body warmth.
1. Among Orthodox Jews, the dead person i generally buried before sundown.
2. Some Asian Indians regard seeing the deceased as adding to the suffering of the fam ily. Hindus and Buddhists believe that the soul lives on and that the dead body withou the soul is but an empty shell, and therefore may not want to see the body.
3. Muslims prefer burial rather than cremation.

17. 2, p. 132
Rationale:
2. Malignant hypertension is found more fre quently in African-Americans.
1. Native Americans have a higher incidence o tuberculosis and diabetes mellitus.
3. Hispanics have a higher incidence of lactos intolerance.
4. Lactose intolerance also is frequently observed among Asians.

18. 4, p. 123
Rationale:
4. The overall treatment in Western culture is specialty specific.
1. Some non-Western cultures use a naturalistic approach for the method of diagnosis.
2. The treatment in some non-Western cultures is herbal.
3. The treatment in non-Western cultures is holistic in nature.

19. 4, p. 133
Rationale:
4. Jewish clients who follow a kosher diet will avoid meat from carnivores, pork products, and fish without scales or fins. Therefore shellfish should not be included in the menu of a client who is an Orthodox Jew and maintains a kosher diet.
1. Beef may be included in a kosher diet.
2. Eggs may be included in a kosher diet.
3. Milk may be included in a kosher diet.

20. 4, p. 132
Rationale:
4. Many Buddhists are vegetarians. The nurse should ensure that a sufficient quantity of vegetables is included in the menu when caring for a Buddhist who maintains a traditional diet.
1. Beef is not a traditional component of a Buddhist's diet.
2. A sufficient quantity of milk is not necessary for the traditional Buddhist's diet.
3. A sufficient quantity of fish is not necessary for the traditional Buddhist's diet.

Chapter 9

1. 4, p. 141
Rationale:
4. The number of people living alone is expanding rapidly and represents approximately 26% of all households.
1. People are marrying later, not earlier.
2. The rate of divorce appears to have stabilized, with approximately 55% of marriages ending in divorce.
3. Couples are choosing to have fewer children or none at all.

2. 1, p. 142
Rationale:
1. Homelessness is identified as one of the greatest health care challenges to nurses.
2. The trend of single-parent families is not the greatest current health care challenge to nurses.
3. The trend of a "sandwiched" or middle generation is not the greatest current health care challenge to nurses.
4. The trend of alternate relationship patterns is not the greatest current health care challenge to nurses.

3. 2, p. 142
Rationale:
2. When the nurse views the family as context, the primary focus is on the health and development of an individual member existing within the client's family. The client's ability to understand and manage his or her own dietary needs is an example of viewing the family as context.
1. The family's ability to support the client's dietary and recreational needs is an example of viewing the family as client.
3. The family's demands on the client based on his or her role performance is an example of viewing the family as client.
4. The adjustment of the client and family to changes in diet and exercise is an example of viewing the family as system.

4. 3, pp. 146-147
Rationale:
3. A healthy family has a flexible structure that allows adaptable performance of tasks and acceptance of help from outside the family system. The structure is flexible enough to allow adaptability but not so flexible that the family lacks cohesiveness and a sense of stability.
1. The healthy family is able to integrate the need for stability with the need for growth and change. It does not view change as detrimental to family processes.
2. The healthy family demonstrates control over the environment and does not passively respond to stressors.

4. The healthy family exerts influence on the immediate environment of home, neighborhood, and school.

5. 4, p. 148
Rationale:
4. The nurse begins the family assessment by determining the client's definition of and attitude toward family and the extent to which the family can be incorporated into nursing care. The nurse also assesses family form and membership.
1. Gathering health data from the family members is not the starting point for a family assessment.
2. Testing a family's ability to cope is not where the nurse should begin a family assessment.
3. Evaluating communication barriers would not be an initial action of the nurse when completing a client's family assessment.

6. 4, p. 150
Rationale:
4. When implementing family-centered care, the nurse adopts the role of educator and offers information about necessary self-care abilities.
1. In family-centered care, the nurse guides the family in problem solving without providing his or her own beliefs.
2. In family-centered care, the nurse assists clients to assume independent roles by increasing family members' abilities in certain areas.
3. In family-centered care, the nurse guides the family in problem solving, not in helping them to accept blame.

7. 3, p. 150
Rationale:
3. The nurse should first find out if anyone else in the family or neighborhood would or could assist with the colostomy care.
1. Informing the client that management of the colostomy must be learned will not change the fact that the client has arthritis and needs assistance.

2. The nurse should first determine whether someone else could perform the task. If not, the nurse arranges for a home care service referral.
4. A colostomy self-help support group may provide emotional support but will not meet the client's need for assistance with colostomy care.

8. 1, pp. 145, 146
Rationale:
1. The optimal goal of effective communication within the family is to be able to problem solve and provide psychological support for its members.
2. Role development is not the optimal goal of effective communication within the family.
3. Socialization among individual family members is not the optimal goal of effective communication within the family.
4. Improving financial conditions for the family is not the optimal goal of effective communication within the family.

9. 4, p. 142
Rationale:
4. It is true that social support systems for the elderly are likely to be different from those for clients in younger age groups.
1. Members of later-life families must be working on developmental tasks.
2. Caregivers for the elderly are usually either spouses or middle-aged children.
3. Accepting shifting of generational roles is often difficult for the elderly client.

10. 1, p. 148
Rationale:
1. Asking, "Who decides where to go on vacation?" enables the nurse to determine the power structure and patterning of roles and tasks of the family.
2. This question does not assess the roles and power structure of the family.
3. This question may be used to help determine family form, not the power structure and roles of the family.

4. This question may provide information on the interactive processes of the family and how time is spent, but does not assess the roles and power structure of the family.

11. 1, p. 142
Rationale:
1. The nurse must consider caregiver strain and work with the family on delegating responsibility.
2. Nursing home placement should not be the nurse's initial response to caregiver strain.
3. Arranging for the client to remain in the medical center is not always feasible and does not address the problem of caregiver strain. It should not be the nurse's initial response in this situation.
4. The nurse should not make decisions for the family, but rather work with the family to problem solve.

12. 2, p. 143
Rationale:
2. In recognition of the pattern of family violence, the nurse knows that spouses are the most frequent abusers.
1. Emotional, physical, and sexual abuse occurs across all social classes.
3. Child abuse is increasing, not decreasing.
4. Mental illness may increase the incidence of abuse within a family but is not a major cause of abuse.

Chapter 10

1. 1, p. 166
Rationale:
1. Kohlberg developed a theory on moral development.
2. Gould developed a theory on psychosocial development.
3. Freud developed a theory on psychosexual development.
4. Erikson developed a theory on psychosocial development.

2. 2, p. 161
Rationale:
2. According to Erikson, the young adult is in the intimacy versus isolation stage of development. This is the time in which the young adult can become fully participative in the community, enjoying adult freedom and responsibility.
1. Coping with physical and social losses is found in Erikson's integrity versus despair stage (old age) of development.
3. Applying themselves to learning productive skills is consistent behavior found in Erikson's industry versus inferiority stage (age 6 to 11 years) of development.
4. According to Erikson, overcoming a sense of guilt or frustration is in the initiative versus guilt stage (age 3 to 6 years) of development.

3. 4, p. 159
Rationale:
4. Freud's theory of personality development approaches development by looking at psychosexual aspects.
1. Piaget's theory approaches development by looking at cognitive development.
2. Kohlberg's theory approaches development by looking at moral reasoning.
3. Gould's theory approaches development by looking at logical maturity.

4. 2, pp. 164, 165
Rationale:
2. According to Piaget, the preoperational child (age 2 to 7 years) is learning to think with the use of symbols and mental images.
1. According to Piaget, the child explores the environment in the sensorimotor stage (birth to 2 years) of cognitive development.
3. Cooperation and sharing are seen in Piaget's concrete operations (age 7 to 11 years) stage of cognitive development.
4. Organization of thoughts and far-reaching problem solving are noted in Piaget's formal operations (age 11 years to adulthood) stage of cognitive development.

5. 4, p. 163

Rationale:

4. A common behavioral task of the older adult client is adjusting to decreasing physical strength.

1. Selecting a mate is a developmental task commonly seen in the early adult.

2. Rearing children is a developmental task of the middle-early adult.

3. Finding a congenial social group is a developmental task of the middle-early adult.

6. 1, p. 162

Rationale:

1. Gould's theory of psychosocial development specifically focuses on the adult years.

2. Piaget's theory focused on cognitive development throughout the life span.

3. Freud's psychosexual theory focused on personality development throughout the life span.

4. Chess and Thomas' theory focused on development from childhood to early adulthood.

7. 3, pp. 156, 157

Rationale:

3. "Developmental tasks are age-related achievements" is a correct statement about growth and development.

1. Human growth and development are orderly, predictable processes beginning with conception and continuing until death.

2. Growth refers to quantitative events. Development refers to qualitative events.

4. Cognitive theories focus on reasoning and thinking processes.

8. 3, p. 166

Rationale:

3. At Level II, Conventional Thought, the person sees moral reasoning based on his or her own personal internalization of societal and others' expectations.

1. In Stage 1, the child's response to a moral dilemma is in terms of absolute obedience to authority and rules.

2. At Level I, Preconventional Thought, the person reflects on moral reasoning based on personal gain.

4. In Stage 6, according to Kohlberg, a person has self-chosen ethical principles, universality, and impartiality.

9. 1, p. 164

Rationale:

1. According to Piaget, the infant is in the first period of development, which is characterized by sensorimotor intelligence.

2. According to Piaget, children aged 7 to 11 years are in the concrete operations period of development, which is characterized by having the ability to perform mental operations.

3. Identity versus role confusion is a developmental stage (puberty) according to Erikson.

4. According to Piaget, children aged 2 to 7 years are in the preoperational period of development, which is characterized by the child learning to think with the use of symbols and mental images.

10. 3, p. 165

Rationale:

3. During Piaget's concrete operations stage of cognitive development, the child is able to understand that objects or quantities remain the same despite a change in their physical appearance, such as when ice becomes water.

1. During Piaget's sensorimotor stage of cognitive development, the child is exploring the environment but is unable to understand the concept of ice becoming water.

2. During Piaget's preoperational stage of cognitive development, the child is learning to think with the use of symbols and mental images but is not able to understand the concept of ice becoming water.

4. According to Piaget's formal operations stage of cognitive development, the individual's thinking moves to abstract and theoretical subjects.

11. 1, p. 166
Rationale:
1. According to Kohlberg's developmental theory of moral development, at Level I, the Preconventional Level, the child's reasoning is based on personal gain. The moral reason for acting relates to the consequences the person believes will occur. The child who makes sure not to be late for school may do so out of fear of punishment.
2. Cleaning the blackboards after school for the teacher is an example of Kohlberg's Stage 3, Good Boy–Nice Girl Orientation. The child desires to win the teacher's approval.
3. Running for school council to change policies is an example of Kohlberg's Stage 5, Social Contract Orientation.
4. Staying away from school gangs that harass other children is an example of Kohlberg's Stage 4, Society-Maintaining Orientation.

12. 4, p. 163
Rationale:
4. During the fifth theme (50s), Gould finds a realization of mortality with a concern for one's state of health.
1. During the first theme (20s), Gould finds individuals wanting to get away from their parents.
2. During the second theme (30s), Gould finds young adults working to accept who they are and to accept their growing children as being unique and separate.
3. During the fourth theme (40s), Gould finds resignation and the belief that possibilities are limited.

13. 1, p. 159
Rationale:
1. According to Freud, disruption in the physical or emotional availability of the parent for the newborn (e.g., undergoing surgery) will affect the oral stage of development.
2. According to Freud, the anal stage is 12 to 18 months to 3 years, when the child is indergoing toilet training.
3. According to Freud, the phallic stage is from ages 3 to 6 years, when the child becomes interested in the genital organs.

4. According to Freud, the latent stage is from ages 6 to 12 years, when the child represses sexual urges and channels them into productive activities that are socially acceptable.

14. 4, p. 161
Rationale:
4. In accordance with Erikson's theory, the middle adult client is involved in the process of expanding personal and social involvement. Middle-aged adults should be able to see beyond their needs and accomplishments to the needs of society.
1. Developing a sense of identity is in accordance with Erikson's identity versus role confusion (puberty) stage of development.
2. Searching for meaning in life is in accordance with Erikson's integrity versus despair (old age) stage of development.
3. Enhancing one's capability to love others is in accordance with Erikson's intimacy versus isolation (young adult) stage of development.

Chapter 11

1. 1, p. 175
Rationale:
1. During the second trimester, between 16 and 20 weeks' gestation, the mother begins to feel fetal movement.
2. During the second trimester, the uterus should be above the level of the symphysis pubis.
3. Confirmation of the desire to breast- or bottle-feed is more likely to take place during the third trimester.
4. Morning sickness is most likely to occur during the first trimester.

2. 1, p. 178
Rationale:
1. The Babinski reflex is a normal reflex found in a 6-month-old infant.
2. Before age 6 months, the extrusion reflex causes food to be pushed out of the mouth. It is normally present from birth to 4 months.
3. The startle reflex is seen in the newborn.
4. The Moro reflex is seen in the newborn.

3. 1, p. 180
Rationale:
1. Height increases an average of 1 inch during each of the first 6 months and 1/2 inch during the next 6 months.
2. The anterior fontanel closes at about 12 to 18 months.
3. The head and chest circumference are equal at age 1 year.
4. Birth weight doubles in approximately 5 months and triples by 12 months.

4. 3, p. 183
Rationale:
3. A 6-month-old infant is able to roll over.
1. A 9-month-old infant is able to attain a sitting position independently.
2. A 9-month-old infant is able to pull self to a standing position.
4. A 9-month-old infant is able to creep on all four extremities.

5. 1, p. 190
Rationale:
1. A 2-year-old child uses short sentences to express independence and control.
2. The 2-year-old may engage in solitary play and begin to participate in parallel play. The preschool child may initiate play with other children.
3. A 2-year-old child does not understand the concepts of right and wrong.
4. A 2-year-old child has a vocabulary of up to 300 words.

6. 2, p. 190
Rationale:
2. During toddlerhood, the child begins to participate in parallel play, which is playing beside rather than with another child.
1. The preschool child may have imaginary playmates.
3. Peer pressure is seen with the school-age child.
4. A fear of the preschool child is bodily harm.

7. 3, p. 194
Rationale:
3. Preschool children may cooperate if they are allowed to manipulate the equipment.
1. A preschool child is unable to take responsibility for his or her own preoperative hygienic care.
2. Leaving the preschooler alone may increase the child's anxiety.
4. Magazines and puzzles would be more appropriate activities for the older child. The preschool child likes to engage in pretend play by using the imagination and imitating adult behavior.

8. 2, p. 194
Rationale:
2. During times of stress or illness, preschoolers may revert to bed-wetting or thumb-sucking and want the parent to feed, dress, and hold them. Reassuring the parent that this is normal coping behavior may help alleviate their concern.
1. Disciplining the child would not be a correct response. The child should be provided with experiences he or she can master. Such successes help the child to return to the prior level of independent functioning
3. Reverting to a prior level of functioning, such as a child who was potty trained now refusing to use the toilet, does not indicate the child was unready to be potty trained. The behavior more likely demonstrates that the child is experiencing stress, and this is a coping behavior.
4. Reverting to a prior level of functioning, such as a child who was potty trained now refusing to use the toilet, does not indicate the child is feeling neglected. The behavior demonstrates that the child is experiencing stress, and this is a coping behavior.

9. 3, pp. 193, 194
Rationale:
3. This response by the nurse informs the child what he or she can do, and involves an age-appropriate familiar toy to provide comfort.
1. Telling the child not to move when in pain is unlikely to be effective. A preschool child may have difficulty in understanding the request.

2. Telling the child he or she is going to get a shot may increase the anxiety, as the child fears bodily harm.
4. It would not be appropriate to give a child a needle. Instead, the child could hold a cotton ball or band-aid, or manipulate play medical equipment. If a child is allowed to determine the site for administration of an injection, specific sites should be offered as choices. However, the nurse must avoid allowing procrastination by the child.

10. 4, p. 183
Rationale:
4. Bibs should be removed at bedtime to avoid suffocation.
1. Placing gates or fences at stairways is an appropriate safety measure to prevent falls of the 8- to 12-month-old infant.
2. Keeping bathroom doors closed is an appropriate safety measure to prevent drowning of the 8- to 12-month-old infant.
3. Caution should be exercised when giving teething biscuits to a 4- to 7-month-old infant because large chunks may be broken off and aspirated. Teething biscuits are typically not given to a 3-month-old.

11. 2, p. 181
Rationale:
2. Two- and 3-month-old infants begin to smile responsively rather than reflexively.
1. By age 1 year, infants have two- or three-word vocabularies such as Da-da.
3. By 8 months, most infants can differentiate a stranger from a familiar person.
4. By 9 months, infants play simple social games such as patty-cake and peekaboo.

12. 1, p. 174
Rationale:
1. During the first trimester of pregnancy, the organ systems are beginning to develop.
2. During the second trimester of pregnancy, fingers and toes are differentiated.
3. During the second trimester of pregnancy, the sex of the fetus can be determined.
4. During the second trimester of pregnancy, fine hair, called lanugo, covers most of the body of the fetus.

13. 4, p. 204
Rationale:
4. Plain popcorn, fresh fruit, raw vegetables, cheese, skim-milk pudding, and hot chocolate are appropriate after-school snacks.
1. Candy bars should be discouraged as a snack because they are high in fat and calories, are low in nutrition, and are cariogenic.
2. Thick milk shakes would be high in fat and calories; better food choices are available for after-school snacks.
3. Potato chips should be discouraged as a snack because they are high in fat and low in nutritional value.

14. 1, p. 198
Rationale:
1. During the school-aged years, the child will grow an average of 1 to 2 inches per year.
2. During the school-aged years, the child will gain an average of 4 to 7 pounds a year. Many children double, not triple, their weight during these middle childhood years.
3. Growth accelerates at different times for different children. Many physical differences are apparent among children at the end of middle childhood.
4. The school-age child appears slimmer as a result of changes in fat distribution and thickness.

15. 1, p. 198
Rationale:
1. Providing a 6-year-old with crayons and a book to color in would be an age-appropriate activity to help the child with the crisis of hospitalization. Painting, drawing, playing computer games, and modeling allow children to practice and improve newly refined skills.
2. A 1000-piece puzzle would be too much for a 6-year-old to complete.
3. A cassette player with soothing tapes would not be an age-appropriate activity for a 6-year-old.
4. Throwing a nerf football around the room may not be appropriate for a hospitalized child with asthma.

16. 4, p. 205

Rationale:

4. The preadolescence developmental stage (puberty) signals the development of secondary sex characteristics.

1. Physical changes often begin 2 years earlier in girls than in boys.

2. Preadolescents usually develop "best friends" with whom they share intimate feelings.

3. New interest in the opposite sex develops in the preadolescence developmental stage.

17. 4, p. 210

Rationale:

4. A warning sign that a teenager is considering suicide includes verbalization of suicidal thoughts.

1. Appetite disturbances, usually a decrease in appetite, may be a warning sign that a teenager is considering suicide.

2. A decrease in school performance and loss of initiative are possible warning signs that a teenager is considering suicide.

3. Sleep disturbances, such as the inability to sleep, are a warning sign for suicide.

18. 3, p. 211

Rationale:

3. The nurse can be proactive by using the interview process and open-ended questions, such as this one, to identify risk factors in the adolescent. Once identified, the risk factors should lead to strategies for prevention.

1. This question does not obtain the most information.

2. This question does not address the individual and does not obtain the most information about the health behaviors of the client.

4. This question may be answered with a "yes" or "no" response and therefore does not obtain the most information.

19. 2, p. 176

Rationale:

2. Heart rate is scored as 1; respiratory effort, 1; muscle tone, 1; reflex irritability, 2; and color, 1; for a total Apgar score of 6.

1. The neonate's Apgar score is not 4.

3. The neonate's Apgar score is not 8.

4. The neonate's Apgar score is not 10.

20. 1, p. 177

Rationale:

1. The expected values for the newborn's vital signs are heart rate, 120 to 160 beats per minute; blood pressure, 74/46 mm Hg; and respiratory rate, 30 to 50 breaths per minute. This option demonstrates values within the normal range.

2. In this option, the heart rate and respiratory rates are too low, and the blood pressure is too high for a newborn. These would be normal vital signs for a toddler.

3. In this option, the heart rate and respiratory rate are too low, and the blood pressure is too high for a newborn. These vital signs are more consistent with the normal range for a preschooler.

4. In this option, the heart rate and respiratory rate are too low, and the blood pressure is too high for a newborn. These vital signs are more consistent with the normal findings for a school-age child.

21. 4, p. 174

Rationale:

4. Foods rich in folic acid include green leafy vegetables, liver, kidney, and asparagus. More limited amounts may be found in milk, poultry, and eggs.

1. Ice cream is not a rich source of folic acid but does provide calcium.

2. Beef is not a rich source of folic acid but does provide protein.

3. Orange juice is not a rich source of folic acid but does provide vitamin C.

22. 3, p. 177

Rationale:

3. To reduce the newborn's loss of heat through evaporation, the nurse should immediately dry the newborn after delivery and wrap the baby in a blanket.

1. To reduce the newborn's loss of heat through radiation, the nurse should use a radiant warmer until the newborn's temperature stabilizes.

2. To reduce the newborn's loss of heat through conduction, the nurse should warm objects that have direct contact with the newborn and cover the newborn's head.

4. Moving the newborn quickly to the nursery would not help reduce the newborn's heat loss.

23. 3, p. 181
Rationale:
3. A 12-month-old child should have the fine motor ability to place objects into a container.
1. A 9-month-old infant should have the gross motor ability to creep on all four extremities.
2. An 18-month-old child should have the gross motor ability to walk alone.
4. A 6-month-old infant should have the fine motor ability to use a palm grasp with fingers encircling an object.

24. 1, p. 199
Rationale:
1. A 6-year-old child should have the gross motor skills to hop and jump onto small squares.
2. An 8- to 10-year-old child should possess the gross motor skills to catch and throw a ball accurately.
3. An 11- to 12-year-old child should possess the gross motor skills to play ice hockey.
4. An 11- to 12-year-old child should possess the gross motor skills to perform a standing high jump of 3 feet.

25. 2, p. 185
Rationale:
2. The introduction of cereals and fruits after 6 months of life provides iron and additional sources of vitamins.
1. The introduction of solid foods is not recommended before age 6 months because the gastrointestinal tract is not sufficiently mature to handle these complex nutrients, and infants are exposed to food antigens that may produce food protein allergies.
3. Honey should not be used in infants because of the potential for infant botulism poisoning.
4. All types of cow's milk are not recommended in the first year because of the infant's decreased ability to digest the contained fat. An iron-fortified commercially prepared formula should be used instead.

26. 3, p. 193
Rationale:
3. The expected values for vital sign measurements in the preschooler are a heart rate of 60 to 100 beats per minute, a blood pressure averaging 92/56 mm Hg, and a respiratory rate of 23 to 25 breaths per minute. The vital sign measurements in this option would be within normal limits for the preschool-age child.
1. These are not normal vital sign values for a preschooler.
2. These are not expected values for a preschooler's vital signs.
4. These vital sign measurements are more consistent with those of a school-age child, not a preschooler.

Chapter 12

1. 1, p. 225
Rationale:
1. Amenorrhea and nausea are physiologic changes that may indicate pregnancy in the first trimester.
2. Braxton-Hicks contractions are noted during the second trimester of pregnancy.
3. Increased urinary frequency is commonly seen in the third trimester of pregnancy.
4. Edematous ankles and dyspnea may be experienced during the third trimester of pregnancy.

2. 4, p. 224
Rationale:
4. This could be a situational crisis for a single-parent family. The nurse should assess environmental and familial factors, including support systems and coping mechanisms commonly used.
1. Asking the client whether she has ever been married does not assess her ability to cope with the pregnancy.
2. Asking the client where she works may help determine if any environmental factors may place her pregnancy at risk but does not assess her ability to cope with the pregnancy.

3. This would not be the most opportune time to discuss contraception with the client and may convey a message of disapproval, nor does asking the client about contraception assess her ability to cope with the pregnancy.

3. 3, p. 227
Rationale:
3. A physiologic change related to normal aging in the middle adult would be decreased strength of abdominal muscles.
1. The middle adult should have normal auditory structures and acuity.
2. The middle adult should have a normal sense of smell.
4. The middle adult should have normal functioning of the cranial nerves.

4. 2, p. 230
Rationale:
2. Mood changes and depression are common phenomena during menopause, and this client is in the expected age range to be experiencing menopause.
1. Depression is not uncommon during menopause.
3. Depression is not something to expect, although it can occur.
4. Asking the client about weight loss may be an indication to verify depression; however, it is not the best initial response.

5. 3, p. 229
Rationale:
3. Exercise on a routine basis can be an effective strategy to reduce the stress experienced by young and middle adults. Exercise is a positive health habit for this age group.
1. Clients do not have to abstain from all alcohol consumption. Teaching clients to abstain from excessive alcohol consumption is important, but it is not a proactive positive health habit to help reduce stress.
2. Monitoring one's blood pressure may be important, but it is not a proactive positive health habit to help reduce stress.
4. Teaching clients about types of medication used for treating depression does not help the client develop positive health habits for reducing stress.

6. 3, p. 218
Rationale:
3. Young adults generally are quite active, experience severe illnesses less commonly than older age groups, tend to ignore physical symptoms, and often postpone seeking health care.
1. Young adults generally do not continue their physical growth.
2. Young adults experience severe illnesses less commonly than older age groups.
4. Young adults often postpone seeking health care.

7. 2, p. 222
Rationale:
2. Violence is the greatest cause of mortality and morbidity in the young adult population. Deaths and injury from motor vehicle accidents is significant among this age group.
1. Unplanned pregnancies may be a source of stress but are not the major cause of mortality and morbidity in the young adult population.
3. Exposure to work-related hazards or agent may cause diseases and cancer, but it is not the major cause of mortality and morbidity in this age group.
4. Developing healthy habits to prevent heart disease later in life is important, but heart disease is not the leading cause of mortality and morbidity for the young adult.

8. 2, p. 218
Rationale:
2. The young adult client may benefit from a personal lifestyle assessment to help identify habits that increase the risk for cardiac, malignant, pulmonary, renal, or other chronic diseases.
1. Assessing a client's marital status does not offer much information about the client's health or risk for future illnesses.
3. Assessing a client's experience with chronic disease is less appropriate for this age group.
4. Assessing the client's history of childhood accidents does not offer much information about the client's current health or risk for future illnesses.

9. 3, p. 231

Rationale:

3. A few examples of the problems experienced by clients in whom debilitating chronic illness develops during adulthood include role reversal, changes in sexual behavior, and alterations in self-image.
1. Chronic illness would result in increased health care tasks.
2. Family roles are often changed with chronic illness, not reinforced.
4. Strained family relationships may result from chronic illness.

10. 3, p. 227

Rationale:

3. A slow, progressive decrease in skin turgor appears in the middle adult.
1. Pupillary reaction to light and accommodation should not change in the middle adult.
2. The thyroid lobes should not be palpable in the middle adult.
4. A normal change in the middle adult is a decreased range of joint motion.

11. 1, p. 223

Rationale:

1. A common stressor for the young adult is job stress.
2. Health-related matters are not common stressors for the young adult.
3. Coping with cognitive changes is not a common stressor for the young adult.
4. Caring for older adult parents is more often seen with the middle adult, not the young adult.

12. 2, p. 223

Rationale:

2. Persons who work in dry-cleaning establishments are exposed to solvents that may cause dermatitis or liver disease.
1. Asbestos is more likely to be found as an occupational hazard for automobile workers and insulators.
3. Tendonitis may result from repetitive wrist motion, as seen in office computer workers.
4. Raynaud's phenomenon may result from vibration, as seen with jackhammer operators.

13. 2, p. 227

Rationale:

2. The visual acuity by Snellen chart should be less than 20/50.
1. Hepatomegaly is not an expected finding and would be considered abnormal.
3. Temperature should be 36.1 to 37.6 degrees Celsius.
4. The expected finding would be a slow, progressive decrease in skin turgor.

Chapter 13

1. 2, p. 242

Rationale:

2. A common physiologic change in the older adult client is an increased sensitivity to glare.
1. Increased tactile responsiveness would not be an expected finding in the older adult client.
3. An expected physiologic change in the older adult client is a loss of hearing acuity for high-frequency tones (presbycusis).
4. The older adult has decreased thoracic expansion during ventilation because of musculoskeletal changes.

2. 1, p. 242

Rationale:

1. Although hypertension is not a normal physiologic change of aging, older adults often experience hypertension because of vascular changes and accumulation of plaque on arterial walls, both of which reduce contractility. Vascular changes include thickening of vessel walls, narrowing of vessel lumen, and loss of vessel elasticity.
2. Hypertension is not caused by a reduction in physical activity.
3. Older adults with hypertension should be counseled on limiting fat and salt in their diets. However, ingestion of processed foods high in salt is not the reason that older clients often experience hypertension.
4. Myocardial damage is not the reason for older adults commonly experiencing hypertension.

3. 1, p. 244

Rationale:

1. Delirium is a potentially reversible cognitive impairment that is often due to a physiological cause such as an electrolyte imbalance, cerebral anoxia, hypoglycemia, medications, tumors, cerebrovascular infection, or hemorrhage.
2. Dementia is not an inevitable outcome of aging.
3. Delirium is not always easily distinguishable from irreversible dementia. Because of the close resemblance between delirium and dementia, the presence of delirium must be ruled out whenever dementia is suspected.
4. The cause of senile dementia (i.e., Alzheimer's disease) is not known. Medications and drug effects can cause delirium.

4. 1, p. 244

Rationale:

1. Alzheimer's disease usually progresses gradually, with a deterioration in function.
2. No cure is known for Alzheimer's disease, but medications can be given to slow the progression of symptoms.
3. Medications, not diet and exercise, can slow the process of Alzheimer's disease considerably.
4. Clients may live years after the diagnosis of Alzheimer's disease.

5. 4, p. 252

Rationale:

4. This is a true statement. Approximately two thirds of older adults use prescription and nonprescription drugs, with one third of all prescriptions being written for older adults.
1. Approximately 90% of adults older than 65 have at least one chronic health condition. Approximately 70% of older adults have multiple chronic conditions with arthritis, hypertension, heart disease, vision impairment, and diabetes mellitus the most common in noninstitutionalized older adults.
2. Heart disease is the leading cause of death in older adults.
3. Nutritional needs of older adults are affected by their levels of activity and by clinical conditions.

6. 4, p. 236

Rationale:

4. This is a true statement.
1. The majority of older adults live with a spouse or have other living arrangements such as living with a family member.
2. Most older adults live in noninstitutional settings.
3. Most older adults are able to care for themselves.

7. 2, p. 251

Rationale:

2. Clients in the older adult age group should be advised to exercise their joints regularly to their level of tolerance.
1. Shoulder pain is not a normal finding in the older adult. It may indicate a condition such as arthritis.
3. Periodic and thorough review of all medications being used is important to restrict the number of medications used to the fewest necessary. Concurrent use of medications increases the risk for adverse reactions.
4. Exercise programs should begin conservatively and progress slowly.

8. 2, p. 252

Rationale:

2. The nurse should encourage the older adult to question the physician and/or pharmacist about all prescribed drugs and over-the-counter drugs.
1. The older adult should be taught the names of all drugs being taken, when and how to take them, and the desirable and undesirable effects of the drugs.
3. The hepatic system is not the only system responsible for the pharmacotherapeutics of medication. Older adults are at risk for adverse reactions because of age-related changes in the absorption, distribution, metabolism, and excretion of drugs. Changes in the GI system may affect absorption, distribution may be affected by changes in body composition and by reduced serum albumin levels, and changes in kidney functioning may impair excretion.

4. The nurse should teach the client how to avoid adverse side effects and to report them to the care provider if they occur. If the client is disturbed by minor side effects, it could be an indication of beginning drug toxicity. Another possibility is that the client may become noncompliant with the medication because of dislike of how the side effects make him or her feel.

9. 3, p. 239
Rationale:
3. Some older adults may deny functional declines associated with aging and refuse to ask for assistance with tasks that place their safety at great risk.
1. Some older adults find it difficult to accept themselves as aging and attempt to conceal physical evidence of aging with cosmetics.
2. Spending more time with other older adults is indicative of the older adult's acceptance of personal aging. Those who find it difficult to accept themselves as aging may avoid activities designed to benefit older adults, such as senior citizens' centers and senior health promotion activities.
4. Older adults who find it difficult to accept themselves as aging may understate their age when asked.

10. 4, p. 242
Rationale:
4. Normal physiologic changes of aging include increased airway resistance in the older adult.
1. The older adult would be expected to have decreased perspiration and drier skin because of glandular atrophy (oil, moisture, sweat glands) in the integument system.
2. A normal physiologic change of the older adult related to hearing, is a loss of acuity for high-frequency tones (presbycusis).
3. The older adult would be expected to have a decrease in saliva.

11. 3, p. 244
Rationale:
3. Older adults who exercise regularly do not lose as much bone and muscle mass or muscle tone as do those who are inactive.

1. Postmenopausal women have a greater problem with osteoporosis than do older men.
2. Muscle fibers are reduced in size with aging.
4. Muscle strength diminishes in proportion to the decline in muscle mass.

12. 4, p. 249
Rationale:
4. The majority of older adults are interested in their health and are capable of taking charge of their lives.
1. Most older adults do not require institutional care.
2. The majority of older adults have social or family support. Most older adults live with a spouse or have other living arrangements, such as living with a family member.
3. Most older adults receive social security benefits and are able to afford medical treatment.

13. 1, p. 247
Rationale:
1. Many older adults use prescription medications that depress sexual activity such as antihypertensives, antidepressants, sedatives, or hypnotics. Some drugs increase libido in older adults. For example, phenothiazines increase sexual desire in women, and levodopa has a similar effect in men.
2. Physiological changes may have an adverse influence on sexual activity. The older man may experience decreased firmness in his erection, a decreased need for ejaculation with orgasm, or a longer recovery period between episodes of intercourse. The older woman may experience vaginal dryness.
3. It is a common misconception that older adults are not interested in sex. The older adult's libido does not decrease, although frequency of sexual activity may decline.
4. Information about the prevention of sexually transmitted diseases should be included when appropriate.

14. 4, p. 250
Rationale:
4. Good nutrition for older adults includes a limited intake of refined sugars.

1. Fiber should not be reduced, as it has benefits of aiding bowel elimination and lowering cholesterol.
2. Protein should not be reduced. Protein intake may be lower than recommended if older adults have reduced financial resources or limited access to grocery stores. Difficulty chewing meat also may limit protein intake.
3. Vitamin A does not need to be reduced in the older adult. Vitamin intake may be less than recommended if shopping for fresh fruits and vegetables is difficult.

15. 1, p. 244
Rationale:
1. Grilled chicken would be a good source of protein that is also low in fat.
2. A hamburger and French fries are high in fat content and calories, making them a less desirable food choice.
3. A hot dog with pickle relish is high in fat and sodium. Good nutrition for the older adult includes a limited intake of fat and salt.
4. A baked potato with cheese and bacon bits is higher in calories and fat. A plain baked potato would be a more healthful food choice.

16. 4, p. 245
Rationale:
4. Delirium is characterized by short, diurnal fluctuations in symptoms, worse at night, in darkness, and on awakening.
1. Delirium lasts hours to less than 1 month, seldom longer. Dementia may last months to years.
2. Delirium is characterized by fluctuating alertness; may be lethargic or hypervigilant. Alertness is generally normal with dementia.
3. Delirium has an abrupt onset. Dementia has a slow progression.

Chapter 14

1. 4, pp. 265, 273
Rationale:
4. The nurse educator is asking the student to synthesize critical thinking skills by encouraging the student to examine alternatives to meet the client's unique needs within the context of the nursing process.

1. Drawing inferences is a specific critical thinking competency used in diagnostic reasoning. The educator who tells the student not to draw inferences is not allowing the student to practice competencies necessary for specific critical thinking in clinical situations.
2. The critical thinker will look beyond a single solution to a problem.
3. Intuition develops as one's clinical experience increases. The nursing student should examine rationales to make good decisions.

2. 2, p. 270
Rationale:
2. Experience is the second component of critical thinking in the "critical thinking model."
1. The third component of the "critical thinking model" is competencies.
3. Specific knowledge base is the first component of the "critical thinking model."
4. Diagnostic reasoning is a specific critical thinking competency in clinical situations.

3. 1, p. 264
Rationale:
1. Intuition is an inner sensing that something is so, as in this example.
2. Reflection is the process of purposefully thinking back or recalling a situation to discover its purpose or meaning.
3. Knowledge of the nurse includes information and theory from the basic sciences, humanities, behavioral sciences, and nursing.
4. Scientific method is an approach to seeking the truth or verifying that a set of facts agrees with reality.

4. 3, pp. 270, 271
Rationale:
3. This is an example of the critical thinking attitude of risk taking. A critical thinker is willing to take risks in trying different approaches to solving problems.
1. To be accountable means to be answerable for the outcomes of your actions.
2. To think independently, one questions others' ways of interpreting knowledge and looks for rational and logical answers to problems.

4. Humility is a critical thinking attitude with which a person admits what he or she does not know and tries to acquire the knowledge needed to make proper decisions.

5. 2, p. 266
Rationale:
2. This is an example of the critical thinking strategy of problem solving. The nurse gathers information from the client and combines that information with what the nurse already knows about ostomy care to find a solution. Effective problem solving involves the examination of alternatives.
1. Inference is the process of drawing conclusions.
3. Management is not a critical thinking strategy.
4. Diagnostic reasoning is a process of determining a client's health status after the nurse assigns meaning to the behaviors, physical signs, and symptoms presented by the client.

6. 4, p. 266
Rationale:
4. This statement reflects using the scientific method in the nursing process. The nurse identified a problem of pain, hypothesized that it was greater than that the day before, and collected data to evaluate its reality.
1. This statement reflects intuition.
2. This statement reflects intuition.
3. This statement reflects information gathering, which may be used in diagnostic reasoning.

7. 4, p. 268
Rationale:
4. Taking appropriate action demonstrates the implementation step of the nursing process.
1. Assessment involves the gathering of data.
2. When formulating a nursing diagnosis, the nurse critically examines and analyzes the data and identifies the client's response to a problem. The nurse may then determine priorities.
3. Planning involves establishing goals and expected outcomes of care.

8. 1, pp. 268, 272
Rationale:
1. The nurse who assigns priorities to action and determines to see this client first because of a lower than normal blood pressure for a post-operative patient is using scientifically and practice-based criteria for making clinical judgment. This is an example of following standards. The nurse uses criteria such as the clinical condition of the client, Maslow's hierarchy of needs, and risks involved in treatment delays to determine which clients have the greatest priority for care.
2. This client is not reported to be having any problems and therefore is not the priority.
3. This client is not the priority.
4. This client is not the priority.

9. 3, p. 265
Rationale:
3. Discussing alternative pain-management techniques is an example of critical thinking at the complex level. The nurse analyzes and examines alternatives more independently.
1. Following a procedure step by step is an example of the basic level of critical thinking.
2. Giving medication at the time ordered is an example of the basic level of critical thinking.
4. Reviewing the client's medical records thoroughly is an example of gathering data and may be used in evaluation of a client's care.

10. 3, p. 266
Rationale:
3. The nurse who observes the absorbency of different brands of dressing is demonstrating testing of possible options.
1. This is not an example of defining the problem.
2. The nurse is not examining pros and cons, and therefore is not considering consequences.
4. The nurse has not yet made a final decision.

11. 4, p. 271
Rationale:
4. Reporting client difficulties demonstrates the critical thinking attitude of responsibility and authority. Asking for help if uncertain and following standards of practice also demonstrate the critical thinking attitudes of responsibility and authority.
1. Offering an alternative approach would demonstrate the critical thinking attitude of risk taking.
2. Looking for a different treatment option demonstrates the critical thinking attitude of creativity.
3. Sharing ideas about nursing interventions demonstrates the critical thinking attitude of thinking independently.

12. 4, p. 269
Rationale:
4. Use of the intellectual standard of critical thinking implies that the nurse approaches assessment logically and consistently.
1. Questioning the physician's order is an example of the critical thinking attitude of risk taking.
2. Recognizing conflicts of interest demonstrates the critical thinking attitude of integrity.
3. Listening to both sides of the story demonstrates the critical thinking attitude of fairness.

13. 2, p. 270
Rationale:
2. Having worked for many years and being able to adapt a procedure to meet the client's needs is an example of the second component of the critical thinking model, experience.
1. Curiosity is a critical thinking attitude in which the nurse asks why, and continues to learn more about the client to make appropriate clinical judgments.
3. Perseverance is a critical thinking attitude in which the nurse does not readily accept the easy answer but does look further to find necessary information and appropriate solutions.
4. Scientific knowledge is knowledge acquired from the study of science. It may be acquired through education such as course work, or in reading nursing literature to remain current in nursing science.

Chapter 15

1. 4, p. 285
Rationale:
4. The three phases of an interview are orientation, working, and termination.
1. These are not the three phases of an interview.
2. These are not the three phases of an interview.
3. These are not the three phases of an interview.

2. 1, pp. 283, 290
Rationale:
1. A client's database originates with the client perception of a symptom or health problem. If an illness is present, the nurse gathers essential and relevant data about the nature and onset of symptoms. The problem-seeking technique takes the information provided in the client's story more fully to describe and identify the client's specific problems.
2. Habits and lifestyle patterns such as smoking and exercise may be assessed in an admission history. However, it is not the first question the nurse should ask when obtaining data for a problem-oriented database after the client reports having a health problem.
3. Information regarding family history, such as members who had heart disease, may be obtained in an admission history. However, if a client reports a problem, the nurse should first follow up with questions relevant to the nature and onset of symptoms.
4. The nurse may inquire about changes in other body systems during an admission history; however, if the client reports a problem, the nurse should first follow up by using a problem-oriented approach. This would include asking specific questions about the client's health problem, such as the nature and onset of symptoms.

3. 4, p. 283
Rationale:
If a client appears in the emergency department with chest pain, the nurse should first ask the client about the severity and duration of the chest pain. In an emergency situation, the client's current health problem becomes the priority assessment.

1. Initially, the nurse should not ask questions regarding family history. Gathering data about the problem currently affecting the client has greater priority.
2. Asking the client about medications taken at home is appropriate, but not at this time. The priority is to assess the symptoms the client is experiencing.
3. Asking the client about concerns regarding hospitalization is not the priority.

4. 1, p. 293
Rationale:
1. Clustering data means the nurse organizes the information obtained into meaningful clusters. A cluster is a set of signs or symptoms grouped together in a logical order. When clustering data, the nurse identifies relations between factors and symptoms.
2. Validating data means to compare the data obtained with another source to ensure its accuracy.
3. After validating data and clustering data, the nurse may formulate a problem statement, usually in the form of a nursing diagnosis.
4. Peer review is the evaluation of the quality of the work effort of an individual by his or her peers.

5. 2, p. 284
Rationale:
3. Subjective data are client's perceptions about his or her health problems. The statement by the client regarding his feeling hot is an example of subjective data.
1. A pulse rate of 88 per minute is an example of objective data. Objective data are observations or measurements made by the data collector.
2. A blood pressure of 168/80 is something that can be measured and therefore is an example of objective data.
4. Becoming febrile can be determined by measurement and therefore is an example of objective data.

6. 3, p. 288
Rationale:
3. An open-ended question prompts the client to describe a situation in more than one or two words. This option demonstrates the open-ended question technique.
1. This question limits the client's answers to one or two words. It is an example of a closed-ended question.
2. The question in this option limits the client's answer to one or two words, such as "yes" or "no." It is an example of a closed-ended question.
4. This option basically consists of two questions, both of which only require a few words to form an answer. It is does not use the open-ended question technique.

7. 2, p. 291
Rationale:
2. The psychosocial history reveals the client's support system, if any recent losses or stressful events exist, and how the individual copes with such stressors. Loss of a job would fit the psychosocial history category.
1. Family history is used to obtain data about immediate and blood relatives to determine whether the client is at risk for illnesses of a genetic or familial nature. It also provides information about the family itself.
3. The environmental history provides data about client's home and working environments.
4. The biographical history provides factual demographic data about the client.

8. 4, p. 285
Rationale:
4. Completion of the admission history is scheduled for a time when interruptions by other staff or visiting family members are minimal. The nurse should create an environment in which the client feels comfortable. Conducting the admission history after the client's orientation to the room and completion of lunch would be optimal because the client will not be distracted by hunger, and the interview will less likely be interrupted.

1. The admission history should be scheduled for a time when interruptions by other staff are minimal. During the physician's visit would not be an optimal time.
2. The nurse should provide an environment private enough to allow the client to be comfortable when providing personal information. Inclusion of family members should be left up to the client to decide. Information obtained should remain confidential.
3. Immediately before a client's testing would not be an optimal time for obtaining a nursing history. The client may feel more anxious about the upcoming test, impeding communication, and sufficient time may not exist to gather all of the information.

9. 3, p. 291
Rationale:
3. By utilizing Gordon's functional health patterns format, the nurse organizes information and makes an assessment identifying functional patterns (client strengths) and dysfunctional patterns (such as an activity and exercise abnormality).
1. The review of systems is a systematic method for collecting data on all body systems. The nurse asks the client about the normal functioning of each body system and any noted changes.
2. A nursing health history is more broad, including information about the client's current level of wellness, a review of body systems, family and health history, sociocultural history, spiritual health, and mental and emotional reactions to illness.
4. A biographic information database provides factual demographic data about the client, such as age, address, occupation, marital status, etc.

10. 2, p. 284
Rationale:
2. Objective data are observations or measurements made by the data collector, such as a blood pressure reading.
1. Subjective data are clients' perceptions about their health problems, such as pain.

3. Fear of surgery would be subjective data because it is the client's perception and not something the data collector can measure.
4. Subjective data are clients' perceptions about their health problems, such as discomfort or breathing. A respiratory rate would be an example of objective data.

11. 1, p. 284
Rationale:
1. A client is usually the best source of information. The client who is oriented and answers questions appropriately can provide the most accurate information about health care needs, lifestyle patterns, present and past illnesses, perception of symptoms, and changes in activities of daily living.
2. The physician may have knowledge of the client's medical problem, but the client is the primary source of information for completing an assessment.
3. Family members can be interviewed as primary sources of information about infants or children and critically ill, mentally handicapped, disoriented, or unconscious clients. Usually, however, they are secondary sources of information and can confirm findings provided by the client. The client in this situation is capable of being the primary source of information.
4. An experienced nurse on the unit may offer insight into a client's health care needs and care but is not the primary source of information for a client assessment.

12. 2, p. 285
Rationale:
2. The first step in establishing the database is to collect subjective information by interviewing the client.
1. The physical examination follows the client interview so that data can be verified.
3. A review of medical records is not the first step the nurse should take in the process of data collection. The medical record is a valuable tool for checking the consistency and congruency of personal observations made during the client interview.

4. Discussion with other health team members may provide additional information and be used to relay information, but it is not the first step in the process of data collection.

13. 3, p. 289
Rationale:
3. Using closed-ended questions helps the nurse to acquire specific information about health problems such as symptoms, precipitating factors, or relief measures in an efficient manner.
1. Channeling occurs when the nurse uses active listening techniques such as "all right," "go on," or "uh-huh," to indicate that the nurse has heard what the client said and to encourage the client to elaborate further.
2. Using open-ended questions prompts the client to describe a situation in more than one or two words. Because it allows the client the opportunity to tell his or her story and reveal what is important, it is not the most efficient method of obtaining specific information regarding a client's signs and symptoms of a health problem.
4. In problem-seeking technique, the nurse takes the information provided in the client's story more fully to describe and identify the client's specific problems. Using closed-ended questions would be the most efficient method for obtaining specific information about the signs and symptoms of a client's health problem.

14. 4, p. 292
Rationale:
4. In this option, the nurse is seeking further clarification of information by asking the client to provide an example. Clarification helps the nurse to gain accurate understanding of a client's situation.
1. This is not an example of clarifying information.
2. This response provides information. The nurse is not using the clarifying technique of communication.
3. In this option, the nurse describes his or her observations. It does not seek clarification.

15. 2, pp. 293, 294
Rationale:
2. With the functional health pattern format, the nurse clusters data that pertain to a functional health category. Fatigue on ambulating short distances and requiring frequent periods of rest are examples of data belonging to the category of activity and exercise.
1. "Respiratory" would be found in a systems approach of health assessment, not a functional health pattern assessment.
3. The functional health pattern category of sleep and rest would focus more on the number of hours of sleep the client obtains, use of sleep aids, and any difficulties associated with sleep.
4. Self-care deficit: activities of daily living would include such aspects as bathing, feeding, and dressing self. The symptoms described would be clustered more accurately under the functional health pattern category of activity and exercise.

16. 4, p. 284
Rationale:
4. Subjective data are clients' perceptions about their health problems. Feeling anxious and tense is information that only the client can provide.
1. Objective data are observation or measurements made by the data collector. In this example, the data collector is making the observation that the client appears sleepy.
2. "No distress noted" is an example of objective data because it is an observation made by the data collector.
3. "Abdomen soft and nontender" is an example of objective data because it is an observation made by the data collector, not a client's perception.

Chapter 16

1. 4, p. 303
Rationale:

4. After completing the client assessment, the nurse develops nursing diagnoses based on the data obtained. Nursing diagnoses distinguish the nurse's role from that of the physician, and nursing diagnoses help nurses to focus on the role of nursing in client care.
1. Nursing diagnoses may facilitate communication among health professionals, but they do not necessarily make all client problems more quickly and easily resolved.
2. Medical problems are identified with medical diagnostic statements to treat a disease condition. Nursing diagnoses describe the client's actual or potential response to a health problem that the nurse is licensed and competent to treat. Nursing diagnoses distinguish the nurse's role from that of the physician.
3. Although most state nurse practice acts include nursing diagnosis as part of the domain of nursing practice, nursing diagnoses are not required for accreditation purposes.

2. 3, p. 304
Rationale:

3. The nurse used scientific knowledge and experience to analyze and interpret data collected about the client. This includes comparing the data with norms.
1. The nurse is comparing data to determine whether a problem exists. A problem has not yet been identified.
2. The nurse is not recognizing gaps in data assessment. An example of a gap in data assessment would be if the client's weight had not been measured.
4. The nurse has not drawn a conclusion about the client's response. The nurse must first compare the data with normal health problems to be able to come to a conclusion.

3. 3, pp. 307, 312
Rationale:

3. This nursing diagnosis is written correctl[y] defines a problem and its possible cause this case, the problem is the client's respo to a diagnostic test.
1. A medical diagnosis should not be recorde an etiology because nursing interventi cannot change the medical diagnosis would be appropriate to state *Acute* related to impaired skin integrity secondar mastectomy incision.
2. This nursing diagnosis is written incorre because it uses supportive data of the prob as an etiology.
4. This nursing diagnosis does not identify problem and etiology. It identifies the clie goal rather than the problem. It could reworded as *Imbalanced nutrition: less t body requirements related to inadequate pro intake.*

4. 3, p. 311
Rationale:

3. This nursing diagnosis is written appro ately. It identifies a problem by usin, NANDA International diagnostic statem and connects it to its etiology.
1. This nursing diagnosis is written incorrec The etiology is not treatable.
2. This nursing diagnosis is written incorrec It identifies the nurse's problem and not client's.
4. This nursing diagnosis is written incorrec It uses a medical diagnosis for the etiology

5. 3, p. 311
Rationale:

3. Because the medical diagnosis requires m ical interventions, it is legally inadvisable use it in the nursing diagnosis. Rather, nurse should identify the client's respor such as decreased mobility. The nurse sho be able to provide nursing interventions t will treat the etiology.
1. Poor fiber intake would be an appropriate ology for the problem of altered eliminatic
2. Limited fluid intake would be an appropri etiology for the nursing diagnosis of alte elimination.

4. Lower abdominal discomfort is an appropriate etiology for the nursing diagnosis for altered elimination.

6. 2, pp. 304, 305
Rationale:
2. A potential etiology for impaired gas exchange may be atelectasis.
1. Atelectasis would not be an etiology for ineffective airway clearance. Increased tenacious sputum production would be a possible etiology for ineffective airway clearance.
3. Atelectasis would not support the diagnostic label for decreased cardiac output.
4. Impaired spontaneous ventilation would not be an appropriate diagnostic label for atelectasis.

7. 3, p. 307
Rationale:
3. This is a true statement. Related factors are causative or other contributing factors that have influence the client's actual or potential response to the health problem and can be changed by nursing interventions.
1. The etiology or cause of the nursing diagnosis must be within the domain of nursing practice and a condition that responds to nursing interventions, not those of the entire health care team.
2. The nursing diagnosis does not have to remain constant during the client's hospitalization. It should change according to changes in the patient.
4. The nursing diagnosis does not identify a "cause and effect" relation; rather it indicates that the etiology contributes to or is associated with the client's problem.

8. 3, p. 311
Rationale:
3. A nursing diagnosis should identify the client's response, not the medical diagnosis. Because the medical diagnosis requires medical interventions, it is legally inadvisable to include it in the nursing diagnosis.
1. A nurse should validate assessment data for accuracy and understanding.

2. Using the NANDA list of diagnoses as a source helps to ensure accuracy.
4. One purpose of the nursing diagnosis is to distinguish the nurse's role from that of the physician. Another purpose is to help nurses focus on the role of nursing in client care. Nursing diagnoses promote understanding between nurses regarding clients' health problems.

9. 4, p. 304
Rationale:
4. Defining characteristics are assessment findings that support the nursing diagnosis. In this example, the inability to speak in complete sentences supports the nursing diagnosis of altered speech.
1. "Altered speech" is the diagnostic label identifying the problem.
2. "As evidenced by" is a connecting statement for the problem and the defining characteristics.
3. "Recent neurologic disturbances" is the etiology.

10. 3, p. 300
Rationale:
3. The primary purpose of a nursing diagnosis is to recognize the client's response to an illness or situation. The nurse can then use the nursing diagnosis to select appropriate nursing interventions to achieve positive client outcomes.
1. A nursing diagnosis is based on the client, not on the medical plan of care.
2. Although nursing diagnoses may facilitate communication, it does not mean that they provide a standardized approach for all clients. Nursing diagnoses are individualized to meet the client's needs.
4. The primary purpose of nursing diagnoses is not to offer the nurse's subjective view of the client's behaviors. Nursing diagnoses are based on subjective and objective client data and should not include the nurse's personal beliefs and values.

11. 3, p. 307

Rationale:

3. "Increased airway secretions" is a condition that responds to nursing interventions and therefore would be an appropriate etiology for a nursing diagnosis.

1. Abnormal blood gas levels would not be an appropriate etiology for a nursing diagnosis because it is not a causative factor, but rather is a defining characteristic of a problem.

2. Myocardial infarction would not be an appropriate etiology for a nursing diagnosis because it is a medical diagnosis. Nursing interventions will not alter the medical diagnosis of myocardial infarction.

4. Cardiac catheterization is a diagnostic procedure and would not be an appropriate etiology for a nursing diagnosis. The client's response to the procedure would be the area of nursing concern.

12. 1, p. 307

Rationale:

1. Incisional pain is an appropriate etiology for a nursing diagnosis. It is a condition that identifies the cause of a client's response to a health problem that a nurse can treat or manage.

2. "Poor hygiene practices" would not be an appropriate etiology for a nursing diagnosis because it insinuates a nurse's prejudicial judgment.

3. "Needs bedpan frequently" is not an appropriate etiology because it identifies a nursing intervention, not an etiology.

4. "Inadequate prescription of medication by the physician" is not an appropriate etiology because it identifies the nurse's problem, not the client's problem. The nursing diagnosis should center attention on client needs.

13. 1, pp. 307, 312

Rationale:

1. This is a correctly written nursing diagnosis. It consists of a problem related to an etiology and is a condition that nursing interventions can treat or manage.

2. This nursing diagnosis is not written correctly because it is a circular statement. It would be appropriate to state *Ineffective breathing pattern related to incisional pain.*

3. This nursing diagnosis is not written correctly because it uses a nurse's prejudicial judgment. It would be more appropriate and professional to state *Risk for impaired skin integrity related to knowledge about perineal care.*

4. This nursing diagnosis is not written appropriately because it identifies a nursing problem, not a client's problem. It would be appropriate to state, *Risk for infection related to presence of invasive lines.*

14. 1, pp. 307, 312

Rationale:

1. This is an example of an appropriately written nursing diagnosis. It consists of a diagnostic label and the associated etiology. Nursing interventions can be directed at treating or managing the behavior of insufficient medication use.

2. This nursing diagnosis is not written correctly. What could be a defining characteristic is used as an etiology. This nursing diagnosis could be rewritten more appropriately as *Impaired mobility related to pain as evidenced by difficulty ambulating,* or it could be an inaccurate diagnostic label and could be rewritten as *Anxiety related to difficulty in ambulating.*

3. This nursing diagnosis is written incorrectly because it identifies the equipment rather than the client's response to the equipment. It would be appropriate to state *Deficient knowledge regarding the need for cardiac monitoring.*

4. This nursing diagnosis is written incorrectly because it identifies a nursing intervention, not the client's problem. It could be reworded, *Diarrhea related to food intolerance.*

15. 3, p. 311

Rationale:

3. The defining characteristics of abnormal breath sounds, dyspnea, an intermittent cough, and variable respiratory rate cue the nurse to the nursing diagnosis of ineffective airway clearance.

1. The nursing assessment data do not support the diagnostic label of risk for injury.
2. The nursing assessment data do not support the diagnostic label of excess fluid volume. Other defining characteristics would be noted, such as edema, weight gain, and an elevated blood pressure.
4. The nursing assessment data do not most accurately describe impaired spontaneous ventilation. Other characteristics, such as apnea, would better support the diagnostic label of impaired spontaneous ventilation.

16. 1, p. 302
Rationale:
1. "Risk for impaired parenting" is a NANDA nursing diagnosis label.
2. "Abnormal hygienic care practices" is not a NANDA nursing diagnosis label. It incorrectly implies a nurse's prejudicial judgment.
3. "Coughing and dyspnea" are symptoms, not a NANDA nursing diagnosis label.
4. "Frequent urination" is a symptom, not a NANDA nursing diagnosis label.

Chapter 17

1. 1, p. 319
Rationale:
1. The client's request would be of low priority because it is not directly related to a specific illness or prognosis.
2. "An unmet need" is not the most appropriate label for the client's request.
3. The client's request is not an intermediate priority. An intermediate priority is one that involves the nonemergency, non–life threatening needs of the client.
4. The client's request is not a safety and security need; the outcome does not threaten her well-being.

2. 1, p. 322
Rationale:
1. Long-term goals focus on prevention, rehabilitation, discharge, and health education. An appropriate long-term goal for this client would be rehabilitation and the client's return to occupation.

2. Preventing ocular infection is a short-term goal. A short-term goal is expected to be achieved within a short time, usually in less than a week. In a week's time, the client's risk for infection should be greatly reduced.
3. Performing independent hygienic care in the hospital is a short-term goal. Long-term goals are usually made for problem resolution after discharge; especially from an acute care setting.
4. Administering eyedrops on time in the hospital is a short-term goal. Long-term goals are usually designed for problem resolution after discharge, especially from an acute care setting.

3. 3, p. 323
Rationale:
3. This option would be the most appropriate outcome criterion. It is client centered, singular, observable, measurable, time limited, and realistic.
1. This option does not allow the nurse to be able to determine whether change has taken place. It would be more measurable to state the client will rate pain below 4 on a scale of 0 to 10 by 24 hours.
2. This option is not time limited.
4. This option is not time limited or singular.

4. 4, p. 324
Rationale:
4. Preparing a client for a diagnostic test is an example of a physician-initiated intervention.
1. Teaching a client to administer his or her insulin injection is an example of a nurse-initiated intervention.
2. Assisting a new mother with breast-feeding is an example of a nurse-initiated intervention.
3. Notifying a nutritionist of a client's dietary preferences is a collaborative intervention.

5. 3, p. 330
Rationale:
3. The intervention statement does not include how frequently the warm soaks should be applied.
1. The method is applying warm wet soaks to the patient's leg while the patient is awake.

2. The quantity is warm wet soaks.
4. The qualification of the person who will perform the action is the designation of "the nurse."

6. 4, p. 323
Rationale:
4. This is a correctly written outcome statement. It is client centered, singular, observable, measurable, time limited, and realistic.
1. This outcome statement is not time limited.
2. This outcome statement is not observable or time limited. "The client will state the purpose of the breathing treatments by 4/10" would be more appropriate.
3. This outcome statement is not client centered. A correct outcome statement would be "Client will ambulate in the hall 3 times a day."

7. 3, p. 330
Rationale:
3. Critical pathways allow staff from all disciplines to develop integrated care plans for a projected length of stay or number of visits for clients with a specific case type.
1. The nursing Kardex is a card-filing system that allows quick reference to the particular needs of the client for certain aspects of nursing care.
2. A computerized care plan is a standardized care plan on the computer.
4. A standardized care plan is a prewritten plan created for a specific nursing diagnosis or clinical problem. The nurse individualizes the care plan for the client's needs.

8. 2, p. 335
Rationale:
2. Consultation is appropriate when the nurse has identified a problem that cannot be solved by using personal knowledge, skills, and resources, or when the exact problem remains unclear. A consultant objectively entering a situation can more clearly assess and identify the exact nature of the problem.
1. The person requesting the consult usually identifies the problem area.

3. The nurse should not bias the consultant with subjective and emotional conclusions about the client and problem.
4. The whole problem is not turned over to the consultant. The consultant is not there to take over the problem but is there to assist the nurse in resolving it.

9. 3, p. 319
Rationale:
3. Difficulty breathing would be the highest priority client need. In general, priorities that protect clients' basic needs of safety, adequate oxygenation, and comfort are considered high priority.
1. An impending divorce is a low-priority client need. It is a need that is not directly related to a specific illness or prognosis but may affect the client's future well-being.
2. A nutritional deficit is an intermediate priority client need. It involves a non–life threatening need of the client.
4. Financial problems are a low-priority client need. Financial problems are not directly related to a specific illness or prognosis but may affect the client's future well-being.

10. 4, p. 323
Rationale:
4. This outcome statement is client centered, singular, observable, measurable, time limited, and realistic.
1. This outcome criterion is not measurable (i.e., guidelines for normal are not stated), and it not time limited (i.e., by when?).
2. This outcome statement is not client centered.
3. This outcome statement is not singular and is not time limited.

11. 4, p. 324
Rationale:
4. The nurse sets realistic goals that can achieved. This increases the client's motivation. The nurse also takes available resources into consideration to set realistic goals.
1. Being client-centered means that the goal should reflect the client behavior and responses expected as a result of nursing interventions.

2. Being observable means the nurse must be able to determine through observation whether change has taken place.
3. Being measurable means the goal is written so the nurse has a standard against which to measure the client's response to nursing care.

12. 1, p. 324
Rationale:
1. Health teaching is an example of a nurse-initiated intervention.
2. Administering medication is a physician-initiated intervention.
3. Ordering a computed tomography (CAT) scan is a physician-initiated intervention.
4. Referring a client to physical therapy is a collaborative intervention.

13. 3, p. 324
Rationale:
3. Changing a dressing is a physician- or prescriber-initiated intervention.
1. Taking vital signs is a nurse-initiated intervention.
2. Providing support to a family is a nurse-initiated intervention.
4. Measuring intake and output is a nurse-initiated intervention.

14. 4, p. 326
Rationale:
4. Interventions to maintain or restore tissue integrity are classified as Level 2, Domain 2 (Physiological: Complex).
1. Maintaining regular bowel elimination is classified as Level 2, Domain 1 (Physiological: Basic).
2. Promoting the health of the family is classified as Level 2, Domain 5 (Family).
3. Managing restricted body movement is classified as Level 2, Domain 1 (Physiological: Basic).

15. 1, p. 330
Rationale:
1. Critical pathways are multidisciplinary. They allow staff from all disciplines, such as medicine, nursing, pharmacy, and social work, to develop integrated care plans for a projected length of stay or number of visits for clients with a specific case type.
2. Nursing interventions are included in critical pathways and in the traditional nursing care plan.
3. Client outcomes are included in both critical pathways and traditional nursing care plans.
4. Client assessment is necessary for developing and evaluating critical pathways and traditional nursing care plans.

16. 4, p. 329
Rationale:
4. This is the most appropriate intervention statement. It includes the action, frequency, quantity, and method.
1. This intervention statement lacks the component of quantity.
2. This intervention statement fails to indicate the frequency or method (i.e., what is the observer specifically looking for?).
3. This intervention statement omits the method.

17. 1, p. 329
Rationale:
1. This intervention statement is the most appropriate. It identifies the action, frequency, quantity, and method.
2. This intervention statement fails to state an accurate frequency or precisely to indicate the nursing actions.
3. This intervention statement fails to indicate the frequency and completely fails to indicate nursing actions (i.e., what are the parameters to notify the physician?).
4. This intervention statement fails to indicate completely the nursing interventions (i.e., what type of therapist?).

18. 4, p. 329
Rationale:
4. An aspect of a nursing care plan that is usually included in the student's care plan, but not in the client's record, is scientific rationales.
1. Nursing diagnoses are included in student care plans and the client's record.
2. Client outcomes are included in both student care plans and the client's record.
3. Nursing interventions are a component of both student care plans and a nursing care plan in the client's record.

19. 4, p. 333
Rationale:
4. A concept map is a diagram of client problems and interventions that shows their relations to one another.
1. The use of a concept map promotes critical thinking and helps nurses to organize complex client data, process complex relationships, and achieve a holistic view of the client's situation. The purpose is not quality assurance in the health care facility.
2. Multidisciplinary communication is enhanced with the use of critical pathways, not concept maps.
3. Standardized or computerized care plans provide a standardized format for client problems, not the concept map. A concept map is highly individualized.

20. 4, p. 322
Rationale:
4. This option is the most appropriate outcome statement. It addresses the nursing diagnosis by identifying a singular outcome the client can realistically achieve, is observable, and provides a time frame.
1. This is not an appropriate outcome statement. It does not specify a time frame.
2. This is not an appropriate outcome statement. No specific behavior is observable for "will appear."
3. This is not an appropriate outcome statement. It does not provide a standard against which to measure the client's response to nursing care, and therefore is not measurable.
It also is not time limited.

Chapter 18

1. 3, p. 345
Rationale:
3. Making rooms free of clutter is an example of manipulating the environment to create safe surroundings.
1. Delegating ambulation of clients to the nursing assistant is an example of organizing personnel (resources) for care delivery.
2. Providing pain medication before a dressing change is an example of organizing care delivery specific to the client. Before beginning to perform interventions, the nurse should make the client as physically and psychologically comfortable as possible.
4. Repositioning the client q2h is an example of organizing care delivery to promote client comfort and prepare the client for nursing intervention.

2. 4, p. 349
Rationale:
4. Nursing actions that control adverse reactions reduce or counteract the reaction, such as administering an antihistamine after an allergic reaction to a medication.
1. Preventive measures, such as immunizations, health teaching, and risk appraisal, promote health and prevent illness to avoid the need for acute or rehabilitative care.
2. Assisting with activities of daily living (ADLs) is a direct care measure with which the nurse provides the client with assistance in activities that are usually performed in the course of a normal day, such as eating, bathing, dressing, grooming, and ambulating.
3. Preparing for special procedures is a direct care measure involving physical care techniques and possible teaching.

3. 2, p. 344

Rationale:

2. The nurse is modifying the nursing care plan. Data have been updated to reflect the client's current status of an elevated partial thrombo- plastin time (PTT), and nursing diagnoses and specific interventions are revised. In this case, the revised intervention is withholding the warfarin (Coumadin).

1. The nurse is doing more than reassessing the client. The nurse modifies the nursing care plan based on new data obtained.

3. Withholding the warfarin reflects modifica- tion of the nursing care plan. The client may require a new or additional nursing diagnosis to address the problem of a risk for deficient fluid volume.

4. By gathering further assessment data and revising nursing interventions, the nurse is modifying the nursing care plan. Withholding the warfarinin is not an example of stating an expected outcome.

4. 1, p. 346

Rationale:

1. If a nurse does not know how to perform a procedure, he or she should seek assistance. Information about the procedure is obtained from the literature and the agency's procedure book. All equipment necessary for the proce- dure is collected. Finally, another nurse who has completed the procedure correctly and safely provides assistance and guidance.

2. Reassessing the client is a partial assessment that may focus on one dimension of the client or on one system. It provides a way to deter- mine whether the proposed nursing action is still appropriate for the client's level of well- ness.

3. Interpersonal skills are used to develop a trust- ing relationship, express a level of caring, and communicate clearly with the client, family, and health care team.

4. Critical decision making is used when the nurse implements the care plan by using the knowledge bases necessary for care planning and for then completing the planned inter- ventions most effectively. In this case, the nurse lacks the necessary knowledge and experience and should seek assistance.

5. 1, p. 346

Rationale:

1. Cognitive skills involve the application of nursing knowledge. Being able to identify a client's discharge needs is a cognitive skill.

2. Interactive skills are interpersonal skills such as developing a trusting relationship and communicating effectively.

3. Psychomotor skills involve the integration of cognitive and motor skills such as in adminis- tering an injection.

4. Effective communication is an interpersonal skill. The nurse communicates with the client and family when providing client teaching and emotional support. The nurse communi- cates with the health care team to achieve client outcomes.

6. 4, p. 346

Rationale:

4. Cognitive skills involve the application of nursing knowledge. Understanding normal and abnormal physiological and psychologi- cal responses is a cognitive skill, as in recog- nizing the potential complications of a blood transfusion.

1. Providing a soothing bed bath involves both interpersonal skills and psychomotor skills. The nurse who provides a soothing bed bath is expressing a level of caring, which is an interpersonal skill. The nurse who provides a soothing bed bath also is using a psychomo- tor skill in performing the bed bath correctly.

2. Communicating with the client and family is an example of an interpersonal skill.

3. Giving an injection to the client is a psy- chomotor skill.

7. 4, p. 346

Rationale:

4. Psychomotor skills involve the integration of cognitive and motor activities, such as in pro- viding ostomy care.

1. Cognitive skills involve the application of nursing knowledge. Knowing the rationale for therapeutic interventions, understanding nor- mal and abnormal physiological and psycho- logical responses, and being able to identify client learning and discharge needs all require cognitive skills.

2. Interpersonal skills are used when the nurse interacts with clients, their families, and other health care team members. Effective communication is an example of an interpersonal skill.
3. Affective means pertaining to an emotion or mental state.

8. 4, p. 347
Rationale:
4. A client with bilateral arm casts has a temporary need for assistance with ADLs.
1. Counseling is a direct care method that helps the client use a problem-solving process to develop new attitudes and feelings. It does not meet the physical need for assistance with ADLs.
2. Teaching is an implementation method used to present correct principles, procedures, and techniques of health care to clients and to inform clients about their health status.
3. Compensating for adverse reactions means the nurse takes action to reduce or counteract the reaction, such as with administering an antihistamine when a client has an allergic reaction to a medication. Assisting with ADLs would be compensating for the client's impaired mobility.

9. 1, p. 348
Rationale:
1. Restraining a violent client is an example of a lifesaving measure to protect the client. The purpose of a lifesaving measure is to restore physiological or psychological equilibrium.
2. Administering analgesics is an example of physical care techniques. It is not a lifesaving measure.
3. Initiating stress-reduction therapy is an example of a counseling technique.
4. Teaching the client how to take his or her pulse is an example of the nursing intervention of teaching. The focus is for the client to obtain new knowledge or psychomotor skills.

Chapter 19

1. 3, p. 361
Rationale:
3. This is an example of a negative evaluation. During evaluation, the nurse is able to determine that the client has not met the expected outcome of decreasing smoking by one cigarette each week, but rather has increased his smoking.
1. This is not an example of a realistic goal. It is an example of the evaluation step of the nursing process.
2. The client is noncompliant.
4. The goal is measurable. During evaluation, the nurse determines whether expected outcomes are met to ascertain whether goals have been met.

2. 2, p. 362
Rationale:
2. The client is showing changes but does not yet meet criteria set; therefore the goal is partially met.
1. The client's response, being able to state three symptoms, does not meet or exceed the outcome criterion of being able to state five symptoms.
3. If the client were showing no progress, then the goal would be not met. However, this client's response does indicate some change.
4. The client's response, being able to list three symptoms, demonstrates some change. If the client were showing no progress, then the goal would be not met.

3. 4, p. 365
Rationale:
4. The nurse who stops auscultating lung sounds to take measures to stop noticeable bleeding is analyzing data presented, as demonstrated by the nurse setting priorities, and is effectively implementing the safest nursing action.
1. The nurse is doing more than performing a nursing assessment. The nurse is taking action based on new assessment data.
2. The nurse is not reorganizing nursing diagnoses. The nurse is implementing the priority nursing action.

3. This is not an example of setting realistic goals and implementing nursing interventions. Applying direct pressure to a wound site to stop bleeding demonstrates critical analysis of the data and implementation of the safest nursing action.

4. 3, p. 362
Rationale:
3. This is the best example of an objective evaluation of the client's goal attainment. It uses the same evaluative measures gathered during assessment and clearly describes objective data.
1. This statement does not use the same evaluative measure gathered during assessment. The assessment measure concerned respiratory changes during ambulation, not pain. If the client's pain level were going to be used as an evaluative measure, it would be optimal to have the client report the pain by using a pain scale to make it more measurable for comparison.
2. This statement is not the best example of an objective evaluation of the client's goal attainment. It does not use the same evaluative measure gathered during assessment. The assessment measure concerned respiratory changes during ambulation, not nausea. Nausea also is more subjective.
4. This is not the best example of an objective evaluation. It includes the nurse's interpretation rather than documentation of objective data.

5. 3, p. 363
Rationale:
3. A complete reassessment of all client factors relating to the nursing diagnosis and etiology is necessary when modifying a plan.
1. After reassessment, the nurse will determine what components of the care plan are accurate for the situation. It may not require redoing the entire care plan.
2. The nurse should focus not only on the nursing diagnoses and goals that have changed. Interventions may also need revising to meet new goals.

4. Adding more nursing interventions may or may not be necessary. The nurse adjusts interventions on the basis of the client's response and previous experience with similar clients. Standards of care are used to determine whether the right interventions have been chosen or whether additional ones are required.

6. 2, p. 361
Rationale:
2. The nurse should compare the established outcome criteria with the client's behavior or response. In this case, the client is expected to complete independently the necessary assessments before administration of digoxin. The client should be able to palpate the radial pulse as an assessment before administration of digoxin.
1. The outcome criterion does not state anything about exercise. During evaluation, the nurse is to judge the degree of agreement between the outcome criterion and the client's behavior.
3. The outcome criterion does not state anything about diet. Evaluating whether the client reviews dietary habits would not be comparable to necessary assessment before medication administration.
4. The outcome criterion does not state anything about the skin. The nurse, who knows that digoxin is a cardiotonic, knows the client should be assessing the heart rate.

7. 3, p. 361
Rationale:
3. Erythema is reddening of the skin; therefore the evaluation should specifically focus on inspection of the color of the skin, as stated in the outcome criterion.
1. The outcome criterion states that the erythema will reduce, not the size of the ulceration. During the evaluation step of the nursing process, the client's behavior or response should be compared with the outcome criterion and judged for degree of agreement between the two.

2. The outcome criterion does not state anything about drainage. Noting the color and amount of drainage may be a part of reassessment of the client but is not what the nurse is evaluating, according to this outcome criterion.
4. Selection of appropriate wound care is an intervention, not an evaluation of a client's behavior or response.

8. 2, p. 361
Rationale:
2. Auscultating lung sounds is the best way to determine whether airways are clear. A positive evaluation is that they are clear, as expected in the outcome statement.
1. Having the ability to perform incentive spirometry does not determine whether the airways are clear. It is an intervention that may help achieve clear airways.
3. A complaint of chest pain would be a negative outcome, and it is not the focus for determining whether airways are free of secretions, as written in the outcome statement.
4. Respiratory rate may be an indicator of respiratory status, but it is not the best way to determine whether airways are free of secretions.

Chapter 20

1. 2, p. 380
Rationale:
2. When delegating, the nurse should always provide unambiguous and clear directions by describing a task, the desired outcome, and the period within which the task should be competed.
1. Tasks should be delegated to those who are capable, not necessarily to those who are willing.
3. A laissez-faire style of leadership is not a requirement for delegation.
4. The nurse manager does not necessarily have to work alongside staff to evaluate their care. The nurse manager can often evaluate staff performance in client outcomes.

2. 2, p. 377
Rationale:
2. To manage time, the nurse must anticipate when care will be interrupted for medication administration, any diagnostic testing, and when is the best time for planned therapies such as dressing changes, client education, and client ambulation.
1. This would be an unrealistic. Some activities have specific time limits in terms of addressing client needs, and some activities follow scheduled routines according to hospital policy. The nurse also may have to work around other schedules, such as if the client had a test ordered for the morning. Therefore the nurse cannot expect to meet all of the client's needs at a specified time of day.
3. Time management involves using client goals as a way to identify priorities. The nurse, in reviewing the care requirements, organizes his or her time so the activities of care and client goals can be achieved. A nurse should complete the activities started with one client before moving on to another.
4. Because the nurse has a limited amount of time with clients, it is essential to remain goal oriented and make a plan for using time wisely.

3. 2, p. 372
Rationale:
2. Functional nursing is task focused, not client focused. In this model, tasks are divided, with one nurse assuming responsibility for specific tasks.
1. Total patient care is a model of care where a RN is responsible for all aspects of care for one or more clients. The RN may delegate aspects of care, but retains accountability for care of all assigned clients.
3. In team nursing, an RN leads a team that is composed of other RNs, LPNs or LVNs, and nurse assistants or technicians. The team members provide direct client care to groups of clients, under the direction of the RN team leader. Nurse assistants are given client assignments rather than being assigned particular tasks.

4. Primary nursing is a model of care delivery whereby an RN assumes responsibility for a caseload of clients over time. Typically the RN selects the clients for his or her caseload and cares for the same clients during their hospitalization or stay in the health care setting.

4. 4, p. 374
Rationale:
4. In decentralized management, decision making is moved down to the level of staff. It requires workers to be empowered to accept greater responsibility for the quality of client care provided. This means that each staff member is accountable for evaluating the plan of care.
1. If decentralized decision making is in place, professional staff have a voice in identifying the RN role. Each RN on the work team is responsible for knowing his or her role and how it is to be implemented on the nursing unit.
2. In decentralized management, autonomy exists (freedom to decide and act). The nurse manager does not necessarily handle the difficult decisions. Those staff members who are best informed about a problem or issue make decisions on the basis of knowledge.
3. Communication pathways are not simplified.

5. 3, p. 384
Rationale:
3. A quality indicator for evaluating the manner in which care is delivered is a process indicator.
1. Structure indicators evaluate the structure or systems for delivering care; an example is adherence in checking whether emergency carts are adequately stocked.
2. There is no team indicator.
4. Client indicators would actually be outcome indicators. Outcome indicators evaluate the result of care delivered.

6. 4, p. 384
Rationale:
4. Wound infections are exceeding the designated threshold, indicating a need for further review of the quality improvement plan.
1. Waiting time for clinic appointments has decreased, meeting the threshold.
2. Satisfaction with care meets the threshold.
3. Expressions of pain have decreased, meeting the threshold.

7. 1, p. 373
Rationale:
1. In team nursing, an RN leads a team that is composed of other RNs, LPNs or LVNs, and nurse assistants or technicians. The team members provide direct client care to groups of clients, under the direction of the RN team leader. Nurse assistants are given client assignments rather than being assigned particular tasks.
2. Primary nursing is a model of care delivery whereby an RN assumes responsibility for a caseload of clients over time. Typically the RN selects the clients for his or her caseload and cares for the same clients during their hospitalization or stay in the health care setting.
3. Functional nursing is task focused, not client focused. In this model, tasks are divided, with one nurse assuming responsibility for specific tasks.
4. Total patient care is a model of care in which an RN is responsible for all aspects of care for one or more clients. The RN may delegate aspects of care, but retains accountability for care of all assigned clients.

8. 3, p. 375
Rationale:
3. Accountability refers to individuals being answerable for their actions. It involves follow-up and a reflective analysis of one's decisions to evaluate their effectiveness.
1. Selecting the medication schedule for the client is an example of taking responsibility.
2. Implementing discharge-teaching plans that meet individual needs is an example of autonomy.

4. Promoting participation of all staff members in unit meetings is an example of decentralized management and of promoting authority.

9. 2, p. 376
Rationale:
2. Second-order priority needs are actual problems for which the client or family has requested immediate help, such as a full bladder.
1. An obstructed airway is a first-order priority need because it is an immediate threat to a client's survival or safety.
3. Side effects of a medication is an example of a third-order priority need. It is a relatively urgent actual or potential problem that the client or family does not recognize.
4. Activities of daily living in the home environment is a fourth-order priority need. It is an actual or potential problem with which the client or family may need help in the future.

10. 1, p. 380
Rationale:
1. An institution's policies and procedures and job description for assistive personnel provide specific guidelines in regard to what tasks or activities can be delegated. The nurse should match tasks to the delegate's skills, such as delegating vital signs to a nurse assistant.
2. It would not be appropriate to delegate an admission history on a new client to a nurse assistant. The RN should perform this task.
3. Initial transfer of a postoperative client should not be delegated to a nurse assistant, as the client would be considered unstable. The RN should perform this task.
4. The nurse should not delegate medication administration to a nurse assistant, even if the nurse prepared it. The nurse assistant is not licensed to administer medication.

Chapter 21

1. 2, p. 393
Rationale:
2. A value is a personal belief about the worth of a given idea, attitude, custom, or object that sets standards that influence behavior. The client is expressing her value of health-promotion activities.

1. A belief is a conviction of the truth of a thin The client's statement does not indicate th she believes in, or has fear of, having a hea attack.
3. A belief is a conviction of the truth or reali of a thing. The client does not state that sl believes these health-promotion activities w keep her from becoming sick.
4. These are not unrealistic expectations.

2. 3, p. 393
Rationale:
3. Individual experience influences what come to value. The client who experienced gunshot during a robbery of his business m value gun control and verbalize a desire have his attacker prosecuted for the viole crime.
1. The individual who has actively picketed f gun control is unlikely to desire the use guns. The individual would be more likely believe that if gun control were legislated, need for guns would exist.
2. The client who has picketed for gun contr and who was shot is unlikely to value firear in our society.
4. The individual who has actively picketed f gun control is unlikely to desire the use guns. The individual would be more likely believe that if gun control existed, no gu would be needed.

3. 1, p. 394
Rationale:
1. The teacher is demonstrating prizing h choice. She cherishes her choice of bei treated like everyone else despite her medic condition and publicly affirms the choice teaching from a wheelchair and insisting th she be treated the same as her colleagues.
2. At this point, the teacher is not choosing fro alternatives. She could have chosen to qu teaching, but she did not. She has alrea made her choice.
3. The teacher is not demonstrating considerir all consequences. She has already made h choice.
4. At this point, the teacher is not demonstra ing acting with a pattern of consistency. She not repeating a behavior.

452   Test Bank Answer Key

4. 2, p. 394

Rationale:

2. Values clarification can help clients gain an awareness of personal priorities, identify ambiguities in values, and resolve major conflicts between values and behavior.
1. Values clarification for nurses can help nurses strengthen their ability to advocate for a client because nurses are better able to identify personal values and accurately to identify the values of the client. Values clarification is not necessarily beneficial for the client when the client and nurse have different beliefs.
3. Values clarification for the client will not necessarily help the nurse who is unsure of the client's values. Values-clarification interventions for the client will help the client and not the nurse to gain awareness.
4. The values that an individual holds reflect cultural and social influences, relationships, and personal needs. Values vary among people and develop and change over time. Therefore it may be inappropriate to state that a client has rejected "normal" values when value systems vary among people. What is considered normal to one person may not be to another.

5. 2, p. 393

Rationale:

2. Values clarification is a process of self-discovery that the nurse should assist the client through. The goal of values clarification with a client is effective nurse-client communication. As the client becomes more willing to express problems and feelings, the nurse can better establish an individualized plan of care. The character of a nurse's response to a client can motivate the client to examine personal thoughts and actions. When the nurse makes a clarifying response, it should be brief and nonjudgmental.
1. Values clarification is a process of self-discovery that the nurse should assist the client through. The character of a nurse's response to a client can motivate the client to examine personal thoughts and actions. When the nurse makes a clarifying response, it should be brief and nonjudgmental. The client is being judgmental in this response.

3. The nurse should not influence the client with his or her own values, even if they are similar.
4. This statement is therapeutic in that it is reflective of a client's feeling and offers information. However, it does not encourage the client to examine his or her values.

6. 1, p. 391

Rationale:

1. The term responsibility refers to the characteristics of reliability and dependability. In professional nursing, responsibility includes a duty to perform actions well and thoughtfully. When the nurse provides competent care, the nurse is demonstrating ethical responsibility.
2. Formation of interpersonal relationships is not an ethical responsibility.
3. Application of the nursing process is not an ethical responsibility.
4. Evaluation of new computerized technologies is not an ethical responsibility.

7. 4, p. 391

Rationale:

4. Accountability refers to the ability to answer for one's own actions. The goal is the prevention of injury to the client. The student nurse who informs her instructor of an error is being accountable for her actions and has a goal to prevent injury to the client.
1. The student nurse would not be described professionally as confident (i.e., sure of oneself).
2. The student is not best described as trustworthy. To be trustworthy, one is worthy of trust or confidence and is reliable. In this case, the student was not reliable to administer medication correctly.
3. This student nurse is not best described professionally as compliant. The student is not acting in accordance with wishes, commands, or requirements.

8. 3, p. 392

Rationale:

3. Veracity in general means accuracy or conformity to truth. The nurse is encouraging the client to be truthful with the client's family.

Test Bank Answer Key 453

1. Confidentiality means not to impart private matters.
2. Fidelity refers to the agreement to keep promises.
4. Justice refers to fairness.

9. 3, pp. 398, 399
Rationale:
3. The correct sequence for resolving ethical problems is recognizing the dilemma, gathering facts, examining one's own values, verbalizing the problem, considering actions, negotiating the outcome, and evaluating the action.
1. This is not the correct sequence for resolving ethical problems.
2. This is not the correct sequence for resolving ethical problems.
4. This is not the correct sequence for resolving ethical problems.

10. 3, p. 398
Rationale:
3. The first step in processing an ethical dilemma is determining whether the problem is an ethical one. The nurse who cannot figure out what is right is stating a characteristic of an ethical dilemma, which is that the problem is perplexing. The next step is to gather as much information as possible that is relevant to the case.
1. The nurse who wants to know the legalities of the living will of a client is collecting some, but not all, data pertaining to the problem.
2. The nurse in this option is stating her own beliefs.
4. The nurse is stating the problem according to her feelings.

11. 3, p. 395
Rationale:
3. Deontology defines actions as right or wrong based on their right-making characteristics such as fidelity to promises, truthfulness, and justice. Deontology does not look to consequences of actions to determine rightness or wrongness. Fidelity to promises and beneficence may be principles on which this statement is based on determining wrongness.

1. This statement does not reflect the deontological ethical theory. Because it reflects a relation between disease and a supreme being, it follows the feminist ethical theory.
2. This statement does not best illustrate the deontological ethical theory because it is citing a consequence. It follows the utilitarian ethical theory.
4. This statement does not best illustrate the deontological ethical theory because it cites a consequence. It follows the utilitarian ethical theory.

12. 2, p. 390
Rationale:
2. Beneficence refers to taking positive actions to help others, as in providing emergency care at an accident scene.
1. Respect for persons has to do with treating people equally despite their social standing, etc.
3. Nonmaleficence is the avoidance of harm or hurt.
4. Triage is the screening and classification of casualties to make optimal use of treatment resources and to maximize the survival and welfare of clients.

13. 3, p. 400
Rationale:
3. Ethics committees serve as a resource to support the processing of ethical dilemmas. Ethics committees serve several purposes: education, policy recommendation, and case consultation or review.
1. Although an ethics committee may gather further information, ethics committees do not interview all persons involved in a case; rather, they offer consultation or case review.
2. This is not a purpose of an ethics committee.
4. This may be part of data gathering to help process an ethical dilemma or for policy recommendation, but it is not the purpose of an ethics committee.

14. 1, p. 390

Rationale:

1. Justice refers to treating people fairly. Allocation of resources and access to health care involve the ethical principle of justice. The client without medical insurance should not have to wait longer to receive health care than do those with insurance.
2. Autonomy refers to a person's independence. Autonomy represents an agreement to respect another's right to determine a course of action.
3. Beneficence refers to taking positive actions to help others.
4. Nonmaleficence refers to the avoidance of harm or hurt.

15. 4, p. 390

Rationale:

4. Following the ethical principle of autonomy, the nurse allows a client to make the decisions regarding care and then supports that decision.
1. Learning how to do a procedure safely and effectively is a nurse's use of ethical responsibility.
2. Returning to speak to a client at an agreed-on time demonstrates the ethical principle of fidelity.
3. Preparing the client's room for comfort and privacy is a nurse's use of ethical responsibility.

16. 3, p. 392

Rationale:

3. This statement reflects the application of the ethical principle of confidentiality. Information is not to be shared with others without specific client consent.
1. This statement reflects a concern regarding allocation of resources. It is not a confidentiality issue.
2. The nurse who makes sure a client has gained understanding is being ethically responsible.
4. This statement reflects data gathering. Information gathered is to be used for the purpose of providing competent health care. It should not be shared with others without specific consent of the client.

17. 4, p. 390

Rationale:

4. Nonmaleficence is the avoidance of harm or hurt. The discomforts of treatment have to be considered: are they benefiting the client, or are they worse than the disease itself. The health care professional tries to balance the risks and benefits of a plan of care while striving to do the least harm possible.
1. Veracity refers to truthfulness. This situation is not questioning truthfulness.
2. Fidelity refers to the agreement to keep promises. This situation does not question fidelity.
3. Justice refers to fairness. This situation is not a matter of justice.

Chapter 22

1. 1, p. 407

Rationale:

1. Civil laws protect the rights of individual persons within our society and encourage fair and equitable treatment among people. Generally, violations of civil laws cause harm to an individual or property, and damages involve payment of money. Administering an incorrect dosage of morphine sulfate would fall under civil law because it could cause harm to an individual.
2. Criminal laws prevent harm to society and provide punishment for crimes (often imprisonment).
3. Common law is created by judicial decisions made in courts when individual legal cases are decided (e.g., informed consent).
4. Administrative law is created by administrative bodies, such as State Boards of Nursing when they pass rules and regulations (e.g., the duty to report unethical nursing conduct).

2. 3, p. 409

Rationale:

3. A living will is an advance directive, prepared when the individual is competent and able to make decisions, regarding that person's specific instruction about end-of-life care. Living wills allow people to specify whether they would want to be intubated, treated with pressor drugs, shocked with electricity, and fed or hydrated intravenously.

1. A living will specifies what interventions the client does not want, so that his or her life will not be prolonged.
2. If his wife had power of attorney, she would be able to make decisions regarding the client's care.
4. Assisted suicide, such as a lethal injection, is not a function of a living will. A living will defines a client's wishes for withholding of treatment that would prolong his or her life.

3. 2, p. 418
Rationale:
2. Student nurses are expected to perform as professional nurses (i.e., as an RN would) in providing safe client care.
1. Students are not working in the same capacity as an unlicensed person and therefore are not compared with the standard of an unlicensed person.
3. This is not a true statement. Staff nurses may serve as preceptors, but that does not excuse the student from performing at the level of a RN.
4. If a client is harmed as a direct result of a nursing student's actions or lack of action, the liability for the incorrect action is generally shared by the student, instructor, hospital or health care facility, and university or educational institution.

4. 3, p. 418
Rationale:
3. It would be important to know the time frames of the employer's malpractice coverage. In other words, is the nurse covered only during the times he or she is working within the institution? It would be important to know the individual liability, meaning if sued, what financial responsibility would the nurse have?
1. The amount of the malpractice insurance provided by the employer is not the most important factor in deciding whether to carry private insurance. Generally, the employer's malpractice insurance coverage is much greater than private insurance coverage.
2. The area of nursing in which the nurse is employed is not the most important factor in deciding whether to carry malpractice insurance. Lawsuits can occur anywhere.

4. The nurse should be aware of Good Samaritan laws, but this would not be sufficient coverage for most nursing practice. Therefore it is not the most importance factor in determining whether to purchase private malpractice insurance.

5. 4, pp. 416, 417
Rationale:
4. In emergency situations, if it is impossible to obtain consent from the client or an authorized person, the procedure required to benefit the client or save a life may be undertaken without liability for failure to obtain consent. In such cases, the law assumes that the client would wish to be treated.
1. Telephone consents usually require two witnesses. This is not the case in this situation.
2. In an emergency, it is not necessary to contact the institutional review board. Doing so would take up valuable time.
3. A family member or acquaintance that is able to speak a client's language should not be used to interpret health information. An official interpreter must be available to explain the terms of consent (except in an emergency situation).

6. 1, p. 419
Rationale:
1. A nurse carrying out an inaccurate or inappropriate order may be legally responsible for any harm suffered by the client.
2. Good Samaritan laws will not protect the nurse in this situation. Good Samaritan laws are for providing care at the scene of an accident. The nurse should refuse to administer the medication when he or she knows it is wrong.
3. Developing a good relationship with the client is important but will not protect the nurse from legal liability for providing incompetent care.
4. Having malpractice insurance is not the answer, as it does not protect the client from harm. The nurse practitioner should refuse administer the medication.

4, p. 419

tionale:

A nurse carrying out an inaccurate or inappropriate order may be legally responsible for any harm suffered by the client. The nurse should clarify the order with the physician if unable to read the order.

The attending physician could be included in a lawsuit, but nurse would be ultimately responsible for the error.

The assisting resident would not be ultimately responsible for the error. The assisting resident did not carry out an inaccurate order.

The pharmacist could be included in a lawsuit, but the nurse would ultimately be responsible for the error because the nurse was the individual who carried out an inaccurate order.

2, p. 419

tionale:

Nurses who float should inform the supervisor of any lack of experience in caring for the types of clients on the nursing unit. They also should request and be given orientation to the unit. Asking to work with another general surgery nurse would be an appropriate action.

A nurse who refuses to accept an assignment may be considered insubordinate, and clients will not benefit from having fewer staff available.

A nurse can make a written protest to nursing administrators, but it should not be the nurse's initial recourse.

Notifying the state board of nursing should not be the nurse's initial recourse. The nurse should first notify the supervisor and request appropriate orientation and training. If problems continue, the nurse should attempt using the usual chain of command within the institution before contacting the state board of nursing.

4, p. 409

tionale:

Competent clients have the right to refuse treatment. This includes lifesaving hydration and nutrition.

1. This is not a true statement. Furthermore, physician-assisted suicide is legal in the state of Oregon.
2. In 1997 the Supreme Court ruled that no fundamental constitutional right exists to assisted suicide.
3. Organ donation does not have to be attempted to save a recipient's life.

10. 4, p. 407

Rationale:

4. The Joint Commission on Accreditation of Healthcare Organizations requires that accredited hospitals have written nursing policies and procedures.
1. Standards of care help define the limits of professional liability. The Joint Commission on Accreditation of Healthcare Organizations does not require an institution to have limits of professional liability.
2. Nurse Practice Acts establish educational requirements for nurses.
3. Nurse Practice Acts define the scope of nursing practice. The rules and regulations enacted by the state board of nursing define the practice of nursing more specifically. The American Nurses Association has developed standards for nursing practice that delineate the scope, function, and role of the nurse and establish clinical practice standards.

11. 3, p. 411

Rationale:

3. Because a license is viewed as a property right, due process must be followed before a license can be suspended or revoked. Due process means that nurses must be notified of the charges brought against them and that the nurses have an opportunity to defend against the charges in a hearing.
1. Hearings for suspension or revocation of a license do not occur in court but are usually conducted by a hearing panel of professionals.
2. Due process must be followed. They do not have to be waived by the nurse.
4. Some states, not the federal government, provide administrative and judicial review of such cases after nurses have exhausted all other forms of appeal.

12. 3, p. 414

Rationale:

3. An unintentional tort is an unintended wrongful act against another person that produces injury or harm. An example of an unintentional tort would be leaving the side rails down, and the client falls and is injured.
1. Restraining a client who refuses care would be an example of assault and battery.
2. Taking photos of a client's surgical wounds without the client's permission is an example of invasion of privacy.
4. Talking about a client's history of sexually transmitted diseases would fall under the category of invasion of privacy. Personal information should be kept confidential.

13. 1, p. 416

Rationale:

1. An emancipated minor, one who is younger than 18 years but who is a parent, may legally give informed consent for the care of her newborn. An emancipated minor can also be someone younger than 18 years who is legally married.
2. A person who has been sedated cannot legally give informed consent. Consent should be obtained before a sedative is administered.
3. If the 84-year-old client were unable to give consent, then the client's wife would be the person legally authorized to do so on the client's behalf. For a friend to be legally able to give consent, he or she would have to possess power of attorney or legal guardianship of the client.
4. If a client does not understand the proposed treatment plan, the nurse must notify the physician or nursing supervisor and must make certain that clients are informed before signing the consent.

14. 3, p. 416

Rationale:

3. The nurse's signature witnessing the consent means that the client voluntarily gave consent, that the client's signature is authentic, and that the client appears to be competent to give consent.

1. It is the physician's responsibility to make sure the client fully understands the procedure. If the nurse suspects that the client does not understand, the nurse should notify the physician.
2. The nurse's signature does not indicate that the client agrees with the procedure, but that the client has voluntarily given consent and is competent to do so. Clients also have the right to refuse treatment, which also is signed and witnessed.
4. The nurse's signature does not verify that the client has authorized the physician to continue with treatment. It verifies only that the consent was given voluntarily, the client is competent to give consent, and the signature is authentic.

15. 2, p. 410

Rationale:

2. If the client is unable, and no surrogate is available to give consent, the do-not-resuscitate (DNR) order can be written but only if the physician is reasonably medically certain that the resuscitation would be futile.
1. A DNR order is not legally required for terminally ill patients.
3. DNR orders are not necessarily maintained throughout the client's stay because a client's condition may warrant a change in DNR status. The attending physician must review the DNR orders every 3 days for hospitalized clients or every 60 days for clients in residential health facilities.
4. No nationally consistent standard exists for DNR implementation. States have their own statutes regarding DNR orders.

16. 4, p. 409

Rationale:

4. The Patient Self-Determination Act requires health care institutions to provide written information to clients concerning the clients rights under state law to make decisions including the right to refuse treatment and formulate advance directives.
1. The Patient Self-Determination Act does not require clients to designate a power of attorney

. The Patient Self-Determination Act does not require that DNR orders meet standard criteria.
. The Patient Self-Determination Act does not require organ donation on death. It is the client's decision whether he or she wants to participate in organ donation.

7. 4, p. 411
ationale:
. The Health Insurance Portability and Accountability Act (HIPAA) requires all hospitals and health agencies to have specific policies and procedures in place to ensure that reasonable safeguards protect written and verbal communications about clients.
. HIPAA does not require insurance coverage for all clients. It limits the extent to which health plans may impose preexisting condition limitations and prohibits discrimination in health plans against individual participants and beneficiaries based on health status.
. HIPAA does not require policies on how to report communicable diseases. It does require safeguards to protect written and verbal information about clients.
. HIPAA does not require limits on information and damages awarded in court cases.

8. 2, p. 413
ationale:
. Battery is any intentional touching without consent. An example of battery is a nurse giving a medication after the client has refused.
. Assault is any intentional threat to bring about harmful or offensive contact. No actual contact is necessary.
. Invasion of privacy exists when the client has unwanted intrusion into his or her private affairs. This case is not an example of invasion of privacy.
. Malpractice is negligence committed by a professional such as a nurse or physician. This case is not an example of malpractice.

9. 1, p. 414
ationale:
. A nurse can be held liable for slander if he or she shares private client information that can be overheard by others.

2. Assault is any intentional threat to bring about harmful or offensive contact. No actual contact is necessary. The nurse in this situation has not committed assault.
3. Malpractice is negligence committed by a professional such as a nurse or physician. Nursing malpractice results when care falls below the standard of care. This case is not an example of malpractice.
4. Invasion of privacy exists if the client has unwanted intrusion into his or her private affairs. This case is not an example of invasion of privacy. This instance falls under the category of defamation of character.

Chapter 23

1. 4, p. 428
Rationale:
4. This response is an example of feedback. Feedback is the message returned by the receiver.
1. The referent motivates one person to communicate with another, such as a time schedule. This is not an example of a referent.
2. The receiver is the person who receives and decodes the message. This question is asking not about the receiver, but rather the response.
3. Channels are means of conveying and receiving messages through visual, auditory, and tactile senses. This response is not an example of a channel.

2. 1, p. 439
Rationale:
1. Clarifying exists when the nurse checks whether understanding is accurate by restating an unclear message to clarify the sender's meaning, or by asking the other person to restate the message, explain further, or give an example of what the person means. This response indicates that the nurse wants to clarify what the client is saying so he or she can have an accurate understanding of what the client means.
2. This is an example of providing information, not clarification.
3. This is an example of focusing, not clarification.
4. This is an example of sharing empathy.

3. 4, p. 438

Rationale:

4. This response is an example of using the therapeutic communication technique of sharing empathy.

1. This response is an example of a nontherapeutic communication technique of asking for explanations.

2. This response is an example of a nontherapeutic communication technique of giving false reassurance.

3. This is an example of a nontherapeutic communication technique of giving disapproval.

4. 4, p. 431

Rationale:

4. Nurses often have to enter a client's personal space to provide care. The nurse should convey confidence, gentleness, and respect for privacy. This response demonstrates respect and provides information so the client may understand the need for personal contact.

1. Telling the client that the blood pressure can be taken at a later time does not promote effective communication.

2. Rotating the nurses who are assigned to take the client's blood pressure impedes the nurse's ability to form a therapeutic, helping relationship.

3. Continuing to perform the procedure quickly and quietly may send a negative nonverbal message. It also does not promote effective communication.

5. 1, p. 437

Rationale:

1. Active listening means to be attentive to what the client is saying both verbally and nonverbally. A nonverbal skill to facilitate attentive listening is to sit facing the client. This posture gives the message that the nurse is there to listen and is interested in what the client is saying.

2. For active listening, the arms and legs should be uncrossed. This posture suggests that the nurse is "open" to what the client says.

3. For active listening, the nurse should lean toward the client. This posture conveys that the nurse is involved and interested in the interaction.

4. For active listening, the nurse should establish and maintain intermittent eye contact. This conveys the nurse's involvement in and willingness to listen to what the client is saying.

6. 1, p. 434

Rationale:

1. An extremely breathless person must use oxygen to breathe rather than to speak.

2. Urinary frequency may interrupt conversation, but is not a communication problem.

3. Chronic stomach pain would not be a communication problem. The patient with chronic pain is, to some degree, used to the pain.

4. A lack of appetite is not a communication problem.

7. 4, p. 429

Rationale:

4. The connotative meaning is the shade of interpretation of a word's meaning influenced by the thoughts, feelings, or ideas people have about the word. "Slipping a little" in reference to hemodynamic pressures is an example of using connotative meaning.

1. Brevity means that communication is simple, brief, and direct. This is not an example of using brevity.

2. Relevance means the message is relevant or important to the situation at hand. This is not an example of using relevance.

3. Pacing and control means speaking slowly enough to enunciate clearly and not changing subjects rapidly. This is not an example of using pacing and control.

8. 3, p. 430

Rationale:

3. Territoriality is the need to gain, maintain, and defend one's right to space. The client who moves away from the nurse during a conversation is demonstrating the influence of space and territoriality on communication.

1. This not an example of gender influencing communication.

This is not an example of environment influencing communication. Noise, temperature extremes, distractions, and lack of privacy are examples of environmental factors that may influence communication.

Although people do maintain varying distances between each other depending on their culture, this is not an example of sociocultural background influencing communication, as cultural orientation is not mentioned in this situation.

. 2, p. 438

ationale:

. Empathy is the ability to understand and accept another person's reality, to perceive feelings accurately, and to communicate this understanding to others.

. This response is asking a question. It does not convey empathy.

. This response is asking a question to clarify the client's meaning. It does not convey empathy.

. This response is asking a relevant question that may focus on a particular topic. It is not an example of empathy.

0. 1, p. 438

ationale:

. The nurse is demonstrating the use of therapeutic communication by sharing hope. The nurse is pointing out that personal growth can come from illness experiences.

. This is a negative statement. The nurse should not state observations that might embarrass or anger the client.

. This response does not demonstrate the use of therapeutic communication. It implies disapproval and is an aggressive, threatening type of response.

. This is not a therapeutic statement. It is negative and aggressive in nature. If it is a true observation, it is one the nurse should not state, as it could anger the client.

11. 2, p. 433

Rationale:

2. This response is an example of trust. Trusting another person involves risk and vulnerability, but it also fosters open, therapeutic communication and enhances the expression of feelings, thoughts, and needs.

1. This statement is not an example of identifying problems and goals.

3. This statement is not clarifying roles of the nurse and client.

4. This statement is not an example of revealing. Although the parent may have provided information that was never before revealed, in this statement, the parent is indicating that there is trust between himself or herself and the nurse practitioner.

12. 3, p. 429

Rationale:

3. Discussing follow-up dietary needs immediately after surgery when the client is experiencing discomfort is an error in timing and relevance. The client is less likely to be able to pay attention and comprehend instruction when feeling pain, and immediately after surgery, discussing follow-up dietary needs would seem irrelevant.

1. Pacing has to do with the speed of conversation. This is not an example of an error in pacing.

2. Intonation is the tone of voice used. This is not an example of an error in intonation.

4. This is not an example of an error in denotative meaning.

13. 2, p. 430

Rationale:

2. The social zone extends the greatest amount from an individual in personal space and touch. It is a distance of 4 to 12 feet. Permission is not needed for touch in the social zone.

1. The personal zone is 18 inches to 4 feet.

3. The consent zone of touch requires permission.

4. The vulnerable zone is in the consent zone of touch. Because the vulnerable zone implies that special care is needed, permission is required.

14. 3, p. 444
Rationale:
3. The nurse and client determine whether the plan of care has been successful by evaluating the client communication outcomes established during planning. This process involves acquiring verbal and nonverbal feedback.
1. Delegation is not the purpose of communication in the evaluation phase of the nursing process. Delegation is more likely to be used in the implementation phase of the nursing process.
2. Validation of the client's needs is not why the nurse specifically uses communication in the evaluation phase of the nursing process. Validation of the client's needs is often determined when data are gathered during the assessment phase of the nursing process.
4. Documenting expected outcomes and planned interventions is part of the planning phase of the nursing process, not the evaluation phase.

15. 1, p. 428
Rationale:
1. Interpersonal variables are factors within both the sender and receiver that influence communication. An example of an interpersonal variable is postoperative discomfort.
2. An extremely warm room is an example of an environmental variable that may affect communication.
3. A talkative roommate is an example of an environmental variable that may affect communication because of the lack of privacy and distraction.
4. Noise, such as a loud television, is an example of an environmental variable that may affect communication.

16. 4, p. 433
Rationale:
4. Common courtesy is part of profession[al] communication. To practice courtesy, th[e] nurse says "hello" and "goodbye," knocks o[n] doors before entering, and uses self-introduc[tion]. Knocking on doors is important i[n] addressing the client.
1. Because using last names is respectful in mo[st] cultures, nurses usually use the client's la[st] name in the initial interaction, and then us[e] the first name if the client requests it.
2. Touching the client right away would not b[e] an appropriate action in establishing a hel[p]ing relationship. It would more likely b[e] interpreted as invading the client's person[al] space.
3. Sitting far enough away from the client i[s] important, in that the nurse should not ente[r] the client's personal space when establishing [a] helping relationship. However, leanin[g] toward the client conveys that the nurse [is] involved and interested in the clien[t]. Knocking on the door before entering th[e] client's room would be the first step i[n] addressing the client properly.

17. 2, pp. 437, 438
Rationale:
2. The nurse who is sharing an observation i[s] using the most therapeutic response. Sharin[g] observations often helps the client communi[cate] without the need for extensive question[ing], focusing, or clarification.
1. This is an example of a nontherapeuti[c] response. It is asking for an explanation. "Why" questions can cause resentment, inse[curity], and mistrust.
3. This is not a therapeutic response. It is givin[g] a personal opinion.
4. Changing the subject is not therapeutic.

18. 2, p. 443
Rationale:
2. Allowing toddlers and preschoolers to touc[h] and examine objects that will come in contac[t] with them is an effective communicatio[n] technique.

1. Toddlers and preschoolers are unable to understand analogies.
3. Sudden movements can be frightening. Children often prefer to make the first move in interpersonal contacts.
4. Focusing on what other children have done is not an effective communication technique for toddlers or preschoolers. Communication should be focused on the child.

19. 1, p. 443
Rationale:
1. The nurse may enhance communication for a client with aphasia by using visual cues (e.g., words, pictures, and objects) when possible.
2. The nurse should not shout or speak too loudly to enhance communication with a person who has aphasia.
3. The nurse should ask simple questions that require "yes" or "no" answers to enhance communication with the client who has aphasia.
4. Using a speech therapist is not the primary way to enhance communication with a client who has aphasia. The nurse can use communication techniques to facilitate communication and to develop a helping relationship with the client. The speech therapist may help the client to learn new ways or to relearn how to communicate.

Chapter 24

1. 3, p. 456
Rationale:
3. Task-mastery motives are based on needs such as achievement and competence. The client who must demonstrate irrigating his colostomy independently to be discharged is displaying the learning motive of task mastery.
1. A physical motive may be seen in the client who desires to return to a level of physical normalcy.
2. A social motive is the need for connection, social approval, or self-esteem.
4. An evaluation stance would be determining whether the outcomes of the teaching-learning process met the client's goal. Evaluation is not a learning motive.

2. 4, p. 459
Rationale:
4. The number of persons being taught, the need for privacy, the room temperature, the room lighting, noise, the room ventilation, and the room furniture are important factors when choosing the setting. The ideal setting helps the client focus on the learning task.
1. Specific ages of all the people involved is not so important for providing education on how to take a blood pressure as is providing an environment conducive to learning.
2. It is not necessary to know the names of employees who are married to teach individuals how to take their blood pressure.
3. Whether the employee has high blood pressure or not should not be so important to the teacher as providing an environment conducive to learning. Having high blood pressure may be a motivating factor for the employees to learn how to take their blood pressure, because of its personal relevance.

3. 4, p. 472
Rationale:
4. The nurse evaluates success by observing the client's performance of each expected behavior. Feedback indicating success in this situation is the client drinking 240 ml of fluid, 5 or 6 times during the shift. This would be a fluid intake of 1200 to 1440 ml, meeting the objective of at least 1000 ml during the designated period.
1. Voiding at least 1000 ml is not the objective. The objective is to have the client drink at least 1000 ml.
2. Verbalizing abdominal comfort without pressure is not an evaluation of the objective regarding specific fluid intake.
3. Having adequate intake and output is not accurate feedback indicating success. The term adequate is not quantified.

4. 4, p. 459
Rationale:
4. Effective teaching methods for the toddler include simple explanations and picture books that describe a story of children in a hospital or clinic.

1. Role playing is an appropriate teaching method for the preschooler.
2. Problem solving is an appropriate teaching method for the adolescent.
3. Independent learning is best used as a teaching method for the young or middle adult.

5. 1, p. 467
Rationale:
1. The telling approach is useful when limited information must be taught. If a client is highly anxious, but it is vital for information to be given, telling can be effective.
2. The entrusting approach provides the client the opportunity to manage self-care. The nurse observes the client's progress and remains available to assist without introducing more new information. This would not be the most effective teaching approach in this situation.
3. Participating involves the nurse and client setting objectives and becoming involved in the learning process together. This would not be the most effective teaching approach in this emergency situation.
4. Group teaching would not be the most effective teaching approach in this situation. A person who is anxious would benefit more from individual instruction.

6. 2, p. 455
Rationale:
2. Application involves using abstract, newly learned ideas in a concrete situation. The client who is taught the clinical manifestations of inflammation and assesses for signs such as redness or edema is using newly learned information in a concrete manner.
1. Attitude has to do with affective learning. The client is not expressing an attitude but is applying new knowledge in a concrete way.
3. Analysis involves breaking down information into organized parts. The client is not demonstrating analysis.
4. Evaluation is a judgment of the worth of a body of information for a given purpose. The client is not expressing judgment.

7. 1, p. 455
Rationale:
1. A guided response is the performance of an act under the guidance of an instructor. The client who is seeking help is demonstrating a guided response.
2. Adaptation occurs when a person is able to change a motor response when unexpected problems arise. The client is not exhibiting adaptation.
3. Perception is being aware of objects or qualities through the use of sense organs. This situation is not an example of perception.
4. Organizing is developing a value system by identifying and organizing values and resolving conflicts. This situation is not an example of organizing.

8. 2, p. 456
Rationale:
2. If a person does not want to learn, it is unlikely that learning will occur. Motivation is the first factor the nurse should assess before teaching.
1. To determine learning needs, the nurse should assess the client's previous knowledge level. However, this would not be the most important factor for the nurse to assess first.
3. Assessing a client's financial resources for obtaining equipment is important; however, it is not the most important factor for the nurse to assess first.
4. Assessing the client's physical and cognitive ability to learn is important. However, it is not the most important factor for the nurse to assess first.

9. 1, p. 465
Rationale:
1. The nurse who stops a demonstration of applying antiembolytic stockings to answer a client's question is following the teaching principle of timing. If the client has a question, it is important to answer the question right away, so the focus may return to the task being taught.
2. Setting priorities is important to conserve the time and energy of the client and nurse. The nurse who stops to answer a question is not setting priorities.

3. A client learns best on the basis of preexisting cognitive abilities and knowledge. This situation is not an example of building on existing knowledge.
4. Organizing teaching material means the nurse considers the order of information to present. This is not an example of organizing teaching materials.

10. 4, p. 455
Rationale:
4. Determining whether the client is able to demonstrate a newly learned skill is an example of an evaluation of a psychomotor skill. Psychomotor learning involves acquiring skills that require the integration of mental and muscular activity, such as walking with a cane.
1. Having the client state side effects of medication is an example of an evaluation of cognitive learning.
2. Determining whether a client responds appropriately to eye contact is an example of evaluation of affective learning.
3. The client who planned an exercise program is demonstrating cognitive learning.

11. 3, p. 451
Rationale:
3. Stress-management techniques for working parents is an appropriate topic for health maintenance/illness prevention.
1. Use of assistive devices, such as canes, is not a health maintenance/illness-prevention topic. It is a coping-with-impaired-function topic.
2. Self-help devices for post–cerebrovascular accident (CVA) clients is not a health-maintenance/illness-prevention topic. It is a coping-with-impaired-function topic.
4. Environmental alterations for clients in wheelchairs is not a health-maintenance/illness-prevention topic. It is a coping-with-impaired-function topic.

12. 1, p. 454
Rationale:
1. The client who is able to explain that the medication should be taken with meals is demonstrating attainment of a cognitive skill.

2. The client who is able to look at the surgical incision without prompting is demonstrating attainment of affective learning.
3. The client who uses crutches appropriately is demonstrating attainment of a psychomotor skill.
4. The client who dresses self after breakfast is most likely demonstrating attainment of psychomotor learning.

13. 3, p. 457
Rationale:
3. Readiness to learn is related to the stage of grieving. This response by the client demonstrates anger. The client is unwilling to learn at this time. The client has not yet reached the acceptance state of grieving, in which learning can occur.
1. This statement indicates that the client is ready to learn and desires to find out more to gain understanding.
2. This statement indicates that the client is willing to learn.
4. The client who requests feedback is expressing readiness to learn.

14. 1, p. 459
Rationale:
1. Keeping teaching sessions short is an appropriate method when teaching an older adult client.
2. The older adult should be taught when the client is alert and rested, not in the early morning or late evening.
3. The teaching session should not be filled with numerous topics.
4. The older adult client is capable of learning and should be the focus. A family member may be included in teaching, but the older adult client should not be excluded.

15. 2, pp. 461, 462
Rationale:
2. Pain, fatigue, or anxiety can interfere with the ability to pay attention and participate. The nursing diagnosis of *Activity intolerance related to pain* indicates a need to postpone teaching. Teaching may be delayed until the nursing diagnosis is resolved or the health problem is controlled.

Test Bank Answer Key   465

1. This nursing diagnosis does not indicate a need to postpone teaching. A knowledge deficit reinforces the need for teaching.
3. This nursing diagnosis does not indicate a need to postpone teaching. Ineffective management of treatment regimen reinforces the need for teaching.
4. This nursing diagnosis does not indicate a need to postpone teaching. The client who is noncompliant may require further teaching.

16. 1, p. 454
Rationale:
1. An independent project such as computer-assisted instruction is an appropriate teaching method for cognitive learning.
2. Demonstration is an appropriate teaching method for psychomotor learning.
3. Modeling of behavior is an appropriate teaching method for psychomotor learning.
4. Discussion of feelings is an appropriate teaching method for affective learning.

17. 3, p. 470
Rationale:
3. When teaching a functionally illiterate client, the nurse should use simple terminology, avoiding medical jargon. The nurse should incorporate familiar terminology to enhance the client's understanding.
1. The nurse should use simple analogies and real-life examples.
2. The nurse should ask for return demonstrations, as this provides the opportunity to clarify instructions and the time to review procedures.
4. Although teaching sessions may be kept short, they should be scheduled at more frequent intervals.

18. 4, pp. 452, 458, 459
Rationale:
4. Adults have a wide variety of personal and life experiences to draw on. Therefore adult learning is enhanced when adults are encouraged to use these experiences to solve problems. Evidence-based information indicates that adult clients prefer interactive, personal communication with nurses or physicians.

1. Evidence-based information indicates that computer-assisted learning is not a preferred method of instruction by many adult learners. As clients become more comfortable with computers, this preference may change.
2. Evidence-based information indicates that not all clients are comfortable in class settings or in support groups. Other educational opportunities should be available.
3. Adult learners prefer short teaching sessions without lots of technical information.

19. 3, p. 466
Rationale:
3. An intervention to promote learning in the affective domain would be encouraging the client to discuss his feelings about his health status.
1. Asking the client what he believes he needs to know about the diagnosis would be an intervention to promote learning in the cognitive domain.
2. Providing brochures on current exercises and nutrition guidelines would be an intervention to promote learning in the cognitive domain.
4. Having the client return demonstration of self-measurement of his blood pressure would be an intervention to promote learning in the psychomotor domain.

20. 4, p. 465
Rationale:
4. The nurse should begin and end each teaching session with important information because clients are more likely to remember information that is taught early in the teaching session, and key points can be summarized at the end. Repetition also reinforces learning.
1. The group should not be moved along at a predetermined pace. Clients may have questions that would go unanswered if there were a predetermined pace. Sometimes teaching sessions have to be stopped after the nurse observes a client's loss of concentration, such as nonverbal cues of poor eye contact or slumped posture.

466   Test Bank Answer Key

. Shorter (approximately 20 minutes), frequent sessions are more easily tolerated and retain the client's interest in the material.
. The nurse should face the client and speak in a low tone of voice for the older adult with a hearing problem.

Chapter 25

. 4, p. 496
Rationale:
4. A change-of-shift report should include instructions given in a teaching plan and the client's response. This should not include detailed content unless staff members ask for clarification.
1. The nurse should relay to staff significant changes in the way therapies are given, but should not describe basic steps of a procedure.
2. The client's diagnosis-related group is not essential background information to be shared in report.
3. The nurse should not review all routine care procedures or tasks.

2. 1, p. 497
Rationale:
1. The nurse who witnessed the incident is the one who completes the report.
2. Details of the incident should be objectively described.
3. An explanation of the possible cause is not included. The sequence of events is described objectively.
4. A notation that an incident report was written is not included in the medical record.

3. 4, p. 482
Rationale:
4. Information within a recorded entry must be complete, containing appropriate and essential information. This notation provides the time and action taken by the nurse, including the reason for doing so.
1. This entry does not indicate what the vital signs were.

2. This entry does not provide a specific amount the client drank. Stating "adequate" is subjective, not objective.
3. This notation does not have the client describe his or her pain or rate it according to a pain scale for comparison later. It also does not indicate whether the client's pain was in the lower left or lower right quadrant, or both.

4. 3, p. 482
Rationale:
3. This is the best example of a late entry. The time is indicated along with the action and an objective observation.
1. This notation is not complete. It does not indicate why the aspirin and oxycodone (Percodan) was given (i.e., what was the client's level of pain?). Where was the pain located?
2. The nurse does not need to document about herself, only about the client. In this option, the nurse does not indicate why the morphine was given (client's level of pain? Location of pain?).
4. This entry is not complete. It does not state the size of the wound, type of dressing used, or the client's tolerance of the procedure.

5. 3, p. 484
Rationale:
3. This datum is an example of the "P" of PIE because it describes the problem.
1. The "S" in SOAP documentation represents subjective data (verbalizations of the client).
2. FOCUS charting does not concentrate on only problems. It is structured according to a client's concerns.
4. The "R" in DAR documentation is the response of the client. This situation describes the client's problem, not the client's response.

6. 4, p. 492
Rationale:
4. A nurse's description of the teaching provided to the client on performance of self-administration of medication is recorded in the discharge summary form.

1. A Kardex is a written form that contains basic client information. A Kardex contains an activity and treatment section and a nursing care plan section that organizes information for quick reference as nurses give change-of-shift report. It does not include a description of teaching that was provided to the client.
2. An incident report concerns any event that is not consistent with the routine operation of a health care unit or routine care of a client (e.g., a client falls).
3. A nursing history form guides the nurse through a complete assessment to identify relevant nursing diagnoses or problems. It provides baseline data about the client.

7. 1, p. 480
Rationale:
1. If a nurse has made an error in documentation, the nurse should draw a single line through the error, write the word *error* above it, and sign his or her name or initials. Then record the note correctly.
2. The nurse should not erase, apply correction fluid, or scratch out errors made while recording because charting becomes illegible. Entries should be made only in ink so it cannot be erased.
3. This is not correct. It may appear as if the nurse was attempting to hide something or deface the record.
4. Footnotes are not used in nursing documentation.

8. 4, p. 480
Rationale:
4. Each entry should begin with the time and end with the signature and title of the person recording the entry.
1. All entries should be recorded legibly and in black ink because pencil can be erased.
2. The nurse should never erase entries or use correction fluid and never use a pencil. The use of correction fluid could make the charting become illegible, and it may appear as if the nurse were attempting to hide something or to deface the record.

3. If the physician made an error, the nurse should not document it in the client's chart. It should be documented in an incident report

9. 1, p. 497
Rationale:
1. A telephone order involves a physician stating a prescribed therapy over the phone to a registered nurse.
2. This is not an appropriate response and not in the client's best interest.
3. It is best to repeat any prescribed orders back to the physician, who can then verify whether it is correct or clarify the order.
4. This is not the appropriate response. A registered nurse must take the verbal order, but it does not have to be the nursing supervisor.

10. 1, p. 484
Rationale:
1. The "R" in FOCUS charting is the client's response. In this case, the nurse would document, "My arm feels better."
2. "Slight hematoma on left forearm" is the "D" referring to data in FOCUS charting.
3. "Infiltrated IV line" would be documented as "D," referring to data in FOCUS charting.
4. "Elevation of left forearm" is the "A" in FOCUS charting. It describes the action or nursing intervention.

11. 2, pp. 480, 481
Rationale:
2. Entries should be concise, factual, and accurate. This is an example of an objective description of a client's behavior.
1. The nurse should not document "physician-made error." Instead, the nurse could chart, "Dr. Green was called to clarify order for medication administration."
3. The nurse should chart only for himself or herself. In this case, nurse Williams should write the charting entry.
4. Only objective descriptions of the client's behavior should be recorded. For example: Client states, "I don't want physical therapy! I want to go home!"

2. 4, p. 495

Rationale:

4. A good system of computerized documentation requires periodic changes in personal passwords to prevent unauthorized persons from tampering with records.

1. All nurses do not use the same access code. Each nurse should have his or her own password.

2. This is not a true statement. Authorized health care providers from any department can access and use the data.

3. Many programs do not have thumbprint identification restrictions.

Chapter 26

1. 4, pp. 502, 505

Rationale:

4. What individuals think and how they feel about themselves affects the way in which they care for themselves. A physical change in the body, such as an amputation, can lead to an altered body image affecting identity and self-esteem. The nurse should assess the client's ideal and perceived self-concept to help the client establish realistic goals and implementation strategies.

1. Assessing a client's interests and past accomplishments may provide information regarding a client's identity. Identity is only one component of self-concept. The nurse must determine the client's ideal and perceived self-concept to get "the big picture," as this will greatly affect his response to the amputation.

2. Intellectual and spiritual strengths may be important when determining a client's ability to cope. However, when developing goals and implementation strategies, the process will begin with the client's perception of self-concept, as this will greatly affect his response to the amputation.

3. When assessing coping behaviors of an individual, involvement with significant others may be an indication of available resources, as well as a source of strength for a client.

2. 2, p. 510

Rationale:

2. A passive attitude is a behavioral characteristic suggestive of a negative self-concept.

1. Avoidance of eye contact would be a behavior suggestive of a negative self-concept.

3. Being excessively dependent is characteristic of a negative self-concept.

4. A lack of interest in what is happening in one's surroundings is characteristic of a negative self-concept.

3. 4, p. 510

Rationale:

4. Being angry, excessively dependent, and having a passive attitude are all behaviors suggestive of an altered self-concept. The older client, who has lost a spouse and is now demanding excessive assistance from a child, is demonstrating an alteration in the integrity stage of his psychosocial development.

1. Accepting one's limitations is not consistent with a disturbance in the integrity stage of psychosocial development.

2. Verbalizing fear about the surgery is not consistent with a disturbance in the integrity stage of psychosocial development.

3. Expressing thoughts about one's care is not consistent with a disturbance in the integrity stage of psychosocial development.

4. 3, p. 513

Rationale:

3. Consultation with significant others, mental health clinicians, and community resources can result in a more comprehensive and workable plan. Clients who are experiencing threats to or alterations in self-concept often benefit from collaboration with mental health and community resources to promote increased awareness.

1. The client's problem of a negative self-concept must be addressed first. As a result, the client may begin to bathe and dress independently.

2. The client needs to express his negative feelings. This would be one step in addressing his self-concept problem. Stating that the client should think positively instead of negatively, at this point, is unrealistic.

4. A long-term goal may be that the client will become more independent and return to prior activities. It is not realistic at this time.

5. 4, p. 506
Rationale:
4. A physical health deficit that prevents role assumption can create a problem in the role-performance component of self-concept.
1. A client who is verbalizing concern about continuing a previous occupation is demonstrating a problem not in body image, but rather in the role-performance component of self-concept.
2. Self-esteem is closely related to self-concept, but is not a component of self-concept.
3. Identity involves the internal sense of individuality, wholeness, and consistency of a person over time and in various circumstances. The client is verbalizing concern about role performance, not necessarily identity.

6. 3, p. 507
Rationale:
3. Role conflict results when a person is required to assume simultaneously two or more roles that are inconsistent, contradictory, or mutually exclusive. The single mother who is having difficulty managing working long hours and trying to raise her children, as she perceives she would like to, is experiencing role conflict.
1. Role ambiguity involves unclear role expectations. The client is not expressing doubt as to what her roles are.
2. Role strain is a feeling of frustration when a person feels inadequate or feels unsuited to a role, such as with gender-role stereotypes.
4. A genderrole stereotype describes an expectation that something is a "man's role" or a "woman's role" because the position has been typically held by a man or woman. The client is not expressing concern about a gender-role stereotype, but rather in managing two contradictory roles.

7. 1, p. 517
Rationale:
1. Encouraging the client's self-exploration i achieved by accepting the client's thought and feelings, by helping the client to clarify interactions with others, and by being empa thetic.
2. Telling the client not to be embarrassed doe not encourage self-exploration. It also assumes that the client is embarrassed, which may not be the case.
3. This response involves the client in a decision making process related to the client's care bu does not support the client's self exploration Self-exploration expands self-awareness.
4. This response is not therapeutic. Telling the client that staff will not try to judge the client's past implies that judgment is due and does not encourage open communication and self-exploration.

8. 3, p. 517
Rationale:
3. This response clarifies the meaning of verba and nonverbal communication. This response also demonstrates acceptance of the client' thoughts and feelings and encourages open communication.
1. This response is not therapeutic. It does no address the client's feelings of anger and conveys a message that feeling angry is not acceptable.
2. This response is not therapeutic. It does not address the cause of the anger but puts limits on how the anger may be expressed.
4. This response is not therapeutic. It does not encourage the client to communicate his or her feelings.

9. 2, p. 503
Rationale:
2. The developmental needs of the early20s to mid-40s age group includes the establishment of intimate relationships with family and significant others, having stable, positive feelings about self, and experiencing successful role transitions and increased responsibilities.

. The self-concept developmental needs of the 12- to 20-year-old age group include accepting body changes, examining attitudes and beliefs, establishing goals for the future, and interacting with those whom he or she finds sexually attractive or intellectually stimulating.

. The self-concept developmental tasks of the mid-40s to mid-60s age group include accepting changes in appearance and endurance, reassessing life goals, and showing contentment with aging.

. The self-concept developmental needs of the late 60s and older age group include feeling positive about one's life and its meaning, and being interested in providing a legacy for the next generation.

10. 1, p. 505
Rationale:

. In the process of substitution, an individual replaces one behavior with another that provides the same personal gratification. The child has learned to substitute one behavior for another for a positive outcome.

. Avoiding unacceptable behavior because it is punished is seen in the process of reinforcement-extinction.

. In the process of identification, an individual internalizes the beliefs, behavior, and values of role models into a personal, unique expression of self.

. In the process of inhibition, an individual learns to refrain from behaviors, even when tempted to engage in them.

11. 2, p. 503
Rationale:

2. The developmental tasks associated with self-concept in the 12- to 20-year-old age group include accepting body changes; examining attitudes, values, and beliefs; and establishing goals for the future.

1. Identifying with a gender is an expected developmental task associated with self-concept in the 3- to 6-year-old age group.

3. Distinguishing oneself from the environment is an expected developmental task associated with self-concept in the 0 to 1-year-old age group.

4. Feeling positive about one's life achievements is an expected developmental task associated with self-concept for the late 60s and older age group.

12. 3, p. 512
Rationale:

3. Asking, "How would you describe yourself?" is an example of a question a nurse could use to assess a client's perception of identity.

1. Asking, "What changes would you make in your appearance?" is an example of a question a nurse could use to assess a client's perception of body image.

2. Asking, "What activities do you enjoy doing?" is an example of a question a nurse could use to assess a client's perception of self-esteem.

4. Asking, "What is your usual day like?" is an example of a question a nurse could use to assess a client's role performance.

13. 4, p. 514
Rationale:

4. An appropriate outcome for the client with situational low self-esteem would be for the client to discuss a minimum of two areas in which he is functioning well.

1. This would not be an appropriate outcome for the client with low self-esteem. The focus should be on his abilities, not inability.

2. This outcome does not address the issue of low self-esteem.

3. Being able to use therapeutic communication is always an asset, but the focus should be on improving his self-esteem by determining his strengths, recognizing his worth as a person, realizing what he is able to control, and providing support from others who are having, or had, the same experience.

Chapter 27

1. 1, p. 524
Rationale:

1. The first step of gender-identity development occurs as the child becomes aware of the differences of the sexes and perceives that he or she is male or female. This is characterized by an interest in his or her genitalia.

2. This is not characteristic of the preschool child. Learning how and why his or her anatomy differs from that of other children would require a higher level of cognitive ability.
3. Children of this age group focus primarily on their parents and family, not on other children.
4. According to Freud, the preschool child identifies with the parent of the same sex and develops a complementary relationship with the parent of the opposite sex. The preschool child does not spend most of his or her time with the parent of the opposite sex.

2. 4, p. 531
Rationale:
4. The nurse should convey a message of acceptance of the client, but not the inappropriate behavior. Reviewing and defining the professional relationship with the client can accomplish this.
1. Matching the gender of the health care worker with the gender of the client may be beneficial when dealing with assessment of sexual needs or sex education. However, in this instance, the client needs to be informed that inappropriate sexual behavior is unacceptable. To turn the client's care over to a male nurse would not resolve the problem and would convey a message of dislike and lack of acceptance of the client.
2. Reporting the incident immediately to the client's physician would not be the nurse's best action. The client needs to be made aware of the problem to discontinue such behavior.
3. Telling the client his behavior is offensive and then leaving the room is not therapeutic. The client needs to be reminded of the professional relationship he shares with the nurse.

3. 3, p. 539
Rationale:
3. In response to identified concerns, the nurse may initiate discussion. This provides an open dialogue enabling the client to talk freely with the nurse to address the concerns.

1. To assist the clients in their situation change, the nurse must explore communication and sexual patterns of the couple. Having similar parenting beliefs will have less impact on their sexual relationship.
2. To assist the couple in adjusting to the change of becoming a family, the nurse should explore communication patterns of the couple. How long they have been married would be less significant.
4. The level of knowledge they have regarding healthy sexual relationships would not affect their sexual relationship as would their ability to discuss their feelings with one another.

4. 4, p. 530
Rationale:
4. Dyspareunia is recurrent or persistent genital pain in either a male or female before, during or after sexual intercourse that is not associated with vaginismus or with lack of lubrication.
1. Orgasmic disorder is the recurrent delay in, or absence of, orgasm after normal sexual excitement.
2. Hypoactive sexual desire disorder is the persistent or recurrent deficiency or absence of sexual fantasies and desire for sexual activity.
3. Vaginismus is an involuntary constriction of the outer one third of the vagina that prevents penile insertion and intercourse.

5. 4, p. 526
Rationale:
4. To be an effective contraceptive method, the diaphragm should be used with a contraceptive cream or jelly. The client is verbalizing understanding.
1. Any act of unprotected intercourse can result in pregnancy. This is not an effective contraceptive method.
2. Any act of unprotected intercourse can result in pregnancy. This statement does not demonstrate understanding of the basal body temperature method of contraception.
3. Using spermicidal foam alone is not recommended. The client should use a condom and foam to be more effective in preventing pregnancy.

472   Test Bank Answer Key

6. 2, p. 527

Rationale:

2. Diseases that are caused by bacteria and that can usually be cured with antibiotics include gonorrhea, chlamydia, syphilis, and pelvic inflammatory disease. All clients need to understand that antibiotics must be taken for the full course of treatment.
1. Chlamydia is caused by bacteria that can be treated, not a virus.
3. Sexually transmitted diseases, such as chlamydia, are transmitted from infected individuals to partners during intimate sexual contact. It is contracted not via blood-borne exchange, but rather through body fluids.
4. Chlamydia is not prevented with the use of spermicidals.

7. 4, p. 539

Rationale:

4. Open communication and positive self-esteem are essential factors in effectively resolving concerns.
1. This statement may only worry the client more.
2. This statement does not focus on the client and therefore does not encourage the client to express his concerns.
3. Telling the client not to worry is nontherapeutic. At this point, not even knowing the outcome of the surgery, the nurse should not predict resumption of sexual activity for the client. Furthermore, this response does not encourage the client to communicate his feelings.

8. 3, p. 525

Rationale:

3. Orgasms may not last as long in the older adult as a result of aging. Older adults may feel more sexually satisfied because they no longer have to be concerned with contraception and are not experiencing the pressures of raising children and working.
1. Decreased levels of estrogen may lead to diminished vaginal lubrication and decreased vaginal elasticity, making intercourse more painful. The couple should not be advised to have sex less frequently, but rather to use a vaginal lubricant and allow more time for caressing.

2. The need to use a lubricant is not due to having sex less often, but is due to decreasing levels of estrogen in the woman.
4. This is not a true statement. Sexual feelings in older adulthood are normal. Sexuality and continued interest in sex throughout late life generally reflects life patterns.

9. 2, p. 536

Rationale:

2. An appropriate expected outcome for the nursing diagnosis of *Sexual dysfunction related to side effects of antihypertensive* would be *Client will relate renewed interest in sex within 1 month.* An appropriate goal would be *Client will express satisfaction with sexual relationship with wife within 1 month.*
1. The client should not avoid taking his antihypertensive medication before intercourse, but should be taught that other available blood pressure medications can maintain blood pressure control and do not negatively affect sexual function. He can then discuss this with his physician.
3. This is not an appropriate expected outcome. Seeing a sexual therapist immediately is not necessary and may only intensify his concern.
4. This is not an appropriate expected outcome. It does not address or resolve the problem.

10. 3, p. 525

Rationale:

3. The perimenopausal and menopausal woman may have diminished vaginal lubrication due to decreased levels of estrogen. Suggestions such as using vaginal lubrication and creating time for caressing and tenderness can help to ease adjustment to normal changes related to aging.
1. Some physical changes with aging may affect sexuality. The client should be educated on the expected changes and how best to address them.
2. If a nurse is uncomfortable discussing sexual issues with a client, then he or she should get another nurse who is comfortable to talk with the client. A sex therapist is not necessary in this situation. Sex therapists address more-complex sexual issues.

4. This is not a true statement. Decreasing the frequency of intercourse would not promote healthy sexual relations.

11. 1, p. 529
Rationale:
1. Sexual abuse may begin, continue, or even intensify during pregnancy.
2. Sexual abuse crosses all gender, socioeconomic, age, and ethnic groups.
3. The abuser may not fit any classic description.
4. Most often sexual abuse is at the hands of a former intimate partner or family member.

12. 2, p. 533
Rationale:
2. Kegel exercises increase the tone and sensation of the pelvic floor (pubococcygeus muscle) for the female client.
1. Sensate-focus exercises do not increase muscle tone.
3. Vaginal dilation will not increase the tone and sensation of the pelvic floor.
4. Stopping urination may help identify proper muscle contraction, but once the muscle is identified, Kegel exercises should not be repeated during urination. Stopping urination midstream may create a backflow of urine into the bladder, predisposing a person to infection.

Chapter 28

1. 2, p. 546
Rationale:
2. Adolescents often reconsider their childlike concept of a spiritual power, and in the search for an identity, they may either question practices and values or find the spiritual power as the motivation to seek a clearer meaning to life.
1. Adolescents do not necessarily have a good concept of a supreme being.
3. Adolescents do not necessarily fully accept the higher meaning of their faith.
4. Older adults, not adolescents, often turn to important relationships and the giving of themselves to others as spiritual tasks.

2. 2, p. 549
Rationale:
2. Knowledge about spirituality begins with nurses' insights into their own spirituality. This self-exploration may occur through reading, religious involvement, or activities such as meditation to understand their own beliefs and values.
1. Researching popular religions may add to the nurse's knowledge, but knowledge of spirituality begins with the nurse examining his or her own beliefs. It is essential for the nurse to be aware of his or her own beliefs so as not to impose them on others, and to be able to recognize and understand a client's spiritual needs.
3. The nurse's knowledge about spirituality does not begin with the nurse sharing his or her faith with clients.
4. Providing prayers and religious articles for clients may be an intervention to meet a client's spiritual needs; however, it is not how the nurse's knowledge about spirituality begins.

3. 4, p. 549
Rationale:
4. After a client has experienced a near-death experience, it is important for the nurse to remain open and give the client a chance to explore what happened.
1. This is not a common experience that can be easily explained. The client should be encouraged to discuss it, as he or she may find meaning from this powerful experience.
2. The nurse should not assume that this was an awful experience for the client. Many people who have had a near-death experience report positive aftereffects, including a positive attitude and spiritual development.
3. This would not be the most appropriate response. It does not help the client explore his or her own experience.

4. 1, p. 552

Rationale:

1. Stating the observation of a client having a Bible opens communication regarding the client's source of strength. Assessing a client's source of strength and faith can direct interaction with him or her, including medical treatment plans.
2. This is not the best response. It does not provide information that would assist the nurse in meeting the client's spiritual needs.
3. This is not the best response. It implies that the client goes to church or should go to church, and assumes that church members are a source of strength for the client. It does not provide assessment information to determine the client's spiritual needs.
4. This is not the best response. It has a negative connotation and does not assess the client's source of strength or beliefs of the client.

5. 1, p. 561

Rationale:

1. Some sects of Hindus are vegetarians. The belief is not to kill *any* living creature.
2. Followers of Judaism may observe the kosher dietary restriction of avoiding pork and shellfish and not preparing and eating milk and meat at the same time.
3. People of Islamic faith do not consume pork and alcohol. Fasting is done during the month of Ramadan.
4. Members of the Sikh religion do not necessarily follow a vegetarian diet.

6. 4, p. 547

Rationale:

4. Hope provides a sense of meaning and purpose. When a person has hope, he or she has an attitude of something to live for and look forward to.
1. Faith is a relationship with a divinity.
2. Religion is a system of organized beliefs.
3. Spirituality provides a cultural connectedness.

7. 4, p. 554

Rationale:

4. While working with a client to assess and support spirituality, the nurse should first determine the client's perceptions and belief system. Exploring the client's spirituality may reveal responses to health problems that require nursing intervention, or it may reveal existence of a strong set of resources that enable the client to cope effectively.
1. Although the agency chaplain may be a source for referral, it is not the first action the nurse should take in assessing and supporting a client's spirituality.
2. The nurse needs first to assess a client's spirituality to determine the client's perceptions and belief system before attempting to assist the client to use faith to get well.
3. Providing a variety of religious literature may be ineffective, as it does not address the client as an individual and does not assess the client's personal spiritual needs. The nurse should first assess the client's perception and belief system before implementing any intervention.

8. 1, p. 553

Rationale:

1. Observance of the Sabbath is important to a client who follows the traditional health care beliefs of Judaism. This client my refuse treatments scheduled on the Sabbath.
2. Followers of the Islamic or Christian faith may use faith healing in response to illness.
3. Ongoing group prayer may be seen with the Islamic faith. Christians also use prayer.
4. Regular fasting may be seen with some Roman Catholics or with followers of the Russian Orthodox Church.

9. 4, p. 561

Rationale:

4. Food practices of Native Americans are influenced by individual tribal beliefs.
1. Some Hindus and Buddhists are vegetarian.
2. Buddhists, Mormons, and some Baptists, Evangelicals, and Pentecostals avoid the use of alcohol and tobacco.

3. Members of Hinduism, Islam, and Judaism may avoid pork products.

10. 2, p. 556
Rationale:
2. Ineffective individual coping is a nursing diagnosis that may apply to clients in need of spiritual care.
1. The nursing diagnosis of altered health maintenance does not indicate the greatest potential need for spiritual care.
3. The nursing diagnosis of impaired memory does not imply the need for spiritual care.
4. The nursing diagnosis of decreased adaptive capacity does not indicate the greatest potential need for spiritual care.

11. 4, p. 555
Rationale:
4. No special rituals are usually performed in the immediate postpartum period with members of the Shinto, Buddhist, or Hindu religions.
1. Many Christians will baptize their infants.
2. Followers of Islam will say special prayers after birth over the child.
3. Navajos make special preparations for the umbilical cord and placenta after the birth of a child.

12. 2, p. 561
Rationale:
2. Mormons and Buddhists both avoid alcohol and tobacco.
1. Hindus and Buddhists may both follow vegetarian diets.
3. Followers of Judaism may avoid eating milk and meat at the same time.
4. Some Roman Catholics and Russian Orthodox members may fast on Fridays.

13. 1, p. 553
Rationale:
1. Females are to be examined by females, according to the Sikh religion.
2. Followers of Judaism view visiting the sick as an obligation. They have no restrictions on gender-related care.

3. Followers of Hinduism view illness as being caused by past sins. Prolonging life is discouraged. No restrictions exist on care related to gender.
4. Buddhists believe in Dharma, which teaches that life is impermanent and all persons have to age and die. No restrictions exist on care related to gender.

14. 2, p. 555
Rationale:
2. After a Navajo child's delivery, the umbilical cord is taken from the newborn, dried, and buried near a place that symbolizes what parents want for the child's future.
1. Catholics do not have special care of the umbilical cord after delivery. They may want their newborn baptized if there is any chance of the newborn not surviving.
3. Shintos have no special rituals related to birth, including the umbilical cord.
4. Hindus have no special rituals related to birth, including the umbilical cord.

C*hapter 29*

1. 4, p. 579
Rationale:
4. A defining characteristic for the nursing diagnosis of hopelessness may include the client stating, "What does it matter?" when offered choices or information concerning him or her. The client's behavior of not eating also is an indicator of hopelessness.
1. This is not an example of social isolation. The client is not avoiding or restricted from seeing others.
2. Spiritual distress is not the most appropriate nursing diagnosis for this client. The focus should be on the client's lack of hope.
3. The client's behavior and verbalization does not indicate denial.

2. 4, p. 571

Rationale:

4. The benefit of anticipatory grief is that it allows time for the process of grief (i.e., to say good-bye and complete life affairs). Anticipatory grief allows time to grieve in private, to discuss the anticipated loss with others, and to "let go" of the loved one. Anticipatory grief can help a person progress to a healthier emotional state of acceptance and dealing with loss.

1. It is not most beneficial for grieving to take place only in private. It is important for grief to be acknowledged by others, and to be able to receive the support of others in the grieving process.

2. Anticipatory grieving can be discussed with others in most circumstances. However, at times, anticipatory grief may be disenfranchised grief as well, meaning it cannot be openly acknowledged, socially sanctioned, or publicly shared, such as a partner dying of AIDS. The benefit of anticipatory grieving is not so much that it can be discussed in most circumstances, as this discussion also can occur with normal grief when the actual loss has occurred.

3. Anticipatory grief is the process of disengaging or "letting go" that occurs before an actual loss or death has occurred. The benefit is not the separation of the ill client from the family as much as it is the process of being able to say good-bye, to put life affairs in order, and as a result, it can help a client or family to progress to a higher emotional state.

3. 4, p. 578

Rationale:

4. When caring for clients experiencing grief, it is important for the nurse to assess his own emotional well-being and to understand his own feelings about death. The nurse who is aware of his own feelings will be less likely to place personal situations and values before those of the client.

1. Although course work on death and dying may add to the nurse's knowledge base, it does not best prepare the nurse for caring for a dying client. The nurse needs to have an awareness of his own feelings about death first, as death can raise many emotions.

2. Being able to control one's own emotions is important; however, it is unlikely that the nurse would be able to do so if he has not first developed a personal understanding of his own feelings about death.

3. Experiencing the death of a loved one is not prerequisite to caring for a dying client. Experiencing death may help an individual mature in dealing with loss, or it may bring up many negative emotions if complicated grief is present. The nurse is best prepared by first developing an understanding of his own feelings about death.

4. 3, p. 588

Rationale:

3. A dying client's family is better prepared to provide psychological support if the nurse discusses with them ways to support the dying person and listen to needs and fears.

1. Demonstration of bathing techniques may help the family meet the dying client's physical needs, not to providing psychological support.

2. Application of oxygen devices may help the family provide physical needs for the client, not to provide psychological support for the client.

4. Information on when to contact the hospice nurse is important knowledge for the family to have and may help them feel they are being supported in caring for the dying client. However, contact information does not help the family provide psychological support to the dying client.

5. 3, p. 584

Rationale:

3. No topic that a dying client wishes to discuss should be avoided. The nurse should respond to questions openly and honestly. As client advocate, the nurse should assist the client to obtain the necessary information to make this decision.

1. The nurse should provide the client with information with which to make such a decision. Although the nurse may suggest that the client discuss this option after having obtained information, it is up to the client to discuss the subject with the family.

2. The nurse should respect the client and provide the necessary information for him or her to make a decision, rather than dismissing the client's question.
4. It is not necessary to contact the physician or the family for consent for organ donation if the client is capable of making this decision.

6. 2, p. 570
Rationale:
2. According to Kübler-Ross, the client is in the denial stage of dying. The client may act as though nothing has happened, may refuse to believe or understand that a loss has occurred, and may seem stunned, as though it is "unreal" or difficult to believe.
1. No stage of anxiety is found in Kübler-Ross's five stages of dying.
3. No stage of confrontation is found in Kübler-Ross's five stages of dying.
4. During depression, the individual may feel overwhelmingly lonely and withdraw from interpersonal interaction.

7. 3, p. 589
Rationale:
3. Some families of Chinese-Americans will prefer to bathe the client themselves. They often believe the body should remain intact; organ donation and autopsy are uncommon.
1. Chinese-Americans do not prefer pastoral care for after-death care of a family member.
2. Organ donation is uncommon for Chinese-Americans.
4. Chinese-Americans may desire time to bathe the client. Quick removal from the hospital is not preferred.

8. 4, p. 580
Rationale:
4. The focus in planning nursing care is to support the client physically, emotionally, developmentally, and spiritually in the expression of grief. When caring for the dying client, it is important to devise a plan that helps a client to die with dignity and offers family members the assurance that their loved one is cared for with care and compassion.

1. Optimism should not be the primary focus when caring for the dying client. The nurse should promote the client's self-esteem and allow the client to die with dignity.
2. The client should be allowed to make choices and perform as many activities of daily living independently as possible. This allows the client to maintain self-esteem and dignity.
3. The client does not need to be left alone. The nurse's or family's presence may indicate to the client that he or she is being cared for and is worthy of attention.

9. 1, p. 588
Rationale:
1. The nurse's role in hospice is to meet the primary wishes of the dying client and to be open to individual desires of each client. The nurse supports a client's choice in maintaining comfort and dignity.
2. Hospice care is for the terminally ill. It is not aimed at offering curative treatment, but rather the emphasis is on palliative care.
3. Hospice care may provide bereavement follow-up for the family after a client's death, but hospice nurses typically do not teach the family postmortem care.
4. Hospice care is primarily for home care, but a client in hospice may become hospitalized.

10. 4, p. 586
Rationale:
4. To promote comfort in the terminally ill client, the nurse should help the client to identify values or desired tasks and then help the client to conserve energy for those tasks.
1. Decreasing the client's fluid intake may make the terminally ill client more prone to dehydration and constipation. The nurse should take measures to help maintain oral intake, such as administering antiemetics, applying topical analgesics to oral lesions, and offering ice chips.
2. The use of analgesics should not be limited. Controlling the terminally ill client's level of pain is a primary concern in promoting comfort.

. Nausea, vomiting, and anorexia may increase the terminally ill client's likelihood of inadequate nutrition. The nurse should serve smaller portions and bland foods, which may be more palatable.

1. 3, p. 587
Rationale:

3. Spending time to let clients share their life experiences, particularly what has been meaningful, enables the nurse to know clients better. Knowing clients then facilitates choice of therapies that promote client decision making and autonomy. Planning regular visits also helps the client maintain a sense of self-worth, because it demonstrates that he or she is worthy of the nurse's time and attention.

. The client should not be left alone to feel abandoned or isolated.

2. Nurses can help clients meet spiritual needs by facilitating connections to a spiritual practice or community and supporting the expression of culturally held beliefs. A client's spiritual advisor also may be called on, but is not the only source of spiritual support. The nurse who turns care over to the spiritual advisor is not promoting the client's sense of self-worth, as it may imply the client is not worthy of the nurse's time or attention.

4. A grief counselor may be requested to visit if the client is experiencing complicated grief. Having a grief counselor visit is not an intervention that will help maintain a client's sense of self-worth.

2. 4, p. 583
Rationale:

4. A nursing intervention to facilitate grief work is to offer the client encouragement to explore and verbalize feelings of grief. This encouragement refocuses the client on current needs and minimizes dysfunctional adaptation behaviors (e.g., not sleeping) by facilitating resolution of grief through problem-solving skills.

1. Administering sleeping medication may help the client get to sleep, but does not resolve the issue of grief. Without addressing the grief, the client may develop another dysfunctional adaptation behavior.

2. It is not necessary to refer the client to a psychologist or psychotherapist at this time. The client needs to be encouraged to verbalize his or her feelings.

3. Having the client complete a detailed sleep-pattern assessment may help the nurse identify the number of hours of sleep the client is obtaining, but it does not address the issue causing the sleep disturbance, which is grief from the loss of the spouse.

13. 2, p. 586
Rationale:

1. Oral care should be provided every 2 to 4 hours.

2. To promote comfort for the terminally ill client specific to nausea and vomiting, the nurse should administer antiemetics, provide oral care at least every 2 to 4 hours, offer clear liquid diet and ice chips, avoid liquids that increase stomach acidity such as coffee, milk, and citrus acid juices, and offer high-protein foods in smaller portions and of a bland nature.

3. Increasing the fluid intake may help prevent constipation.

4. A low-residue diet may help prevent diarrhea.

14. 2, p. 586
Rationale:

2. Positioning the client upright is an independent nursing intervention for the promotion of respiratory function in a terminally ill client.

1. Limiting fluids may not promote respiratory function, and unless a client is on a fluid-restricted diet, the nurse should not do so.

3. Reducing narcotic analgesic use is not a nurse-initiated activity to promote respiratory function. A respiratory rate should be assessed before administering narcotics to prevent further respiratory depression. Management of air hunger involves judicious administration of morphine and anxiolytics for relief of respiratory distress.

4. The administration of bronchodilators would require a physician's order. It is not an independent nursing activity.

15. 1, 570
Rationale:
1. During the "yearning and searching" phase of Bowlby's phases of mourning, the nurse anticipates that the client may have outbursts of tearful sobbing and acute distress.
2. During Bowlby's "disorganization and despair" phase of mourning, the nurse anticipates that the client may express anger at anyone who might be responsible, including the nurse.
3. During the "numbing" phase of Bowlby's phases of mourning, the nurse anticipates that the client may act stunned by the loss.
4. During the "reorganization" phase of Bowlby's phases of mourning, the nurse anticipates that the client may discuss the change in role that will occur.

Chapter 30

1. 1, p. 609
Rationale:
1. A regular exercise program reduces tension and promotes relaxation, increasing one's resistance to stress, and reduces the risk of cardiovascular disease.
2. Support systems may benefit a person experiencing stress but do not reduce the incidence of heart disease.
3. Self-awareness skill development may enable persons to recognize when they are experiencing stress and need to implement stress-reducing strategies, but will not reduce the incidence of heart disease.
4. Time management, including setting priorities, helps individuals identify tasks that are not necessary or can be delegated to someone else. Effective time management will help lower one's level of stress, but does not reduce the incidence of heart disease.

2. 1, p. 611
Rationale:
1. When using a crisis-intervention approach, the nurse helps the client make the mental connection between the stressful event and the client's reaction to it.

2. Because an individual's or family's usual coping strategies are ineffective in managing the stress of the precipitating event in a crisis situation, the use of new coping mechanisms is required.
3. Time-management skills will not help reduce the stress of the precipitating event in a crisis situation.
4. What may have worked in past experiences is ineffective in managing the stress of the precipitating event in a crisis situation.

3. 1, p. 599
Rationale:
1. Displacement is transferring emotions, ideas, or wishes from a stressful situation to a less anxiety-producing substitute.
2. Compensation is making up for a deficiency in one aspect of self-image by strongly emphasizing a feature considered an asset.
3. Conversion is unconsciously repressing an anxiety-producing emotional conflict and transforming it into nonorganic symptoms.
4. Denial is avoiding emotional conflicts by refusing consciously to acknowledge anything that might cause intolerable emotional pain.

4. 2, p. 599
Rationale:
2. Regression is coping with a stressor through actions and behaviors associated with an earlier developmental period, such as an 8-year old child sucking his thumb and wetting the bed.
1. An adult client who exercises to the point of fatigue is not demonstrating regression.
3. An adult client who avoids speaking about health concerns may be using denial as a coping mechanism.
4. An 11-year-old who develops stomach cramps and headaches is an example of conversion.

5. 4, p. 603

Rationale:

4. The nurse learns from the client both by asking questions and by making observations of nonverbal behavior and the client's environment. To determine the amount of anxiety the client is experiencing, the nurse gathers information from the client's perspective.
1. Asking if the client desires for family to be called is not assessing the client's level of anxiety.
2. The nurse should first focus on developing a trusting relationship with the client. If the nurse takes the client to visit someone who had the same surgery, the nurse would not be able to assess the client's current level of anxiety.
3. This is not the best response. It does not assess the amount of anxiety the client is currently experiencing.

6. 2, p.597

Rationale:

2. The reticular formation is primarily responsible for an individual's level of consciousness.
1. The medulla oblongata controls vital functions such as heart rate, blood pressure, and respiration.
3. The pituitary gland supplies hormones that control vital functions. The pituitary gland produces hormones necessary for adaptation to stress (e.g., adrenocorticotropic hormone).
4. The external stress response is not primarily responsible for a person's level of consciousness.

7. 3, p. 600

Rationale:

3. Teaching the client relaxation strategies can help reduce the stress of anxiety-provoking thoughts and events, as seen in PTSD, and reinforces an adaptive coping strategy.
1. Suppression would be a maladaptive coping mechanism.
2. PTSD persists longer than 1 month.
4. The focus should be on developing adaptive coping mechanisms and lowering the individual's anxiety. The focus is not on physical needs for the client who is experiencing PTSD.

8. 4, p. 599

Rationale:

4. Dissociation is experiencing a subjective sense of numbing and a reduced awareness of one's surroundings. The client who is sitting quietly and not interacting with any of the staff may be displaying dissociation.
1. The client who avoids discussion of the problem may be using denial as an ego-defense mechanism.
2. The client who acts like another colleague on the job is using identification as an ego-defense mechanism.
3. The client who experiences headaches and stomachaches is using the ego-defense mechanism of conversion.

9. 2, p. 597

Rationale:

2. The exhaustion stage occurs when the body can no longer resist the effects of the stressor and when the energy necessary to maintain adaptation is depleted.
1. During the resistance stage, the body stabilizes.
3. Reflex pain response is not a stage of GAS.
4. During the alarm reaction, increasing hormone levels result in increased blood volume, epinephrine and norepinephrine amounts, heart rate, blood flow to muscles, oxygen intake, and mental alertness.

10. 3, p. 601

Rationale:

3. The client who recently experienced a loss and does not want to meet new people is an example of a sociocultural indicator of stress.
1. This is not an example of an emotional indicator of stress. The client is not displaying anger or crying.
2. This is not an example of a spiritual indicator of stress. The client is not restless or verbalizing discontent with a higher being.
4. This is not an example of an intellectual indicator of stress.

11. 2, pp. 609, 610

Rationale:

2. Biofeedback can be learned in a training program designed to develop one's ability to control the autonomic (involuntary) nervous system. The client learns to monitor functions such as heart rate, blood pressure, skin temperature, or muscle tension, and learns to relax in response to create desired changes

1. Guided imagery is a relaxed state in which a person actively uses imagination in a way that allows visualization of a soothing, peaceful setting. This is not an example of guided imagery.

3. Time-management techniques include developing lists of tasks to be performed in order of priority. This is not an example of time management.

4. This is not an example of a regular exercise program. It does not improve muscle tone and reduce the risk of cardiovascular disease.

12. 3, p. 610

Rationale:

3. The nurse's focus for a client experiencing a crisis is immediate stress reduction.

1. The client experiencing a crisis is unable to work through independent problem solving.

2. Completing an in-depth evaluation of stressors and responses to the situation would be inappropriate for the client who is experiencing a crisis.

4. A person who has experienced a crisis has changed, and the effects may last for years or for the rest of the person's life. If a person has successfully coped with a crisis and its consequences, he or she becomes a more mature and healthy person, and ongoing therapy may not be necessary.

13. 4, p. 607

Rationale:

4. A priority assessment is to determine if the person is suicidal or homicidal by asking directly.

1. The priority assessment for the client who is experiencing a significant degree of stress is not the client's physical needs. The nurse should first determine if the client is a danger to himself or others.

2. After determining if the client is suicidal or homicidal, the nurse can begin the problem-solving process and assess what else is happening in the client's life.

3. The nurse should first determine if the client is a danger to himself or others. Then the nurse can examine the degree of disruption in the person's life, such as in activities of daily living.

14. 2, p. 602

Rationale:

2. Anxiety disorders are the most prevalent disorders in later life and are continuations of life-long illnesses.

1. Losses in later life may be less stress provoking than generally assumed, partly because certain life transitions are anticipated and people prepare by coping in advance.

3. The effect of psychosocial factors on health status is not altered by age.

4. The timing of stress-inducing events can significantly influence older adults' ability to cope. The fact that older adults may have several stressful events (e.g., loss of a spouse and new medical diagnosis) within a short period can result in detrimental effects on coping.

*C*hapter 31

1. 3, p. 634

Rationale:

3. Wrapping the client's extremities has been recommended to reduce the incidence and intensity of shivering.

1. Hypothermia blankets may be used to reduce fever, but if the client is already shivering, a hypothermia blanket is not used, as further stimulation of shivering should be avoided.

2. Hot packs should not be applied to the client's axilla and groin.

4. Fluids should be not restricted, but increased to replace fluids lost because of the fever.

2. 2, p. 622

Rationale:

2. Confusion is a symptom of heatstroke, along with delirium, nausea, muscle cramps, visual disturbances, and even incontinence.

1. The most important sign of heatstroke is hot, dry skin, not diaphoresis. Victims of heatstroke do not sweat because of severe electrolyte loss and hypothalamic malfunction.

3. A normal temperature is 36° C to 38° C. With heatstroke, the client's body temperature may reach as high as 45° C.

4. The heart rate is increased with heatstroke, not decreased.

3. 1, p. 623
Rationale:

1. The client is exhibiting signs of heat exhaustion (i.e., symptoms of fluid volume deficit).

2. If the client were experiencing heatstroke, the client would have an increased pulse and would not be sweating.

3. Muscle cramps are related to heatstroke. The client is not exhibiting signs consistent with heatstroke.

4. The client is not exhibiting signs of hypothermia such as shivering, loss of memory, or cyanosis.

4. 4, p. 624
Rationale:

4. The nurse should wait 20 to 30 minutes before measuring the oral temperature.

1. The nurse should wait, rather than measuring the child's temperature rectally, as this is not an emergency situation.

2. Taking the oral temperature at this time would result in an inaccurate reading.

3. Rinsing the mouth with warm water also may provide an inaccurate reading of the child's actual body temperature. The nurse should wait 20 minutes and measure the child's oral temperature.

5. 1, p. 623
Rationale:

1. The treatment of heat exhaustion includes transporting the client to a cooler environment and restoring fluid and electrolyte balance.

2. Antibiotic therapy is not warranted.

3. Hypothermia wraps are not used to treat heat exhaustion.

4. Alcohol baths are not recommended.

6. 2, p. 635
Rationale:

2. The brachial or apical pulse is the best site for assessing an infant's or young child's pulse because other peripheral pulses are deep and difficult to palpate accurately.

1. The radial pulse is not the best site for assessing a 2-year-old's pulse.

3. The femoral pulse is not the best site for assessing a 2-year-old's pulse.

4. The pedal pulse is not the best site for assessing a 2-year-old's pulse.

7. 3, p. 618
Rationale:

3. The first action the nurse should take is to assess the client's respiratory rate. The nurse can then determine if it is within normal limits and will be able to compare it with the previous measurement to determine if the client is breathing faster than before.

1. Stress may increase an individual's respiratory rate. The nurse should first make the objective measurement of the client's rate.

2. Having the client lie down may decrease a client's respiratory rate, but the nurse should first assess the client before implementing any nursing measures.

4. The nurse should count the respirations. Based on these findings, the nurse may or may not need to take the client's pulse. Assessing the pulse will not verify whether the client is breathing faster than before.

8. 1, pp, 642, 644, 653
Rationale:

1. The client's vital signs are consistent with the client being in pain. It would be safe and appropriate for the nurse to give the pain medication.

2. Asking if the client is anxious is not the most appropriate action.

3. The client is not demonstrating signs of shock (i.e., decreased blood pressure, increased pulse). The most appropriate action is for the nurse to administer pain medication.

4. This would not be the most appropriate action. The nurse should medicate the client for pain.

9. 4, pp. 661-662

Rationale:

4. When measuring the blood pressure in the legs, systolic pressure is usually higher by 10 to 40 mm Hg than that in the brachial artery, but the diastolic pressure is the same.
1. The systolic pressure, not the diastolic pressure, is 10 to 40 mm Hg higher than in the brachial artery.
2. This is not a true statement.
3. This is not a true statement.

10. 1, pp. 641, 653, 665

Rationale:

1. These measurements are within the expected limits for an older client. An adult's average blood pressure is 120/80. The systolic pressure may increase with age, but the blood pressure should not exceed 140/90. The range for an adult's pulse is 60 to 100 beats per minute. The expected respiratory rate is 16 to 25 breaths per minute.
2. These are not within the expected limits for a client of this age.
3. These are not within the expected limits for a client of this age.
4. These are not within the expected limits for a client of this age.

11. 3, pp. 641, 647, 652, 653

Rationale:

3. These are expected findings of a 10-year-old client. The normal pulse range for a 10-year-old is 75 to 100 beats per minute; the normal respiratory rate is 20 to 30 breaths per minute. The expected blood pressure range for a 7-year-old is 87 to 117/48 to 64; children who are larger (i.e., heavier and/or taller) have higher blood pressures. The average blood pressure for a 10-year-old is 110/65 mm Hg.
1. These are not expected values of a 10-year-old client.
2. These are not expected values of a 10-year-old client.
4. These are not expected values of a 10-year-old client.

12. 2, p. 641

Rationale:

2. The expected pulse range for an adult is 60 to 100 beats per minute. This client's pulse is elevated at 110 beats per minute.
1. This client's temperature is within the normal range of 36°C to 38°C for an adult.
3. This client's respiratory rate is within the normal range of 12 to 20 for an adult.
4. This client's blood pressure reading is within the normal range of less than or equal to 120/80 for an adult.

13. 3, p. 630

Rationale:

3. When assessing a client's axillary temperature with a glass thermometer, the thermometer should be left in place for 3 to 5 minutes.
1. The thermometer should be held at the opposite end of the bulb.
2. The thermometer should be covered with a plastic sheath when in use, and after use, the plastic sheath is discarded. If the thermometer requires cleaning, the nurse should not use hot water, as it could cause the thermometer to break.
4. The parent, not the child, should hold the thermometer. A 1½-year-old client may drop the thermometer, creating a mercury spill.

14. 4, p. 644

Rationale:

4. The nurse should notify the physician, as these are abnormal findings. The client's respirations are becoming dangerously low at 8 (normal, 12 to 20 breaths per minute). The client's pulse is low at 54 (expected, 60 to 100 beats per minute), and the blood pressure should be equal to or less than 120/80, which it is at 110/68. The additional assessment findings also are not normal and should be reported to the physician.
1. The nurse should not wait another 30 minutes to retake vital signs. The present readings warrant notifying the physician.
2. These are abnormal findings. The nurse should not continue with care as planned.

3. The nurse should first notify the physician. Administering a stimulant would require a physician's order and may not be what the client requires. For example, the client may need a narcotic antagonist rather than a stimulant.

15. 3, p. 654
Rationale:
3. The nurse's primary concern should be the patient's safety and preventing an accidental fall. If the client just got up from bed and is complaining of dizziness, the client may be experiencing orthostatic hypotension. The nurse should first assist the client to sit down before performing any other assessment.
1. The nurse should not leave the client and go for help. The nurse should assist the client to a sitting position. If help is required, the nurse can then put on the client's call light.
2. The nurse may take the client's blood pressure after assisting the client to a sitting position to prevent the client from falling.
4. The nurse should first assist the client to sit down to prevent the client from falling accidentally. The nurse may then assess the client. If the nurse finds during the assessment that the client's result from pulse oximetry is low, the nurse may instruct the client to take deep breaths.

16. 1, p. 662
Rationale:
1. If the cuff is wrapped too loosely or unevenly around the arm, the effect on the blood pressure measurement may be a false high reading.
2. A false low systolic and false high diastolic blood pressure reading may occur if the cuff is deflated too quickly.
3. A false high systolic reading may be obtained if the blood pressure assessment is repeated too soon.
4. A false low diastolic reading may be obtained if the stethoscope is applied too firmly against the antecubital fossa.

17. 4, p. 634
Rationale:
4. Blankets cooled by circulating water delivered by motorized units increase conductive heat loss. Cooling blankets are used to reduce a fever.
1. Bathing with an alcohol/water solution is not recommended because it may lead to shivering. Shivering is counterproductive and can increase energy expenditure up to 400%.
2. Ice packs to the axillae and groin are no longer recommended because they may induce shivering (which is counterproductive and increases the client's energy expenditure), and because it has no advantage over antipyretic medications.
3. Tepid sponge baths are no longer recommended because they may lead to shivering and are no more advantageous than administering antipyretics.

18. 4, p. 654
Rationale:
4. Diuretics reduce blood pressure by reducing reabsorption of sodium and water by the kidneys, thus reducing circulating fluid volume.
1. The effects of sympathetic nerve stimulation, such as with anxiety, increase blood pressure.
2. Heavy alcohol consumption has been linked to hypertension.
3. Cigarette smoking has been linked to hypertension.

19. 2, p. 653
Rationale:
2. The diagnosis of prehypertension in adults is made when an average of two or more diastolic readings on at least two subsequent visits is between 80 and 89 mm Hg or when the average of multiple systolic blood pressures on two or more subsequent visits is between 120 and 139 mm Hg. Hypertension is noted with diastolic reading greater than 90 mm Hg and systolic readings greater than 140 mm Hg. According to the newest guidelines, this client's blood pressure reading (130/84) would fall into the prehypertension category.
1. Normal is less than or equal to 120/80; this is a normal blood pressure reading.

3. Normal is less than or equal to 120/80; this is a normal blood pressure reading.
4. Normal is 120/80 or less; this is a normal blood pressure reading.

20. 1, p. 653
Rationale:
1. The normal blood pressure reading is 120/80 or less. This client's blood pressure is significantly higher at 180/100, and may be an indication of hypertension. (One elevated blood pressure measurement dos not qualify as a diagnosis of hypertension; it would have to be elevated on at least two separate occasions). The nurse should retake the blood pressure.
2. The client's temperature is within normal limits for a rectal temperature. The average rectal temperature is 37.5°C.
3. The client should repeat the blood pressure to confirm the reading before reporting the findings.
4. The blood pressure reading is not within normal limits. The pulse, respiratory rate, and temperature are within normal limits.

21. 3, p. 622
Rationale:
3. A remittent fever spikes and falls without a return to normal temperature levels.
1. A sustained fever is a constant body temperature continuously above 38°C (100.4°F) that demonstrates little fluctuation.
2. An intermittent has fever spikes interspersed with usual temperature levels. Temperature returns to acceptable value at least once in 24 hours.
4. A relapsing fever has periods of febrile episodes interspersed with acceptable temperature values.

22. 4, p. 630
Rationale:
4. The axillary site can be used with newborns and uncooperative clients.
1. The rectal site should not be used for routine vital signs in newborns.
2. The oral site should not be used with infants.
3. The tympanic site is questioned as being accurate in newborns.

23. 1, p. 631
Rationale:
1. The nurse's first action is to remove the client from immediate contaminated environment.
2. After removing the client from the area, the nurse may remove any clothing or linen that has been contaminated with mercury.
3. The nurse should perform hand hygiene thoroughly after changing any clothing or linen that has been contaminated with mercury. It is not required that the client be bathed unless skin contact has occurred. The first action of the nurse is to remove the client from the area.
4. After caring for the client, the nurse should notify the environmental services department.

24. 2, p. 651
Rationale:
2. Peripheral vascular disease can reduce pulse volume, which may affect the pulse oximetry reading.
1. The sensor should be placed on an extremity site (such as an earlobe or digit) with adequate local circulation, and the site should be free of moisture.
3. Reduced light in the room will not affect the oximetry reading. Outside light sources can interfere with the oximeter's ability to process reflected light.
4. An increased temperature of the room will not affect the oximetry reading. If the room was very cold, the client's peripheral blood flow may decrease, affecting the oximetry reading.

25. 2, p. 635
Rationale:
2. A conscious client benefits from drinking hot liquids such as soup.
1. Alcohol should be avoided.
3. Caffeinated fluids should be avoided.
4. Extremities should be warmed gradually. Tissue damage could occur if placed under hot water. The entire body should be warmed, such as by putting heating pads next to the head and neck, which lose heat the quickest.

26. 4, 655

Rationale:

4. The client's blood pressure should not be measured after the client has exercised, smoked, or ingested caffeine. The client should wait 30 minutes before assessment of the blood pressure.
1. The cuff should be deflated at a rate of 2 mm Hg per second.
2. When possible, the client should be sitting in a chair.
3. The blood pressure should be assessed at the same time each day.

27. 1., p. 661

Rationale:

1. The popliteal artery, palpable behind the knee in the popliteal space, is the site for auscultation when taking the blood pressure in the leg.
2. This is not the correct site for assessment before measuring the blood pressure in the leg.
3. This is not the correct site for assessment.
4. This is not the correct site for assessment.

28. 3, p. 638

Rationale:

3. An apical pulse should be assessed at the client's PMI. The PMI is located at the intercostal space 4 to 5 at the left midclavicular line.
1. This is not the correct placement for auscultating a client's apical pulse.
2. The PMI is higher and more medial in children younger than 8 years. The client is not identified as being a child.
4. This is not the correct placement for auscultating a client's apical pulse.

29. 1, p. 642

Rationale:

1. Fever and heat may increase a client's pulse rate.
2. Digoxin is a negative chronotropic drug; it will decrease the client's pulse rate.
3. A conditioned athlete who participates in long-term exercise will have a lower heart rate at rest.

4. Unrelieved severe pain increases parasympathetic stimulation, decreasing the heart rate.

30. 4. p. 648

Rationale:

4. Cheyne-Stokes respirations are characterized by an irregular respiratory rate with alternating periods of apnea and hyperventilation. The respiratory cycle begins with slow, shallow breaths that gradually increase to an abnormal rate and depth. The pattern then reverses, breathing slows and becomes shallow, and the pattern climaxes in apnea before respiration resumes.
1. Biot's respirations are abnormally shallow for two to three breaths, followed by an irregular period of apnea.
2. Kussmaul's respirations are abnormally deep, regular, and increased in rate.
3. Hyperpneic respirations are labored, increased in depth, and increased in rate (more than 20 breaths per minute). Occurs normally during exercise.

C*hapter 32*

1. 1, p. 681

Rationale:

1. Sitting upright provides full expansion of lungs and provides better visualization of symmetry of upper body parts.
2. The supine position maximizes the nurse's ability to assess pulse sites.
3. The prone position is used only to assess extension of the hip joint.
4. The dorsal recumbent position is used for abdominal assessment because it promotes relaxation of abdominal muscles.

2. 1, p. 690

Rationale:

1. Pallor is more easily seen in the face, buccal mucosa of the mouth, conjunctiva, and nail beds.
2. The palmar surface of the hands may be used to detect color hues in dark-skinned clients.

3. The ear lobe is not a good site to assess for color changes such as pallor, in the dark-skinned client.
4. The best site to inspect for jaundice, not pallor, is the sclera.

3. 2, p. 684
Rationale:
2. Injuries and trauma that are inconsistent with the reported cause, multiple injuries including bruises, cuts, and burns, and behavioral findings of difficulty sleeping and appearing anxious are all indicators of possible domestic violence.
1. The findings are not consistent with substance abuse. Indicators of substance abuse may include frequent missed appointments or emergency department visits, having a history of changing doctors, history of activities that place them at risk for HIV infections, complaints of insomnia or chest pain, and a family history of addiction. People who abuse substances may have cuts, burns (especially of the fingers), needle marks, homemade tattoos, or increased vascularity of the face.
3. These findings are not indicative of vascular disease. Symptoms of vascular disease may include edema, color changes of the lower extremities, and weakened pedal pulses.
4. These findings are not indicative of mental illness. The client is coherent.

4. 4, p. 703
Rationale:
4. To visualize internal eye structures, the nurse uses an ophthalmoscope to focus on the red reflex.
1. To evaluate the lower eyelids, the nurse asks the client to open the eyes for inspection. A syringe and sterile water are not necessary for this assessment.
2. The lacrimal apparatus is best assessed by inspecting for edema and redness and palpating it gently to detect tenderness. Normally it cannot be felt.

3. Accommodation is tested by asking the client to gaze at a distant object and then at a test object held by the nurse approximately 10 cm from the client's nose. The pupils normally converge and accommodate by constricting when looking at close objects.

5. 1, p. 682
Rationale:
1. In organizing a physical examination, the nurse should perform painful procedures near the end of the examination.
2. The nurse should record quick notes during the examination to avoid keeping the client waiting. Observations can be completed at the end of the examination.
3. The TV or radio should be turned off so as to not distract the client throughout the examination, and to provide an environment conducive to auscultation.
4. Both sides of the body should be assessed for comparison to determine symmetry. A degree of asymmetry is normal in the dominant versus nondominant arm.

6. 2, p. 715
Rationale:
2. During assessment of the thyroid gland, the client holds a cup of water and takes a sip to swallow once instructed by the nurse. As the client swallows, the isthmus of the thyroid gland rises. The nurse should feel whether it is enlarged. Normally the thyroid gland is small, smooth, and free of nodules.
1. Light, gentle palpation is needed to feel any abnormalities.
3. For the posterior approach, both of the nurse's hands are placed around the neck, with two fingers of each hand on the sides of the trachea just beneath the cricoid cartilage.
4. The bell of the stethoscope is best for auscultation of bruits.

7. 3, p. 720
Rationale:
3. Normal vesicular sounds are soft, breezy, and low-pitched. The inspiratory phase is 3 times longer than the expiratory phase.

Medium-pitched blowing sounds with inspiration equaling expiration are bronchovesicular breath sounds.

Loud, high-pitched, hollow sounds with longer expiration are bronchial breath sounds.

Vesicular sounds are created by air moving through smaller airways. Abnormal breath sounds result from air passing through narrowed airways.

2, p. 723

ationale:

By age 7 years, a child's PMI is in the same location as the adults (i.e., the fifth intercostal space, left of the midclavicular line).

The PMI of an 8-year-old child is more likely to be located at the fifth intercostal space, left of the midclavicular line.

The PMI is not located to the right of the midclavicular line.

The PMI of an infant is at the third or fourth intercostal space, left of the midclavicular line.

3, p. 727

ationale:

Leg cramps, numbness or tingling in extremities, sensation of cold hands or feet, pain in legs, or swelling or cyanosis of feet, ankles, or hands is indicative of vascular disease.

Headache, dizziness, and tingling of body parts are more likely associated with a neurologic problem, not vascular disease.

Diplopia, floaters, and headaches are indicative of an eye problem, not vascular disease.

Pain and cramping in the lower extremities are usually worsened with activity in vascular disease.

0. 4, p. 735

ationale:

The best time for a BSE is 2 to 3 days after the menstrual period ends, when the breast is no longer swollen or tender from hormone elevations.

The woman should check her breasts the same time each month, 2 to 3 days after the menstrual period ends.

2. This is partially true. The client should also be informed to perform the BSE 2 to 3 days after the menstrual period ends.

3. This is not the best time for a woman to perform a BSE. The breasts will be enlarged and tender from hormone elevations.

11. 1, p. 692

Rationale:

1. This finding is consistent with the definition of a macule.

2. A papule is a palpable, circumscribed, solid elevation in skin, smaller than 0.5 cm.

3. A vesicle is a circumscribed elevation of skin filled with serous fluid, smaller than 0.5 cm.

4. A nodule is an elevated solid mass, deeper and firmer than a papule, 0.5 to 2.0 cm.

12. 4, p. 763

Rationale:

4. Interpreting abstract ideas or concepts, such as in explaining the meaning of this phrase, reflects the capacity for abstract thinking. The client with altered mentation will likely interpret the phrase literally or merely rephrase the words.

1. An example of assessing knowledge would be asking the client the reason for seeking health care. This example is not designed to measure knowledge.

2. The nurse is not attempting to measure judgment. An example of assessing judgment would be to ask the client what he or she would do if he or she suddenly became ill when alone at home.

3. The nurse is not attempting to measure association. An example of assessing association would be to ask the client to complete a phrase, such as "a dog is to a beagle as a cat is to a _____."

13. 3, p. 764

Rationale:

3. The trigeminal nerve is tested by lightly touching the cornea with a wisp of cotton, by assessing the corneal reflex, and by measuring sensation of light pain and touch across the skin of the face.

1. The optic nerve is tested by using the Snellen chart or asking the client to read printed material.
2. The facial nerve is tested by having the client smile, frown, puff out cheeks, and raise and lower eyebrows while you look for asymmetry. Having the client identify salty or sweet taste on the front of the tongue also tests the facial nerve.
4. The oculomotor nerve is tested by assessing directions of gaze and testing papillary reaction to light and accommodation.

14. 3, p. 692
Rationale:
3. This finding is consistent with the definition of a vesicle.
1. A nodule is an elevated solid mass, deeper and firmer than a papule, 0.5 to 2.0 cm.
2. A macule is a flat, nonpalpable change in skin color, smaller than 1 cm.
4. A wheal is an irregularly shaped, elevated area or superficial localized edema that varies in size.

15. 1, p. 711
Rationale:
1. Normal mucosa in a light-skinned adult is glistening, pinkish-red, soft, moist, and smooth.
2. Oral mucosa may appear more dry in the older adult because of reduced salivation, but is not rough.
3. Cyanotic mucosa with rough nodules would be an abnormal finding.
4. Oral mucosa should not appear deep red with rough edges in a light-skinned adult.

16. 4, p. 755
Rationale:
4. Kyphosis is an exaggeration of the posterior curvature of the thoracic spine (hunchback)
1. Lordosis is an increased lumbar curvature (swayback).
2. Osteoporosis is a metabolic bone disease that causes a decrease in quality and quantity of bone.
3. Scoliosis is a lateral curvature of the spine.

17. 3, p. 726
Rationale:
3. Extra heart sounds or heart murmurs a heard more easily with the client lying on the left side (lateral recumbent) with the stethoscope at the apical site.
1. Sitting upright is used for assessing lun expansion and symmetry of the upp extremities.
2. Standing is not the best position for auscultating a heart murmur.
4. The dorsal recumbent position is best used f abdominal assessment.

18. 3, p. 766
Rationale:
3. The Romberg test assesses the client's balanc
1. The Weber test assesses for unilateral deafnes
2. The Allen test assesses for patency of the arte ies of the hand (usually before arterial pun ture).
4. The Rinne test compares bone-conductio hearing with air-conduction hearing.

19. 3, p. 764
Rationale:
3. To test cranial nerve VIII (auditory), the nur should assess the client's ability to hear th spoken word.
1. To test cranial nerve II (optic), the nur should assess the client's ability to rea printed material.
2. To test cranial nerves III (oculomotor), I (trochlear), and VI (abducens), the nur should assess the client's directions of gaze.
4. To assess cranial nerve X (vagus), the nur should ask the client to say "ah."

20. 2, p. 721
Rationale:
2. Wheezes are high-pitched, continuous mus cal sounds like a squeak heard continuous during inspiration or expiration; usual louder on expiration.
1. Coarse crackles and bubbling are not descri tive of wheezes.
3. Dry, grating noises are heard with a pleur friction rub.
4. Loud, low-pitched rumbling is characterist of rhonchi.

1. 2, p. 752
Rationale:

The nurse instructs the male client that the protocol for testicular self-examination is to use both hands to roll the testicle gently, feeling for lumps, thickening, or a change in consistency (hardening).

All men 15 years and older should perform the testicular self-examination monthly.

The examination should be performed after a warm bath or shower when the scrotal sac is relaxed.

A cordlike structure on the top and back of the testicle is a normal finding. It is the epididymis.

2. 1, p. 678
Rationale:

A sweet, fruity smell noticed in the oral cavity is indicative of diabetic acidosis.

Halitosis of the oral cavity is indicative of gum disease.

Stomatitis is characterized by oral pain, bad breath, inflammation, and oral ulcers in the mouth.

Foul-smelling stools in the infant are indicative of malabsorption syndrome.

3. 1, p. 697
Rationale:

Clubbing of the nails is caused by a chronic lack of oxygen such as in heart or pulmonary disease.

Paronychia is caused by local infection or trauma.

Beau's lines are caused by systemic illness such as severe infection or by injury to the nail.

Splinter hemorrhages are caused by minor trauma, subacute bacterial endocarditis, or trichinosis.

4. 1, p. 699
Rationale:

Myopia is nearsightedness.

Peripheral vision is not reduced with myopia. The client with myopia is able to see close objects, but not distant objects. Peripheral vision may be decreased in open-angle glaucoma.

3. Diminished night vision may occur with cataracts, not myopia.

4. Problems with glare, flashes, and floaters may indicate eye disease, and the client should be referred to a physician.

25. 2, p. 709
Rationale:

2. The nurse should have the child who is experiencing a nosebleed sit up and lean forward to avoid aspiration of blood, apply pressure to the anterior nose with the thumb and forefinger as the child breathes through the mouth, and apply ice or a cold cloth to the bridge of the nose if pressure fails to stop bleeding.

1. The child should not lean backward, as this may cause the child to aspirate blood.

3. A cold cloth will slow bleeding and help blood to coagulate, not a warm cloth.

4. The child should breathe through the mouth. Blowing his nose may only continue the bleeding as it may disturb any clot formation.

26. 2, p. 722
Rationale:

2. Older adults should be counseled to receive annual influenza and pneumonia vaccinations.

1. It is not necessary to receive these vaccinations every 6 months.

3. The influenza and pneumonia vaccines should be taken annually in the older adult because of the greater susceptibility to respiratory infection.

4. It is recommended that older adults receive the influenza and pneumonia vaccines annually because they have a greater susceptibility to respiratory infection.

27. 3, p. 737
Rationale:

3. Normal changes of the breasts during pregnancy include the areola becoming darker and the diameter increasing.

1. Breast tissue becomes softer during menopause, not pregnancy.

2. Nipples become flatter in older adulthood.

4. Superficial veins become more prominent during pregnancy.

28. 2, p. 730
Rationale:
2. The client with risk for or evidence of vascular insufficiency should not wear tight clothing over the lower body or legs, such as knee-length stockings.
1. Walking regularly is recommended for the client with vascular insufficiency.
3. The client with vascular insufficiency should elevate his or her feet when sitting.
4. The client with vascular insufficiency should avoid sitting or standing for long periods.

29. 2, p. 713
Rationale:
2. To assess the client's glands, the nurse should use the pads of the fingers and palpate gently.
1. The dorsum of the hand may be used to detect skin temperature, not to assess the client's glands.
3. The palmar surface of the hand is not used to assess the client's glands.
4. The nurse should not use a fingertip grasp of the tissue when assessing a client's glands.

30. 3, p. 708
Rationale:
3. In conduction deafness, sound is heard best in the impaired ear.
1. Sound that is not heard in either ear is not indicative of conduction deafness.
2. Sound would not be heard best by the client in the left ear if there were conduction deafness in the right ear.
4. This option is describing the Rinne's test, not the Weber's test. In conduction deafness, bone-conducted sound can be heard longer. In sensorineural loss, sound is reduced and heard longer through air.

31. 2, p. 734
Rationale:
2. In the presence of arterial insufficiency, the client has signs resulting from an absence of blood flow, such as pain, pallor, and decreased or absent pulses in the lower extremities. The lower extremities become dusky red when the extremities are lowered. They feel cool to touch because blood flow is blocked to the extremity.

1. Decreased hair growth or the absence of h growth over the legs may indicate arter insufficiency.
3. Marked edema is seen in venous insufficien not arterial insufficiency.
4. Brown pigmentation around the ankles seen in venous insufficiency. Skin changes arterial insufficiency include thin, shiny ski decreased hair growth, and thickened nails.

32. 2, p. 720
Rationale:
2. Sounds heard during auscultation over t trachea should be loud, high-pitched and h low.
1. Soft, low-pitched, and breezy sounds a heard over the lung's periphery.
3. Moist, crackling, and bubbling sounds a adventitious sounds known as "crackles" a are caused by sudden reinflation of groups alveoli and disruptive passage of air. They a most commonly heard in dependent lob right and left lung bases.
4. High-pitched and musical sounds a wheezes. Wheezes can be heard over all lur fields.

33. 4, p. 764
Rationale:
4. In testing cranial nerve III (oculomotor), t nurse determines the client's ability to react light with changes in pupil size. Testir accommodation also will assess cranial ner III.
1. In testing cranial nerve VII (facial), the nur determines the client's ability to smile ar frown.
2. In testing cranial nerve II (optic), the nur determines the client's ability to read print material.
3. In testing cranial nerve IX (glossopharyngea the nurse determines the client's ability identify sweet and sour tastes.

Chapter 33

1. 4, p. 778
Rationale:
4. A sign of an acute inflammatory process is pain. The swelling of inflamed tissues increases pressure on nerve endings, causing pain. Chemical substances such as histamine also stimulate nerve endings, adding to the pain response.
1. The skin is not blanched, but rather with the increase in local blood flow, it is reddened.
2. The symptom of localized warmth results from a greater volume of blood at the inflammatory site.
3. The cellular response of acute inflammation involves WBCs arriving at the site, with an increase in WBCs, rather than a decrease.

2. 1, p. 783
Rationale:
1. The normal erythrocyte sedimentation rate for women is 20 mm/hr. The client's ESR is 35 mm/hr, indicating the presence of the inflammatory process.
2. The normal WBC count is 5,000 to 10,000/mm³. The client is within normal limits at 8,000/mm³. The normal neutrophil count is 55% to 70%. The client is within normal limits at 65%.
4. The normal iron level is 60 to 90 g/100 ml. The client is within normal limits at 75 g/100 ml.

3. 3, p. 780
Rationale:
3. The staff member who places the Foley catheter bag on the bed when transferring the client is placing the client at risk for a nosocomial infection because urine in the catheter or drainage tube may reenter the bladder (reflux).
1. Washing hands before applying a dressing is a correct action to help prevent a nosocomial infection.
2. Taping a plastic bag to the bed rail for tissue disposal is a correct action to aid the client in proper disposal of secretions.

4. Using alcohol to cleanse the skin before starting an intravenous line is a correct action to prevent a nosocomial infection of the bloodstream.

4. 1, p. 797
Rationale:
1. Droplet precautions are instituted when droplets are larger than 5 µm, such as in the case of streptococcal pharyngitis.
2. Contact precautions are instituted for herpes simplex.
3. Airborne precautions are instituted with pulmonary TB.
4. Airborne precautions are instituted with measles.

5. 1, p. 781
Rationale:
1. Burn clients have a very high susceptibility to infection because of the damage to skin surfaces. This would be the individual with the highest risk for infection.
2. Victims of chronic diseases, such as diabetes mellitus and multiple sclerosis, are susceptible to infection because of general debilitation and nutritional impairment.
3. Diseases that impair body-system defenses, such as emphysema and bronchitis (which impair ciliary action and thicken mucus), increase susceptibility to infection.
4. Diseases that impair body-system defenses, such as peripheral vascular disease (which reduces blood flow to injured tissues), increase susceptibility to infection.

6. 4, pp. 797-798
Rationale:
4. A sense of loneliness may develop because normal social relationships become disrupted. The nurse should plan care to control the risk of the client feeling isolated.
1. Denial is not a risk related to isolation.
2. Aggression is not a risk for the client on isolation precautions.
3. Regression is not a risk related to isolation.

7. 1, p. 802
Rationale:
1. Surgical asepsis should be used during procedures that require intentional perforation of the client's skin, such as with the insertion of IV catheters.
2. The nurse is using medical aseptic technique when placing soiled linen in moisture-resistant bags.
3. The nurse is using medical aseptic technique when disposing of syringes in puncture-proof containers.
4. The nurse is using medical aseptic technique when washing hands before changing a dressing.

8. 2, p. 802
Rationale:
2. A sterile object (the packing) remains sterile only when touched by another sterile object. The client's abdomen is not sterile; therefore the nurse should throw the packing away and prepare a new one.
1. The nurse should not add alcohol to the packing and insert it into the incision.
3. The packing is considered contaminated, as it touched a nonsterile surface, and therefore should be discarded.
4. The nurse should not rinse the packing with sterile water and put the packing into the incision, as it is considered contaminated. It touched a nonsterile surface. The nurse should throw the packing away and prepare a new one.

9. 2, p. 777
Rationale:
2. During the illness stage, the client manifests signs and symptoms specific to the type of infection. The client with a viral infection would likely exhibit a fever.
1. No acute symptoms appear during the convalescent period.
3. An example of a client in the incubation period is when the client was first exposed to the infection 2 days ago, but has no symptoms.
4. The client who "feels sick" but is able to continue normal activities is in the prodromal stage of a course of infection.

10. 2, p. 775
Rationale:
2. To prevent the transmission of hepatitis A, the nurse must take special care when handling feces.
1. Hepatitis B and C may be found in blood.
3. Hepatitis A is not found in saliva.
4. Hepatitis A is not found in vaginal secretions.

11. 2, p. 776
Rationale:
2. Varicella zoster virus (chickenpox) is transmitted by droplets carried through the air after sneezing or coughing.
1. Varicella zoster virus (chickenpox) is not transmitted by a vector.
3. Person-to-person contact is not responsible for varicella zoster virus (chickenpox) transmission.
4. The transmission of varicella zoster virus (chickenpox) does not occur by contact with contaminated objects.

12. 3, p. 783
Rationale:
3. An elevated WBC is indicative of an acute infection. The normal WBC count is 5000 to 10,000/mm³.
1. The normal neutrophil count is 55% to 70%. The client is within normal limits at 65%.
2. The normal iron level is 60 to 90 g/100 ml. The client is within normal limits at 80 g/100 ml.
4. The normal erythrocyte sedimentation rate (ESR) is up to 15 mm/hr for men and up to 20 mm/hr for women. The client is within normal limits at 15 mm/hr.

13. 4, p. 788
Rationale:
4. To control or eliminate reservoir sites for infection, the nurse eliminates or controls sources of body fluids, drainage, or solutions that might harbor microorganisms. The nurse also carefully discards articles that become contaminated with infectious material such as in changing soiled dressings.
1. Covering the mouth and nose when sneezing is an intervention to control a portal of exit.

2. Wearing disposable gloves helps protect the susceptible host.

3. Isolating client's articles is an intervention to control transmission.

14. 1, p. 789
Rationale:

1. The most important and most basic technique in preventing and controlling transmission of infections is hand hygiene.

2. Use of disposable gloves may help reduce transmission of infections, but is not the single most important technique to prevent and control the transmission of infections.

3. The use of isolation precautions is not the single most important technique to prevent and control the transmission of infections.

4. Sterilization of equipment is not the single most important technique to prevent and control the transmission of infections.

15. 1, p. 797
Rationale:

1. A client with active tuberculosis requires airborne precautions.

2. A client with active tuberculosis does not require droplet precautions, as the droplet nuclei of tuberculosis are smaller than 5 μm.

3. Contact precautions are not necessary for the client with active tuberculosis.

4. Reverse isolation is not required for the client with active tuberculosis.

16. 3, p. 805
Rationale:

3. Before pouring the solution into the container, the nurse pours a small amount (1 to 2 ml) into a disposable cap or plastic-lined waste receptacle. The discarded solution cleans the lip of the bottle. This action is consistent with sterile asepsis.

1. Sterile forceps should be used to move items on a sterile field when using sterile asepsis.

2. Sterile fields should not be prepared well in advance of a sterile procedure. A sterile object or field becomes contaminated by prolonged exposure to air.

4. Wrapped sterile packages should be opened starting with the flap farthest away from the nurse (i.e., the top flap).

17. 2, p. 783
Rationale:

2. An infection in older adults may not demonstrate typical signs and symptoms. Atypical symptoms such as confusion, incontinence, or agitation may be the only symptoms of an infectious illness. An unexplained increased heart rate, confusion, or generalized fatigue may be the only symptoms of pneumonia in the older adult.

1. Hypotension is not one of the atypical symptoms of an older adult experiencing infection. It may be a symptom of a systemic infection related to an elevation in body temperature (regardless of age).

3. Erythema is a typical symptom of a localized infection.

4. Chills are a typical symptom of a systemic infection.

18. 1, p. 795
Rationale:

1. The correct sequence for putting on protective equipment is to perform hand hygiene, apply the mask and eyewear, apply gown, and then apply gloves.

2. This is not the correct sequence for putting on protective equipment.

3. This is not the correct sequence for putting on protective equipment.

4. This is not the correct sequence for putting on protective equipment.

19. 2, p. 802
Rationale:

2. A sterile object held below a person's waist is considered contaminated. To maintain sterile asepsis, discard packages that may have been in contact with the area below waist level.

1. Sterile gloves are not put on before opening sterile packages, as the outside of the packages are not sterile. The nurse uses hand hygiene and opens sterile packages, being careful to keep the inner contents sterile.

3. After a cap or lid is removed, it is held in the hand or placed sterile side (inside) up on a clean surface. A bottle cap or lid should never rest on a sterile surface, even though the inside of the cap is sterile.

4. The edges of a sterile field are considered to be contaminated. Sterile items should be placed in the middle of the sterile field to maintain sterile asepsis.

20. 3, p. 805
Rationale:
3. A surgical scrub should be maintained for at least 2 to 5 minutes.
1. To avoid contamination during a surgical hand scrub, the nurse holds the hands above the elbows.
2. Several studies suggest that neither a brush nor a sponge is necessary to reduce bacterial counts on the hands, especially when an alcohol-based product is used.
4. For maximal elimination of bacteria, remove all jewelry.

21. 2, p. 796
Rationale:
2. Specimen containers should be placed in plastic bags for transport with a label on the outside of the bag.
1. Linen should be placed in an impervious linen bag and may be removed from the client's room. Bags should be tied securely at the top with a knot.
3. For the person infected with MRSA, equipment remains in the room. After discharge or with the discontinuation of isolation, client care equipment is properly cleaned and reprocessed, and single-use items are discarded.
4. Gloves should be removed first when leaving the client's room.

22. 1, p. 775
Rationale:
1. *Escherichia coli* causes gastroenteritis and urinary tract infections. The client with *E. coli* infection is likely to demonstrate diarrhea.
2. *E. coli* is found in the colon, not the respiratory tract.
3. Cold sores are seen with herpes simplex virus (type I), not with *E. coli*.
4. Discharge from the eyes is not seen with *E. coli* infection. It may be seen with *Neisseria gonorrhoeae*.

Chapter 34

1. 3, p. 832
Rationale:
3. The parenteral route provides a means of administration when oral medications are contraindicated. Onset of action is quicker. Less cause for embarrassment is given than with a rectal suppository.
1. An enteric-coated medication is given orally. Because the client is vomiting, the oral route should not be used.
2. Nausea does not affect the rate of absorption.
4. It is inaccurate to state that a rectal suppository *must* be administered. A rectal suppository is one option. The disadvantage of a rectal suppository is that insertion often causes embarrassment for the client. It is contraindicated if rectal bleeding is present or if the client had rectal surgery. Stool in the rectum can impair absorption.

2. 2, p. 829
Rationale:
2. Toxic levels of morphine may cause severe respiratory depression. Toxic effects may develop after prolonged intake of a medication or when a medication accumulates in the blood because of impaired metabolism or excretion. The client with a decreased urine output is not excreting the morphine.
1. The therapeutic effect is the expected or predictable physiological response a medication causes. Respiratory depression and decreased urine output are not the desired (i.e., therapeutic) effect of morphine.
3. An idiosyncratic effect is when a medication causes an unpredictable outcome, such as when a client overreacts or underreacts to a medication. This is not an example of an idiosyncratic effect.
4. When a client experiences an allergic response to a medication, the medication acts as an antigen, triggering the release of the body's antibodies. The client may experience itching, urticaria, a rash, or in more severe cases, have difficulty breathing. The client's response to morphine is not an example of an allergic effect.

3. 1, p. 831

Rationale:

1. Administration of a medication by the buccal route involves placing the solid medication in the mouth and against the mucous membranes of the cheek until the medication dissolves.
2. Crushing the medication is not necessary, as it is designed to dissolve in the client's cheek.
3. Clients are not to take any liquids with medications given by buccal administration or immediately after.
4. The mouth is not sterile. Sterile technique is not necessary for buccal administration.

4. 2, p. 835

Rationale:

2. To calculate this problem, the nurse should first convert the measurements to one system. Because 1 grain = 60 mg, the nurse may multiply the 1.5 grains by 60 to equal 90 mg. The nurse may then use the formula for calculating a drug dosage.

$$\frac{90 \text{ mg}}{100 \text{ mg}} \times 1 \text{ capsule} = 0.9 \text{ capsules}$$

Because 0.9 of a capsule cannot be administered, it is rounded to **1.** The nurse will administer 1 capsule.

1. This is not a correct dosage calculation. Furthermore, capsules cannot be halved.
3. This is not a correct dosage calculation. Furthermore, capsules cannot be halved.
4. This is not a correct dosage calculation.

5. 3, p. 835

Rationale:

3. The nurse should use the formula to calculate a drug dosage:

$$\frac{6 \text{ mg}}{15 \text{ mg}} \times 1 \text{ ml} = 2/5 \text{ ml}$$

1. This is not a correct dosage calculation.
2. This is not a correct dosage calculation.
4. This is not a correct dosage calculation.

6. 4, p. 837

Rationale:

4. The most accurate method of calculating pediatric doses is based on a child's body surface area.
1. Drug calculations are not most precise when made on the basis of a child's weight. Height and weight do not always correlate with the maturity of the child's organs, such as the liver, for metabolizing a drug.
2. Drug calculations are not most precise when made on the basis of a child's height.
3. Drug calculations are not most precise when made on the basis of a child's age. Children vary widely in size and maturity for chronological age.

7. 3, p. 831

Rationale:

3. The medication is being given 3 times a day, 4 hours apart. The medication the nurse is documenting is diazepam, 5 mg PO tid.
1. Although the medication is being given 4 hours apart, it is not being given every 4 hours. If it were given every four hours, it could be given six times in 24 hours, not three, as with tid administration.
2. Bid means twice a day. The client is receiving the medication 3 times a day.
4. The medication is not spaced apart, as every 8 hours.

8. 2, pp. 847, 849

Rationale:

2. Allowing the child a choice of taking a medication with water or juice may have greater success because the child is involved.
1. The child should not be given the option of not taking a medication.
3. The nurse should explain the procedure to a child, using short words and simple language appropriate to the child's level of comprehension. Long explanations may increase a child's anxiety.
4. This statement is not a motivation for a child to take a prescribed medication. Giving the child a star or token afterward would be more motivating for a child.

9. 3, pp. 674, 879
Rationale:
3. If a vial becomes contaminated with another medication, it should be discarded.
1. Fluid from one vial should not be injected into another, as it would contaminate the second vial.
2. The needle should not be wiped with alcohol. It is considered sterile and does not require to be wiped with alcohol. Wiping the needle would place the nurse at risk for a needle stick.
4. Air should be inserted into both vials, making sure the needle does not touch the solution in the first vial.

10. 4, p. 880
Rationale:
4. The client should be taught to inject air into both vials and withdraw the regular insulin first.
1. Air should be injected into the vial of NPH insulin, and then the vial of regular insulin.
2. The regular insulin should be withdrawn after air has been injected into both vials.
3. Air should be injected into the vial of NPH insulin, and then the vial of regular insulin. The regular insulin should be withdrawn immediately after injecting the air into the vial of regular insulin. Then the NPH insulin is withdrawn.

11. 2, p. 867
Rationale:
2. Spacers are especially helpful when the client has difficulty coordinating the steps involved in self-administering inhaled medications.
1. The use of a spacer is not dependent on the dosage of medication.
3. The use of a spacer is not dependent on the schedule of administration.
4. Spacers are not required with the use of a dry powder inhaler.

12. 3, p. 888
Rationale:
3. Research that has investigated complications associated with IM injection sites indicates that the ventrogluteal site is the preferred site for most injections given to adults and children older than 7 months.
1. The deltoid muscle is not developed enough for an IM injection in the 1-year-old client.
2. The dorsogluteal site is not recommended because of the risk of the needle hitting the sciatic nerve.
4. The vastus lateralis is a preferred site for infants younger than 12 months.

13. 4, p. 890
Rationale:
4. The Z-track method is used to minimize local skin irritation by sealing the mediation in muscle tissue.
1. The Z-track method does not provide faster absorption of the medication.
2. The Z-track method does not reduce discomfort from the needle.
3. The Z-track method does not provide a more even absorption of the drug.

14. 3, p. 860
Rationale:
3. Eye drops should be instilled into the lower conjunctival sac. The conjunctival sac normally holds 1 or 2 drops and provides even distribution of medication across the eye.
1. The cornea is very sensitive. If drops were instilled onto the cornea it would stimulate the blink reflex.
2. The outer canthus would not hold the eye drop, and medication would be wasted, nor would it be distributed evenly across the eye.
4. The opening of the lacrimal duct is not the correct site for eye drops to be instilled. It would not provide even distribution of drops across the eye, and medication would most likely be wasted because this area could not contain the drops.

5. 3, p. 863

Rationale:

. The client should remain in the side-lying position, in this case, the right lateral position, for 2 to 3 minutes after ear drops are administered.

. The prone position is not recommended after administration of ear drops.

. The upright position is not recommended after ear drop administration. The ear drops would run out of the ear canal.

. The dorsal recumbent position with the neck hyperextended is not recommended after the administration of ear drops.

6. 3, p. 859

Rationale:

. ii, 2; gtts, drops; OD, right eye.

. gtts is the abbreviation for drops, not cc's.

. OS, left eye.

. OU, both eyes.

7. 4, p. 842

Rationale:

. To identify a client correctly, the nurse checks the medication administration form against the client's identification bracelet and asks the client to state his or her name to ensure that the client's identification bracelet has the correct information.

. The nurse may ask the client his or her name if the identification bracelet is missing or illegible, and obtain a new identification bracelet for the client. The nurse should ask the client to state his or her full name. The nurse should not merely say the client's name and assume that the client's response indicates that he or she is the right person.

. Checking the name on the chart does not identify the right client.

. Asking other caregivers is not the most effective way to determine a client's identity before administering medications. The nurse should develop the habit of checking the client's name band.

18. 4, p. 841

Rationale:

4. The nurse should question the order if the written order is illegible, the dose seems unusually low or high, or the medication seems inappropriate for the client's condition. The nurse should call the prescriber to clarify the order.

1. The nurse cannot independently change physician's orders. The nurse would have to call the prescriber and receive the order for the change.

2. The nurse should first call the prescriber and clarify the order. If the prescriber does not change the order, the nurse may then refuse to give the medication and notify the nurse manager.

3. The nurse could be held accountable for administering an ordered medication that is knowingly inappropriate for the client.

19. 2, p. 835

Rationale:

2. The nurse should first change the household measurement to a metric equivalent. (5 ml = 1 tsp), and then the nurse should use the formula for calculating a medication dosage:

$$\frac{80 \text{ mg}}{80 \text{ mg}} \times 5 \text{ ml} = 5 \text{ ml}$$

1. This is an incorrect dosage.

3. This is an incorrect dosage. 10 ml would equal 2 teaspoons, in this case, 160 mg.

4. This is an incorrect dosage. 15 ml would equal 3 teaspoons, in this case, 240 mg.

20. 1, p. 884

Rationale:

1. The angle of injection for an intradermal injection is 5 to 15 degrees.

2. This is not the correct angle of injection.

3. Subcutaneous injections may be administered at a 45-degree angle.

4. Subcutaneous or intramuscular injections may be administered at a 90-degree angle.

21. 2, p. 890

Rationale:

2. Intradermal injections are typically given for allergy testing or tuberculin screening.
1. Pain medications are not administered intradermally.
3. Anticoagulants are not administered intradermally. They are typically given subcutaneously.
4. Intradermal injections are not used for low-dose insulin requirements.

22. 2, p. 888

Rationale:

2. The nurse finds the ventrogluteal site by locating the greater trochanter with the heel of the hand, the anterior iliac spine with the index finger, and the iliac crest with the middle finger.
1. The vastus lateralis site is found by locating the middle third of the lateral thigh.
3. The anterior aspect of the thigh may be used for subcutaneous injections; it is not how the ventrogluteal site is located.
4. The acromion process and axilla may be used to locate the deltoid site.

23. 4, p. 886

Rationale:

4. The site most frequently recommended for heparin injections is the abdomen.
1. The scapular areas may be used for subcutaneous injections, but it is not a recommended site for heparin injections.
2. The vastus lateralis is used for intramuscular injections; not subcutaneous injections.
3. The posterior gluteal site is not recommended for heparin injections.

24. 3, p. 897

Rationale:

3. A priority for the nurse before the administration of medication via the IV route is to confirm placement of the IV line. Confirming the placement of the IV catheter and the integrity of the surrounding tissue ensures that the medication is administered safely.
1. The nurse should first confirm placement of the IV line.

2. The nurse should first confirm placement of the IV line before administering a medication by the IV route. The client's mental alertness may be something the nurse monitors after medication administration.
4. The nurse should first confirm placement of the IV line before administering any IV fluids.

25. 2, p. 880

Rationale:

2. Regular insulin reaches its peak in 2 to 4 hours after administration. If the client received regular insulin at 7:00 AM, the nurse should be alert for a possible hypoglycemic reaction from 9:00 AM to 11:00 AM.
1. Regular insulin has an onset in 30 minutes.
3. Intermediate-acting insulin (e.g., NPH insulin) would peak in 6 to 12 hours, but not regular insulin.
4. The client would not be at risk for a hypoglycemic reaction from regular insulin 13 hours after administration. Long-acting insulin would have an effect this much later after administration.

26. 1, p. 856

Rationale:

1. To protect the client from aspiration, the nurse should determine the presence of a gag reflex before administering oral medications.
2. The nurse should first check for a gag reflex. Then, if possible, the client should be allowed to self-administer oral medications.
3. Checking for a gag reflex takes priority over assessing the ability to cough in preventing aspiration.
4. Straws should be avoided because they decrease the control the client has over volume intake, which increases the risk of aspiration. Some clients cannot tolerate thin liquids such as water, and need them to be thickened.

27. 4, p. 856

Rationale:

4. The nasogastric tube should be verified for placement before administering any medication through it.
1. Medications should never be added to the tube feeding.

2. Not all tablets can be crushed, such as sustained release tablets, nor should all capsules be opened. Medications should be reviewed carefully before crushing a tablet or opening a capsule.

3. Medications should be dissolved and administered separately, flushing between 1 and 30 ml of water between each medication.

28. 4, p. 884

Rationale:

4. If blood appears in the syringe, the nurse should remove the needle and dispose of the medication and syringe properly. The nurse should then prepare another dose of medication for administration.

1. The medication should not be injected, as it would be entering a blood vessel.

2. The needle should not be pulled back slightly and then injected, as there is no assurance of the needle being out of the vessel.

3. The medication should not be injected, as there is no assurance of the needle being out of the vessel.

29. 1, p. 849

Rationale:

1. Straws may help children swallow pills. If it is a liquid iron preparation, the straw may help the children, as they are less able to see the medication and may see drinking from a straw as desirable.

2. The child is to receive the medication orally. The oral route is preferred unless contraindicated.

3. The medication should not be mixed with water, as the child may refuse to drink all of the larger mixture, and water does not mask the flavor of the medication. Juice, a soft drink, or a frozen juice bar may be offered after a medication is swallowed.

4. Many 3 year-olds have difficulty swallowing pills, and liquid forms are safer to swallow to avoid aspiration.

30. 2, p. 879

Rationale:

2. U-500 insulin is 5 times as strong as U-100 insulin. Therefore the amount of U-500 insulin should be divided by **5.** Thirty units of U-500 insulin/5 = 6 units of insulin to draw into a U-100 syringe.

1. This is an incorrect dosage.

3. This is an incorrect dosage.

4. This is an incorrect dosage.

Chapter 35

1. 2, p. 921

Rationale:

2. Studies have found that therapeutic touch is effective in reducing headache pain.

1. Clients such as a premature infant, who are sensitive to energy repatterning, may need to avoid therapeutic touch.

3. Clients, such as a pregnant woman, who are sensitive to energy repatterning, may need to avoid therapeutic touch.

4. Persons who are sensitive to human interaction and touch (e.g., those who have been physically abused or have psychiatric disorders) may misinterpret the intent of the treatment and may feel threatened and anxious by the treatment.

2. 3, p. 923

Rationale:

3. The Dietary Supplement Health and Education Act passed in 1994 allows herbs to be sold as dietary supplements as long as no health claims are written on their labels.

1. Herbal medicines have not undergone the same rigorous testing as pharmaceuticals have, and therefore the majority have not received approval for use as drugs.

2. Many herbal medicines are sold as foods or food supplements in health food stores and through private companies because they do not have FDA approval to be sold as a drug.

4. When herbal medicines are developed, concentrations of the active ingredients have been found to vary considerably. Not all companies follow strict quality-control and manufacturing guidelines, which set standards for acceptable levels of pesticides, residual solvents, bacteria, and heavy metals.

3. 1, p. 924
Rationale:
1. Ginseng is believed to have an effect of increased physical endurance, balancing of the body, and increasing resistance to stress.
2. Ginger is known for its effect as an antiemetic.
3. Echinacea is known for stimulation of the immune system, and as an antiinflammatory and antibacterial agent.
4. Chamomile is believed to have an antiinflammatory, antispasmodic, and antiinfective effect.

4. 1, p. 912
Rationale:
1. Between one third and one half of the population in the United States uses one or more forms of complementary or alternative medicine.
2. Insurance coverage of complementary and alternative medicine is increasing, but it is not available at the same amount as for traditional medicine.
3. The interest in complementary and alternative medicine is evident in the increased number of articles about it in respected medical journals and the development of several journals that specifically focus on complementary and alternative medicine.
4. Typically those who use alternative therapies are professional, well educated, and from a higher socioeconomic standing.

5. 3, p. 916
Rationale:
3. The relaxation response is characterized by decreased heart and respiratory rates, blood pressure, oxygen consumption, and increased alpha brain activity and peripheral skin temperature.

1. A cognitive benefit of relaxation therapy is increased receptivity (i.e., the ability to tolerate and accept experiences that may be uncertain, unfamiliar, or paradoxical).
2. Relaxation therapy increases peripheral skin temperature, not decreases it.
4. Relaxation therapy increases alpha brain activity, not decreases it.

6. 2, p. 916
Rationale:
2. Passive relaxation is useful for persons for whom the effort and energy expenditure of active muscle contracting leads to discomfort or exhaustion, such as the person with terminal cancer. Relaxation has been shown to contribute significantly to cancer palliative care.
1. The person with hypertension would not require the passive type of relaxation.
2. The person with work-related stress would not require the passive type of relaxation.
3. The client experiencing dysfunctional grieving would not require the passive type of relaxation. Therapeutic touch has been found effective in improving the mood in bereaved adults.

7. 3, p. 919
Rationale:
3. Biofeedback techniques are used to assist individuals in learning how to control specific autonomic nervous system responses. With Raynaud's disease, clients experience intermittent vasospastic attacks of small arteries and arterioles of the hands (most commonly) and/or the feet. Biofeedback can be used to control this autonomic response.
1. Relaxation therapy is not the best selection of an alternative therapy for the client with Raynaud's disease.
2. Imagery has not been proven to help the client with Raynaud's disease.
4. Acupuncture is not the best selection of an alternative therapy for the client with Raynaud's disease. Acupuncture is more frequently used to treat pain.

4, p. 918

ationale:

A person who has a strong fear of losing control, or who has experienced sensations of loss of control, may perceive meditation as a form of mind control and thus may be resistant to learning the technique. Some clients may uncover repressed emotions or feelings they cannot cope with during relaxation and/or biofeedback sessions.

A benefit of most biobehavioral therapies, such as meditation, is that it reduces irritability. Aggression is an unlikely response.

Delusions are not a result of biobehavioral therapies.

Many biobehavioral therapies, such as meditation, reduce insomnia.

1, p. 921

ationale:

The most important concept of Chinese medicine is the concept of yin and yang, which represent opposing, yet complementary phenomena that exist is a state of dynamic equilibrium. When an imbalance exists in these two paired opposites, then it is thought that disease occurs.

Meridians are the channels of energy that run in regular patterns through the body and over its surface. It is not the primary concept of traditional Chinese medicine.

The six evil senses are external causes of disease according to traditional Chinese medicine. They are wind, cold, fire, damp, summer heat, and dryness. It is not the primary concept that traditional Chinese medicine is based on.

Acupoints are certain points on the body where special needles are inserted to modify the perception of pain, normalize physiological functions, or treat or prevent disease. Acupuncture is just one healing modality used in traditional Chinese medicine. It is not the primary concept that traditional Chinese medicine is based on.

10. 1, p. 918

Rationale:

1. The first step in assisting a client with meditation and breathing is to position the client comfortably.
2. A quiet space is required, not necessarily a warm environment.
3. The first step is not to have the client close his or her eyes, but to get in a comfortable position in a quiet environment. Furthermore, the client does not have to close his or her eyes to meditate and breathe.
4. The first step is to assist the client into a comfortable position, not to note areas of tension or pain.

11. 4, p. 913

Rationale:

4. A macrobiotic diet is predominantly a vegan diet (no animal products except fish). Emphasis is placed on whole cereal grains, vegetables, and unprocessed foods.
1. A macrobiotic diet does not include meats, only fish and plant proteins.
2. The "Zone" is a dietary program that requires eating protein, carbohydrate, and fat in a 30%:40%:30% ratio.
3. Orthomolecular medicine (megavitamin) diet includes an increased intake of vitamin C and beta-carotene.

12. 1, p. 924

Rationale:

1. Chamomile is used for inflammatory diseases of the gastrointestinal and upper respiratory tracts, and for gastrointestinal spasms. It also may be used to treat infections and inflammation of the skin and mucous membranes.
2. St. John's wort is used to treat mild to moderate depression, viral infections, and to aid wound healing.
3. Echinacea is used to treat upper respiratory tract infections, allergic rhinitis, and aid wound healing.
4. Gingko biloba has been used for many health conditions including Alzheimer's disease, dementia, eye disease, heart disease, poor circulation, varicose veins, anxiety, and age-related diseases.

13. 4, p. 925
Rationale:
4. Chaparral is an herb used for an anticancer effect. It has no proven efficacy and may induce severe liver toxicity.
1. No contraindications exist for taking chaparral with coffee or other caffeinated beverages. Ephedra should be avoided with the consumption of caffeine.
2. Chaparral does not induce venoocclusive disease. However, comfrey may do so.
3. Chaparral is not known to contain a carcinogenic substance. Sassafras and Calamus may contain a carcinogenic substance.

Chapter 36

1. 4, p. 932
Rationale:
4. Resistive isometric exercises are those in which the individual contracts the muscle while pushing against a stationary object or resisting the movement of an object. An example of a resistive isometric exercise is pushing against a footboard.
1. Quadriceps setting is an example of an isometric exercise.
2. Gluteal muscle contraction is an example of an isometric exercise.
3. Moving the arms and legs in a circle is an example of isotonic exercise.

2. 2, p. 937
Rationale:
2. The first step in assessing body alignment is to put the client at ease so that unnatural or rigid positions are not assumed.
1. When assessing body alignment, the nurse's first action is to put the client at ease. Later the nurse may assess the client's gait to observe the client's balance, posture, and ability to walk without assistance.
3. Activity tolerance is the kind and amount of exercise or activity a person is able to perform. It is not the first step in assessing a client's body alignment.
4. Assessing ROM is one of the first assessment techniques used to determine the degree of damage or injury to a joint. It is not the first step in assessing a client's body alignment.

3. 4, p. 948
Rationale:
4. The nurse provides support at the waist s that the client's center of gravity remains the midline. The nurse should be on th client's weaker side to assist him with ambu lation.
1. The nurse should hold onto the client's wais not his arm, and should be on his weaker side not his strong side.
2. The nurse should be on the client's weake side.
3. The nurse should hold onto the client's wais to help steady him in maintaining his cente of gravity midline so that he does not lose hi balance and fall.

4. 2, p. 948
Rationale:
2. Two points of support, such as both feet c one foot and the cane, should be on the floc at all times.
1. The cane should be kept on the stronger side the client's right side.
3. The client should keep his or her body uprigh and midline. Leaning can cause the client t lose his or her balance and fall.
4. After advancing the cane, the client shoul move the weaker leg, the client's left leg, for ward to the cane.

5. 1, p. 951
Rationale:
1. The two-point gait requires at least partia weight bearing on each foot. The client move a crutch at the same time as the opposing leg so that the crutch movements are similar t arm motion during normal walking.
2. In a three-point gait, weight is borne on botł crutches and then on the uninvolved leg.
3. The four-point gait gives stability to the clien but requires weight bearing on both legs. Eacł leg is moved alternately with each opposing crutch so that three points of support are or the floor at all times. This client is suppose to use only partial weight bearing, so this gai would not be appropriate.
4. Paraplegics who wear weight-supporting brace on their legs use the swing-through gait. I would not be appropriate for this client.

6. 4, p. 951

Rationale:

4. To descend stairs, the client places the crutches on the stairs, and the client moves the affected leg and then the unaffected leg to the stairs with the crutches.

1. The client should continue to use the crutches for support, not the banister or wall.

2. The client should continue to use both crutches for support when going up or down stairs.

3. When ascending stairs, the client moves the unaffected leg up the stair and then the crutches and affected leg.

7. 3, p. 948

Rationale:

3. If the client has a syncopal episode or begins to fall, the nurse should assume a wide base of support with one foot in front of the other, supporting the client's weight, and then extend the leg, allowing the client to slide against the leg, gently lowering the client to the floor and protecting the client's head.

1. The nurse should not attempt to walk the client quickly back to the room.

2. The nurse should not lean the client against a wall as he or she might fall.

4. The nurse should not leave the client alone and go for help.

8. 1, p.946

Rationale:

1. Flexing the knees and keeping the feet wide apart provides a broad base of support and increases stability.

2. The nurse should position himself or herself close to the client or object being lifted to minimize the force (10 pounds held at waist height close to the body is equal to 100 pounds held at arms' length). Having the client or object close to the center of gravity also helps maintain balance.

3. Twisting should be avoided, as it increases the risk of back injury.

4. The leg muscles should be used for lifting or moving. They are stronger, larger muscles capable of greater work without injury.

9. 3, p. 945

Rationale:

3. Lower-intensity activities should be done more often, for longer periods, or both.

1. The activity does not have to be continuous; benefits can be realized with short bouts of activity over the course of the day.

2. This is inaccurate because 1000 to 1400 calories may be easily expended each week.

4. All types of activity can be applied in an exercise plan; it does not have to be formal exercises.

10. 3, p. 940

Rationale:

3. An appropriate outcome for *Activity intolerance related to increased weight gain and inactivity* is that the client will perform exercise 3 to 4 times over the next 2-week period. This outcome is realistic, measurable, and addresses the problem.

1. A resting heart rate of 90 to 100 beats per minute is too high, and it does not address the need to increase activity.

2. This outcome does not state whether this blood pressure is at rest or after exercising. It also does not address the need to increase activity.

4. A more appropriate outcome is that the client will increase his or her activity (over the next 2-week period).

Chapter 37

1. 3, p. 961

Rationale:

3. Annual inspections of heating systems, chimneys, and appliances should be done in private homes. Carbon monoxide detectors are available but should not be used as a replacement for proper use and maintenance of fuel-burning appliances.

1. Bacterial contamination of foods is controllable. The FDA is a federal agency responsible for the enforcement of federal regulations regarding the manufacture, processing, and distribution of foods, drugs, and cosmetics to protect consumers against the sale of impure or dangerous substances.

2. Motor vehicle accidents are the leading cause of unintentional death, not fire.
4. Temperature extremes can affect the safety of clients in acute care facilities, especially the older adults.

2. 4, p. 969
Rationale:
4. According to the Fall Assessment tool, the greatest indicator of risk is a history of falls.
1. According to the Fall Assessment tool, the second leading risk factor for falls is confusion.
2. According to the Fall Assessment tool, impaired judgment is the fourth leading risk factor for falls.
3. According to the Fall Assessment tool, sensory deficit is the fifth leading risk factor for falls.

3. 1, p. 996
Rationale:
1. The mitigation phase consists of the assessment process to determine hazard vulnerability for the hospital's service area. This includes an identification of the kinds of emergency situations that are most likely to occur and their probable impact.
2. During the preparedness phase, steps are taken to manage the effects of the event, and an inventory of available resources is taken.
3. During the response phase, steps are taken by staff to triage victims.
4. During the recovery phase, steps are taken to restore essential services.

4. 2, p. 970
Rationale:
2. Clinical features of anthrax include flu-like symptoms, gastrointestinal distress, and popular lesions.
1. Abdominal cramping, diarrhea, drooping eyelids, jaw clench, and difficulty swallowing are clinical features of botulism.
3. Fever, cough, chest pain, and hemoptysis are characteristic of plague.
4. Vesicular skin lesions on the face and extremities are seen with smallpox.

5. 4, p. 986
Rationale:
4. A mummy restraint is used in the short term for a small child or infant for examination or treatment involving the head and neck. This would be the most appropriate type of restraint to use for a 1-year-old who is going to receive an IV line.
1. The wrist restraint maintains immobility of an extremity to prevent the client from removing a therapeutic device, such as an IV tube. It would not be the best choice for starting an IV on a 1-year-old.
2. The jacket restraint is often used to prevent a client from getting up and falling. It is not the best choice for starting an IV line.
3. An elbow restraint is commonly used with infants and children to prevent elbow flexion, such as after an IV line is in place.

6. 2, pp. 982, 983
Rationale:
2. Alternatives to restraints should be attempted first. (A physician's order is required for restraints to be applied). The most appropriate intervention is to check on the client frequently.
1. Alternatives to restraints should be attempted first.
3. A radio may help oriente a client to reality. However, the most appropriate intervention for the client who wanders is to check on the client frequently.
4. Clients who wander should be assigned to rooms near the nurse's station and checked on frequently.

7. 4, p. 991
Rationale:
4. If there is a fire and the client is on life support, the nurse should maintain the client's respiratory status manually with an Ambu-bag and move the client away from the fire.
1. The first action of the nurse is not to pull the fire alarm. The workmen could do that.
2. The workman can attempt to extinguish the fire. The nurse should attend to the client who is closest to the fire in the next room.

3. The nurse should not call the doctor to obtain orders to take the client off the ventilator, as this will take valuable time. The client must be moved away from the fire, and the source of oxygen must be discontinued, as it is combustible. The client will need to be manually resuscitated with an Ambu-bag.

8. 1, p. 991
Rationale:
1. Type A fire extinguishers are used for ordinary combustibles such as wood, cloth, paper, and plastic. A trash can fire would require a type A fire extinguisher.
2. Type B fire extinguishers are used for flammable liquids such as gasoline, grease, paint, and anesthetic gas.
3. Type C fire extinguishers are used for electrical equipment.
4. There is no type D fire extinguisher.

9. 2, p. 979
Rationale:
2. Orienting the client to the position of furniture in the room and stairways is the best intervention to help prevent falls for the client with decreased vision.
1. Attempts should be made to reduce glare. Light bulbs that are 60 watts or less may be increased to 75 watts to help improve visibility. The best intervention to prevent falls is first to orient the client to the surroundings.
3. Maintaining complete bed rest is not the best option. Complete bed rest can cause other health problems because of a lack of mobility.
4. The client should not be restrained for poor vision. Attempts should be made to help compensate for the decreased vision to prevent falls.

10. 1, p. 977
Rationale:
1. This statement indicates that further teaching is required. Children weighing less than 80 pounds or younger than 8 years should always be in an age/weight-appropriate car seat that has been installed according to manufacturer's directions. In cars with a passenger air bag, children younger than 12 should be in the back seat.

2. This is an appropriate safety measure to reduce injuries from falling off a bike or being hit by a car.
3. This is an important safety measure, as many adolescents begin sexual relationships.
4. This is an appropriate safety measure that may someday save a child's life.

11. 4, p. 981
Rationale:
4. Restraints must be periodically removed, and the nurse must assess the client to determine if the restraints continue to be needed.
1. This is not a true statement. A physician's order for restraints must have a limited time frame. If the orders are renewed, it should be done so within a specified time frame according to the agency's policy.
2. Restraints are not to be ordered prn (as needed).
3. The use of restraints must be part of the client's medical treatment. An order or consent is necessary for restraints in long-term care facilities.

12. 3, p. 991
Rationale:
3. The next action the nurse should take is to confine the fire by closing doors and windows and turning off oxygen and electrical equipment.
1. The nurse should extinguish the fire by using an extinguisher after closing the doors of the client rooms.
2. After activating the alarm, the nurse should close all the doors, not remove all of the other clients from the unit.
4. This would not be an appropriate action, as the nurse could get burned in attempting to move the trash can.

13. 3, p. 993
Rationale:
3. The first action is to assess for airway patency, breathing, and circulation.

1. After checking the child's airway, breathing, and circulation, the parent should remove any particles of cleanser from the mouth. The parent should identify the type and amount of substance ingested and then call the Poison Control unit.
2. The parent should administer ipecac syrup only if instructed to induce vomiting by the Poison Control unit. Administering ipecac is not the parent's first action.
4. Removing the particles of cleanser is not the parent's first action. The parent may do so after assessing the child's airway, breathing, and circulation.

Chapter 38

1. 1, p. 1009
Rationale:
1. The first action the nurse should take is to assess for further inflammatory reactions to determine if they is localized or systemic.
2. Discussing body-image problems would not be the priority nursing action.
3. Skin should be washed with warm water, not hot, as it may dry the skin. All soap should be rinsed well, so not to leave residue that may cause further irritation.
4. The rash may be caused by moisture; thus moisturizing the skin would not be appropriate. A lotion to help prevent itching may be applied.

2. 2, p. 1010
Rationale:
2. The client who has right-sided paralysis is at increased risk for a pressure ulcer developing because of immobility. When restricted from moving freely, dependent body parts are exposed to pressure, reducing circulation to affected body parts. The inability to turn or change position increases risk for pressure ulcers.
1. Poor nutrition is a risk factor for developing a pressure ulcer, but not for this client.
3. This client is not identified as having reduced hydration.
4. Skin secretions increase the risk for developing a pressure ulcer. However, this client's greatest risk factor is having impaired mobility.

3. 1, p. 1049
Rationale:
1. Clients prone to bleeding, such as the client with thrombocytopenia, must use an electric razor.
2. Clients with congestive heart failure may use a razor blade to shave.
3. Clients with osteoarthritis do not have to use an electric razor to shave.
4. Clients with pneumonia may use a razor blade to shave. If the client is wearing oxygen, an electric razor should not be used, as it could create a spark. Oxygen is flammable.

4. 4, p. 1027
Rationale:
4. To promote venous return, the nursing assistant should use long strokes washing the client's legs from the ankle to the knee and from the knee to thigh.
1. To prevent warping, dentures should be kept covered in water when they are not worn, and they should always be stored in an enclosed, labeled cup, with the cup placed in the client's bedside stand.
2. Nails should clipped with nail clippers, straight across and even with tops of fingers, and then filed. Scissors should not be used.
3. The client's eyes should be washed with plain water, as soap irritates eyes.

5. 2, p. 1038
Rationale:
2. Vascular changes associated with diabetes mellitus reduce the blood supply to the feet. Sensation in the feet also can be reduced as a result of damage to the nerves (i.e., as with diabetic neuropathy). Sensory loss in the feet may result in undetected injuries. These clients are especially at risk for the development of chronic foot ulcers.
1. The best rationale for meticulous foot care for this client is because of the risks associated with the client's diagnosis of diabetes mellitus.
3. No indication if apparent that the client has a history of poor hygienic care.

4. Poor vision may contribute to difficulty in providing foot care, but this client's greatest risk for developing a foot ulcer is diabetic neuropathy.

6. 4, pp. 1038, 1039
Rationale:
4. Wrapping small pieces of lamb's wool around toes reduces irritation of soft corns between toes.
1. Clients with peripheral vascular disease should not soak their feet. Soaking increases risk of infection because of maceration of the skin.
2. Nails should be filed straight across and square.
3. The client with peripheral vascular disease should not cut corns or calluses or use commercial removers. The client should consult a podiatrist.

7. 3, p. 1044
Rationale:
3. For administering oral care, the nurse should place a semicomatose client on the side (Sim's position) with head turned well toward dependent side to facilitate drainage of secretions from the mouth.
1. The semicomatose client should not be placed in reverse Trendelenberg position for oral care.
2. The semicomatose client should not be placed in the high Fowler's position for oral care.
3. The semicomatose client should not be placed supine for oral care, as oral secretions would collect in the back of the pharynx.

8. 1, p. 1046
Rationale:
1. Frequent brushing helps to keep hair clean and distributes oil evenly along hair shafts.
2. A hot comb would not be helpful for straight or oily hair.
3. Braids made too tightly can lead to bald patches.
4. The frequency of shampooing depends on a person's daily routines and the condition of the hair.

9. 4, p. 1051
Rationale:
4. Use of cotton-tipped applicators should be avoided because they can cause ear wax to become impacted within the canal.
1. Warm water, not cool, should be used to irrigate ears.
2. Asking the client to turn his or head toward the nurse is not the best response.
3. Batteries last 1 week with daily wearing of 10 to 12 hours.

10. 2, p. 1009
Rationale:
2. The client with acne should be taught to wash the hair and skin thoroughly each day with very warm water and soap to remove oil.
1. Moisturizing lotions or creams should not be used, as they tend to clog pores and make the acne worse.
3. It is not recommended to use a depilatory to remove excess hair.
4. Adding moisture to the air with the use of a humidifier is an appropriate intervention for the client with dry skin, not acne.

11. 2, p. 1016
Rationale:
2. The client who is unable to complete bathing and grooming independently has a nursing diagnosis of *Self-care deficit.*
1. Being unable to complete bathing and grooming are not defining characteristics for the nursing diagnosis of *Powerlessness.*
3. Being unable to complete bathing and grooming are not defining characteristics for the nursing diagnosis of *Tissue integrity impairment.*
4. No indication is seen this client has a knowledge deficit of hygiene practices.

12. 4, p. 1030

Rationale:

4. The bag bath is intended to reduce the risk of infection. Use of the traditional washbasin may increase the risk of infection because if it is not cleaned and dried completely after use, gram-negative bacteria may contaminate the washbasin. Successive use of a contaminated basin may cause the client's skin to harbor more gram-negative organisms, increasing the client's risk of infection.
1. The bag bath is typically more expensive than the traditional bed-bath method.
2. Using the bag bath does take less time, but it is not the best rationale for using this method.
3. The bag bath does not leave the skin softer than traditional hygienic care.

13. 1, p. 1032

Rationale:

1. To perform female perineal care, the client should be assisted to the dorsal recumbent position.
2. Side-lying is not the position of choice for performing perineal care of the female.
3. The supine position is the position of choice for performing perineal care of the male, not the female.
4. The prone position is not the position of choice for performing perineal care of the female.

14. 4, p. 1038

Rationale:

4. The client with vascular insufficiency of the lower extremities may exhibit diminished pedal pulses.
1. The client with vascular insufficiency of the lower extremities would have decreased hair growth on the legs and feet, not increased hair growth.
2. The client with vascular insufficiency typically has a shiny appearance of the skin of the lower extremities.
3. The client with vascular insufficiency characteristically demonstrates blanching of the skin on elevation.

15. 4, p. 1033

Rationale:

4. If the client has an erection during perineal care, the nurse should defer the procedure until later.
1. The nurse should not continue with the perineal care at this time.
2. Telling the client it's okay may increase the client's embarrassment.
3. If the client is dependent in his care, the nurse should not ask the client to perform care he is unable to do. The nurse should maintain a professional attitude.

16. 3, p. 1043

Rationale:

3. Normal saline rinses (approximately 30 ml) on awaking in the morning, after each meal, and at bedtime can effectively clean the oral cavity. The rinses can be increased to every 2 hours if necessary.
1. Clients with stomatitis should be advised to avoid commercial mouthwash.
2. Clients with stomatitis should be advised to avoid alcohol.
4. Gentle brushing and flossing are important in preventing bleeding of the gums. A soft toothbrush, not a firm toothbrush, should be used.

Chapter 39

1. 3, p. 1070

Rationale:

3. The QRS complex indicates that the electrical impulse has traveled through the ventricles.
1. Stimulating the parasympathetic system would cause the heart rate to decrease, not increase.
2. In the diseased heart, the stretch of the myocardium is beyond the heart's physiological limits.
4. When stroke volume is decreased, an increase in heart rate occurs.

. 2, p. 1079

ationale:

. The nurse should provide a low concentration of oxygen to the client.

. The client should be instructed to use pursed-lip breathing.

. The most effective position for the client with cardiopulmonary disease is the 45-degree semi-Fowler's position, using gravity to assist in lung expansion and reduce pressure from the abdomen on the diaphragm.

. The nurse's first priority should be to attend to the client who is in respiratory distress, not to contact the physician.

. 2, p. 1075

ationale:

. The client is experiencing sinus tachycardia. The rhythm is regular with a normal P wave, normal QRS complex, and a rate of 100 to 180 beats per minute.

. A sinus dysrhythmia has a rate of 60 to 100 beats per minute, slows during inspiration, and increases with expiration. The client is not experiencing a sinus dysrhythmia.

. With supraventricular tachycardia, the heart rate is 150 to 250 beats/minute, the P wave may be buried in the preceding T wave, and the PR interval is variable. This client is not experiencing supraventricular tachycardia.

. With ventricular tachycardia, the rhythm is slightly irregular, at a rate of 100 to 200 beats per minute, the P wave is absent, PR interval is absent, and the QRS complex is wide. This client is not experiencing ventricular tachycardia.

. 2, p. 1074

ationale:

. Cervical trauma at C3 to C5 can result in paralysis of the phrenic nerve, preventing chest expansion.

. Although this is a risk factor, the client's greatest risk is related to the level of his fracture.

. No mention of an abnormal chest shape is seen. This client's greatest risk for developing pneumonia is related to the level of his fracture.

4. If the client were anemic as a result of blood loss from trauma, his oxygen-carrying capacity of blood would be decreased. No mention of excessive blood loss is noted, nor would this place him at great risk for developing pneumonia.

5. 2, p. 1078

Rationale:

2. Pulmonary congestion may be experienced in left-sided heart failure.

1. Jugular neck vein distention is characteristic of right-sided heart failure.

3. Peripheral edema is characteristic of right-sided heart failure.

4. Hepatomegaly (liver enlargement) is characteristic of right-sided heart failure.

6. 3, p. 1077

Rationale:

3. Ventricular tachycardia would be the most disconcerting dysrhythmia of the four options. Ventricular tachycardia results in a decreased cardiac output; it may lead to severe hypotension, loss of pulse, and consciousness.

1. Sinus bradycardia would not be of concern for this client. It is of no clinical significance unless it is associated with signs and symptoms of a decreased cardiac output.

2. Sinus dysrhythmia is of no clinical significance unless dizziness occurs with a decreased rate.

4. Atrial fibrillation is not as detrimental as ventricular tachycardia.

7. 3, pp. 1079, 1140

Rationale:

3. The respiratory system tries to correct metabolic acidosis by increasing ventilation to reduce the amount of carbon dioxide and thereby raise the pH.

1. The respiratory system would compensate for metabolic acidosis with increased respirations, not hypoventilation. Bicarbonate is the renal component of acid/base balance, not the respiratory component.

2. The pH measures hydrogen ion concentration. Alternating deep versus shallow breaths is not a compensating mechanism of the respiratory system for metabolic acidosis.

Test Bank Answer Key   511

4. The respiratory system does not compensate by expanding the lung tissues to their fullest. In metabolic acidosis, the respiratory system compensates by exhaling a greater amount of carbon dioxide.

8. 4, p. 1080
Rationale:
4. With a narcotic overdose, the respiratory center is depressed, reducing the rate and depth of respiration and the amount of inhaled oxygen. The client may display signs of hypoventilation, such as a decreased level of consciousness.
1. A narcotic (heroin) overdose would cause sedation and respiratory depression, not agitation.
2. The client would experience bradypnea, not hyperpnea.
3. A narcotic (heroin) overdose would cause sedation and respiratory depression, not restlessness.

9. 2, p. 1101
Rationale:
2. Nasotracheal suctioning is the preferred route for obtaining a sputum specimen when the client is unable to cough to produce a sputum specimen on his or her own.
1. The nasopharyngeal route for suctioning is used when the client is able to cough, but is unable to clear secretions by expectorating or swallowing. It is not the preferred route for obtaining a sputum specimen.
3. The oropharyngeal route is used when the client is able to cough, but is unable to clear secretions by expectorating or swallowing. It is not the preferred route for obtaining a sputum specimen.
4. The orotracheal route is used when the client is unable to manage secretions by coughing. The nasotracheal route is preferred over the orotracheal route because stimulation of the gag reflex is minimal.

10. 4, p. 1080
Rationale:
4. Central cyanosis is observed in the tongue, soft palate, and conjunctiva of the eye, where blood flow is high. Central cyanosis indicates hypoxemia.
1. Peripheral cyanosis seen in the palms and soles of the feet is often a result of vasoconstriction and stagnant blood flow.
2. Peripheral cyanosis seen in the nail beds is often a result of vasoconstriction and stagnant blood flow.
3. Peripheral cyanosis seen in the earlobes is often a result of vasoconstriction and stagnant blood flow.

11. 4, p. 1117
Rationale:
4. Chest tubes are inserted to remove air and fluids from the pleural space, to prevent air or fluid from reentering the pleural space, and to re-establish normal intrapleural and intrapulmonic pressures. The client who had mitral valve replacement surgery would be expected to have a chest tube postoperatively to prevent excess fluid build-up in the pleural space.
1. Increased oxygen will not prevent excess fluid build-up.
2. Frequent chest physiotherapy may help facilitate removal of secretions, but will not prevent excess fluid build-up.
3. Incentive spirometry is used to promote deep breathing and to prevent or treat atelectasis in the postoperative client. It will not prevent excess fluid build-up.

12. 1, p. 1117
Rationale:
1. The client with a pneumothorax (collapsed lung) will exhibit dyspnea and pain.
2. Eupnea is normal, easy breathing. It would not be expected in the case of a pneumothorax.
3. Fremitis is the vibration felt when the hand is placed on the client's chest and the client speaks (vocal fremitus). Fremitus would be decreased with a pneumothorax.

4. Orthopnea is a condition in which the person must use multiple pillows when lying down or must sit with the arms elevated and leaning forward to breathe. The client with a pneumothorax would be exhibiting dyspnea.

13. 1, p. 1124
Rationale:
1. The nurse caring for the client with a nasal cannula should plan to assess the client's nares and superior surface of both ears for skin breakdown every 6 hours.
2. The nurse should check patency of the cannula every 8 hours.
3. The nurse does not need to check the client's mouth in relation to the client's use of a nasal cannula. The nurse should continue providing oral hygiene and may assess the mouth (i.e., tongue) for cyanosis, along with other assessment measures.
4. Oxygen flow should be checked every 8 hours, not every 24 hours.

14. 2, p. 1098
Rationale:
2. Chest percussion is indicated and appropriate for the client experiencing cystic fibrosis to assist in mobilizing the thick pulmonary secretions.
1. Percussion is contraindicated in clients with bleeding disorders, such as the client with thrombocytopenia.
3. Percussion is contraindicated in the client with osteoporosis.
4. Percussion is contraindicated in the client with a spinal fracture or with fractured ribs.

15. 2, p. 1080
Rationale:
2. Mental status changes are often the first signs of respiratory problems and may include restlessness and irritability.
1. Cyanosis is a late sign of hypoxia.
3. A decreased respiratory rate is not an early sign of hypoxia. The respiratory rate will increase as the body attempts to compensate for the decreased level of oxygen. As the hypoxia worsens, the respiratory rate may decline.

4. During early stages of hypoxia, the blood pressure is elevated unless the condition is caused by shock.

16. 3, p. 1086
Rationale:
3. Central cyanosis is the most serious finding because it indicates hypoxemia.
1. Poor skin turgor indicates dehydration. It is not an indication of the client's decreased oxygenation.
2. Clubbing of the nails is found in clients with prolonged oxygen deficiency, endocarditis, and congenital heart defects. It is a change that occurs over time, and not an indication of the client's current deterioration in oxygenation status.
4. Pursed-lip breathing is used to slow expiratory flow. It is not the most serious indication of a client's decreased oxygenation.

17. 3, p. 1089
Rationale:
3. A cardiac catheterization involves the injection of contrast material to visualize the cardiac chambers, valves, the great vessels, and coronary arteries. It also is used to measure the pressures and volumes within the chambers of the heart.
1. A Holter monitor is a portable ECG worn by the client. It does not require contrast media.
2. Echocardiography is a noninvasive measure that graphically depicts overall cardiac performance.
4. An exercise stress test evaluates the cardiac response to the physical stress of the client on a treadmill. Contrast material is not used for this test.

18. 3, p. 1095
Rationale:
3. Annual influenza vaccine is recommended for clients of any age with a chronic disease.
1. Annual influenza vaccine is recommended for clients older than 65 years, but this is not the only group.

2. Annual influenza vaccine is recommended for any age group, including those age 40 to 60 years, who have a chronic disease of the heart, lung, or kidneys; clients with diabetes; clients with immunosuppression or severe forms of anemia; or those in close or frequent contact with anyone in a high-risk group.
4. Clients with an acute febrile illness should not be vaccinated.

19. 4, p. 1105
Rationale:
4. Intermittent suction for up to 10 to 15 seconds should be applied during catheter removal to prevent injury to the mucosa.
1. The client is not placed in a supine position. The client is usually placed in a semi-Fowler's position. The client's head is turned to the right to help the nurse suction the left main-stem bronchus, and the client's head is then turned to the left to help the nurse suction the right main-stem bronchus.
2. Nasotracheal suctioning is a sterile procedure.
3. The nasotracheal area should be suctioned first, and then the oropharyngeal area. The mouth and pharynx contain more bacteria than the trachea does.

20. 4, p. 1119
Rationale:
4. If the client is in a chair and the tubing is coiled, the tubing should be lifted every 15 minutes to promote drainage. Care should be taken to ensure that the tubing remains secure.
1. This is inaccurate. Clamping a chest tube is contraindicated when the client is ambulating or being transported.
2. In a water-sealed system, gentle bubbling in the suction-control chamber indicates it is functioning. The suction source may be checked to verify that it is on the appropriate setting. In a waterless system, the suction control (float ball) indicates the amount of suction the client's intrapleural space is receiving. The tubing should not be disconnected.

3. The chest tube should be stripped or milke only if indicated (i.e., clotted drainage appea in the tube; check institutional policy). It believed that stripping the tube great increases intrapleural pressure, which coul damage the pleural tissue and cause or worse an existing pneumothorax. Milking causes smaller pressure change.

21. 2, pp. 1103, 1106
Rationale:
2. To promote maximal oxygenation, the nurs should replace the oxygen and allow re between suctioning passes.
1. Suctioning should be intermittent for up t 10 to 15 seconds.
3. Wall suction is set at 80 to 120 mm Hg portable suction, 7 to 15 mm Hg for adult Elevated pressure settings, such as 200 mr Hg, increase the risk of trauma to mucosa an can induce greater hypoxia.
4. The number of suctioning passes is dete mined by client assessment and nee Repeated passes can remove oxygen and ma induce laryngospasm. The client is not suc tioned until the catheter comes back clear.

22. 4, p. 1121
Rationale:
4. If the drainage unit is broken, the end of th chest tube can be quickly submerged in a cor tainer of sterile water to re-establish the seal.
1. Clamping the chest tube may result in a ter sion pneumothorax.
2. In the case of the tubing becoming discor nected, the client should be instructed t exhale as much as possible and to cough. Th client should not hyperventilate.
3. Raising the tubing above the client's ches level will not help the situation.

23. 4, p. 1075
Rationale:
4. The nurse would expect to find the clier experiencing a sinus dysrhythmia at a rate c 82 beats per minute to have no clinical symp toms.
1. The client with atrial fibrillation may con plain of fatigue.

2. The client experiencing a sinus dysrhythmia would not be expected to complain of chest pain.

3. The client with atrial fibrillation may complain of a "fluttering" sensation in the chest.

24. 2, p. 1077
Rationale:

2. The nurse should prepare for CPR for the client experiencing ventricular fibrillation.

1. Atropine is used for sinus bradycardia with hypotension and decreased cardiac output. In this case, the nurse should prepare to administer CPR, not atropine.

3. A pacemaker may be required for the client with sinus bradycardia. It is not the treatment for ventricular fibrillation.

4. The Valsalva maneuver is used to treat supraventricular tachycardia, not ventricular fibrillation.

25. 4, p. 1078
Rationale:

4. Peripheral edema is an expected assessment finding in the client diagnosed with right-sided heart failure.

1. Dyspnea is an expected assessment finding in the client diagnosed with left-sided heart failure.

2. Confusion is a symptom of hypoventilation.

3. Dizziness is an expected assessment finding in the client experiencing hypoxia.

26. 2, p. 1079
Rationale:

2. Epigastric pain is a symptom of a myocardial infarction in women.

1. Visual disturbances are not a symptom of a myocardial infarction in women.

3. Loss of motor function unilaterally is not a symptom of myocardial infarction in women.

4. Right scapular discomfort and stiffness is not a symptom of myocardial infarction in women.

27. 3, p. 1090
Rationale:

3. The normal paCO$_2$ is 35 to 45 mm Hg.

1. The normal SpO$_2$ is 98% to 100%; the client's is low at 88%.

2. The normal pH is 7.35 to 7.45; the client's is high at 7.52.

4. The normal PEFR should increase or remain the same when compared with the prior assessment. A decreased PEFR would indicate airway obstruction. Predicted values are based on age, sex, and height.

28. 4, p. 1087
Rationale:

4. Pale conjunctiva is an assessment finding consistent with the diagnosis of anemia.

1. Xanthelasma is caused by hyperlipidemia.

2. Petechiae appear on the skin in patients with platelet deficiency (thrombocytopenia). Petechiae on the conjunctivae are consistent with a fat embolus or bacterial endocarditis.

3. Corneal arcus is caused by hyperlipidemia in young to middle adults. It is a normal finding in older adults with arcus senilis.

Chapter 40

1. 4, p. 1144
Rationale:

4. An elevated hematocrit would be expected with a deficit of body fluid in the intravascular compartment. When an excess of body fluid exists in the intravascular compartment, a decreased hematocrit would be expected.

1. Crackles (in lungs) are consistent findings with fluid volume excess.

2. An assessment finding associated with fluid volume excess is a bounding pulse.

3. Engorged peripheral veins may be seen with fluid volume excess.

2. 1, p. 1145
Rationale:

1. Metabolic acidosis may be found in cases of starvation. The client's pH is below the normal of 7.35 (at 7.3), the PaCO$_2$ is in the normal range of 35 to 45 mm Hg (at 38 mm Hg), and the HCO$_3$ is below the normal of 22 mEq/L (at 19 mEq/ml). These findings demonstrate metabolic acidosis.

2. These values are consistent with respiratory alkalosis, compensated. This would not be typical of malnutrition.
3. These are normal arterial blood gas results.
4. These values are consistent with metabolic alkalosis, compensated. This would not be an expected finding with extremely poor nutrition.

3. 1, pp. 1139, 1141
Rationale:
1. Because sodium is necessary for nerve-impulse transmission, the priority nursing assessment with hyponatremia is the neurological system.
2. The gastrointestinal system is not the body system for priority assessment.
3. The priority assessment is not the pulmonary system. Neurological changes will occur first.
4. The priority assessment is not the hepatic system.

4. 2, p. 1145
Rationale:
2. These assessment findings (i.e., warm and flushed skin, lethargy, and medical diagnosis of pneumonia) are indicative of respiratory acidosis.
1. Lethargy and flushed skin may be seen with metabolic acidosis, but this child has a respiratory problem with difficulty breathing, which is consistent with respiratory acidosis.
3. Respiratory alkalosis also may be caused with hyperventilation as a result of pneumonia, but this child's assessment findings are not consistent with respiratory alkalosis.
4. The client's diagnosis and assessment findings are not indicative of metabolic alkalosis.

5. 4, pp. 1145, 1154
Rationale:
4. The client's pH is elevated at 7.48 (normal, 7.35 to 7.45), the CO_2 is normal at 42 (normal, 35–45 mm Hg), and the bicarbonate is elevated at 32 (normal, 22–26 mEq/L). The client is experiencing metabolic alkalosis.
1. In metabolic acidosis, the client's pH would be below 7.35, and the bicarbonate would be below 22 mEq/L. The client is not experiencing metabolic acidosis.

2. In respiratory acidosis, the client's pH would be below 7.35, and the CO_2 would be elevated above 45 mm Hg. The client is not experiencing respiratory acidosis.
3. In respiratory alkalosis, the client's pH would be above 7.45, and the CO_2 would be below 35 mm Hg. The client is not experiencing respiratory alkalosis.

6. 3, pp. 1145, 1154
Rationale:
3. The compensating mechanism in the presence of respiratory acidosis is retention of bicarbonate by the kidneys to increase the pH level.
1. Hyperventilation would be the compensating mechanism in metabolic acidosis to decrease CO_2 levels.
2. Hypoventilation would be the compensating mechanism in metabolic alkalosis to increase CO_2 levels.
4. The compensating mechanism in the presence of metabolic alkalosis is excretion of bicarbonate to decrease the pH level.

7. 3, p. 1149
Rationale:
3. The client at greatest risk for a fluid volume deficit is the client who has severe diarrhea. Any condition that results in the loss of GI fluids predisposes the client to dehydration and a variety of electrolyte disturbances.
1. The very young are at risk for a fluid volume deficit because their body-water loss is proportionately greater per kilogram of weight. However, the very young client is not the individual at most risk for fluid volume deficit.
2. A 12-year-old who is moderately active in warm weather will lose body water through sweating, but is not the individual at greatest risk for a fluid volume deficit.
4. The very old are at increased risk for fluid volume deficit, as they have a decreased thirst sensation and a decreased number of filtering nephrons. However, the older adult client is not the individual at greatest risk for a fluid volume deficit.

516   Test Bank Answer Key

8. 1, pp. 1160-1161
Rationale:
1. The client will need a hypotonic solution, such as 0.45% NS. A hypotonic solution has an osmolality that is less than body fluids, so the cells will draw the fluid in, which is the desired effect when the client has experienced a loss of intracellular fluid.
2. 10% dextrose is a hypertonic solution that will draw fluid into the vascular space.
3. 5% dextrose in lactated Ringer's is a hypertonic solution. Hypertonic solutions pull fluid into the vascular space by osmosis.
4. Dextrose 5% in 1/2 NS is a hypertonic solution. Hypertonic solutions pull fluid into the vascular space by osmosis. The client needs a hypotonic solution to rehydrate the cells.

9. 4, p. 1142
Rationale:
4. Flank pain and lower back pain may be indicative of kidney stones from excess calcium. The laboratory value for the nurse to obtain would be a serum calcium level.
1. Flank pain and lower back pain is not indicative of a problem with serum potassium being too high or too low.
2. The client is not having symptoms suggesting an altered serum sodium level.
3. The client is not displaying symptoms consistent with an altered magnesium level.

10. 3, pp. 1175, 1176
Rationale:
3. 1000 ml ÷ 8 hr = 125 ml/hr;

$$\frac{15 \text{ gtt/ml}}{60 \text{ min}} \times 125 \text{ ml} = 32 \text{ gtts/min}$$

1. This is an inaccurate flow rate.
2. This is an inaccurate flow rate.
4. This is an inaccurate flow rate.

11. 4, p. 1167
Rationale:
4. The nurse should avoid veins in an extremity with compromised circulation, such as a dialysis graft.
1. The nurse should use the most distal site in the nondominant arm, if possible.
2. The nurse should avoid hardened cord-like veins.
3. The nurse should use the nondominant arm, if possible.

12. 2, p. 1189
Rationale:
2. Signs of phlebitis may include increased temperature over the vein, erythema, pain, and edema. With phlebitis, the area is warm to the touch; with infiltration, the area is cool to the touch.
1. The intensity of pain is not a differentiating factor between phlebitis and infiltration. Pain may occur with both.
3. The amount of subcutaneous edema is not a differentiating factor between phlebitis and infiltration. Edema may occur with both.
4. Skin discoloration of a bruised nature is not the best way to differentiate phlebitis from infiltration. With phlebitis, the area is typically reddened. With infiltration, the area is typically pale.

13. 2, p. 1192
Rationale:
2. If a blood reaction is suspected, the nurse stops the blood transfusion immediately.
1. The nurse should take the client's vital signs, but the initial action should be to stop the blood transfusion.
3. The nurse should not slow the rate of blood flow. The nurse should stop the blood transfusion.
4. The nurse should first stop the blood transfusion. The nurse may notify the physician and blood bank personnel after the transfusion is stopped.

14. 2, p. 1150
Rationale:
2. Hypertension is a symptom of fluid volume excess.
1. A weak, thready pulse is associated with fluid volume deficit. A bounding pulse is a symptom of fluid volume excess.
3. Dry mucous membranes are symptomatic of fluid volume deficit, not excess.
4. Flushed skin is a symptom of fluid volume deficit.

15. 1, p. 1141

Rationale:

1. Furosemide (Lasix) is a non–potassium-sparing diuretic. Without a potassium supplement, the client may become hypokalemic. Hypokalemia increases the risk for digoxin toxicity. Both hypokalemia and digoxin toxicity can cause cardiac dysrhythmias.
2. Clients with hypokalemia from diuretic use may experience intestinal distention and decreased bowel sounds. Severe diarrhea may be a cause, not a result, of hypokalemiahypokalemia.
3. Clients with hyperactive reflexes may have hypocalcemia. Furosemide (Lasix) and digoxin do not predispose a client to hypocalcemia.
4. Peripheral cyanosis is not a potential problem related to the client's medication regimen.

16. 3, p. 1142

Rationale:

3. Chvostek's sign is seen with hypocalcemia. Rapid administration of blood transfusions containing citrate may cause hypocalcemia. Citrate solution is used to prevent clotting of the blood so that it can be stored in the refrigerator until it is needed for transfusion. If cold blood is administered too rapidly, it may cause cardiac dysrhythmias. If a client receives a rapid blood transfusion, the kidneys may not be able to excrete phosphorus quickly enough, and the phosphorus level increases while the calcium level decreases. Sepsis also may increase the risk for developing hypocalcemia.
1. The client who has a rapid blood transfusion of citrated blood would not be expected to experience excessive sweating. The client who experiences an anaphylactic reaction or sepsis typically has cool, clammy skin.
2. Anxiety may be related to an anaphylactic or febrile, nonhemolytic reaction to a blood transfusion. However, it is not the best indication of a possible reaction, as the client may be anxious because of receiving a blood transfusion, having nothing to do with a physiological reaction to the transfusion.
4. Nausea and vomiting may or may not indicate a reaction to a blood transfusion.

17. 4, p. 1145

Rationale:

4. A salicylate overdose may cause respiratory alkalosis due to hyperventilation.
1. Metabolic acidosis may occur with salicylate poisoning, but the pH demonstrates an alkalotic state.
2. Metabolic alkalosis is not consistent with aspirin overdose.
3. An aspirin overdose does not cause respiratory acidosis.

18. 4, p. 1158

Rationale:

4. Daily weights are the single most important indicator of fluid status.
1. Skin turgor is a measure of hydration, but it is not the single best indicator of a client's fluid status.
2. Intake and output measurements are an important nursing intervention for monitoring fluid status; however, daily weights are the best indicator.
3. Serum electrolytes help monitor fluid status. Daily weights are the single best indicator of a client's fluid status.

19. 3, p. 1176

Rationale:

3. $\dfrac{60 \text{ gtt/ml}}{60 \text{ min}} \times 125 \text{ ml} = 125 \text{ gtt/min}$
1. This calculation is incorrect.
2. This calculation is incorrect.
4. This calculation is incorrect.

20. 3, p. 1141

Rationale:

3. A cause of hyponatremia is an adrenal insufficiency. The client with hyponatremia may experience diarrhea, abdominal cramping, and nausea and vomiting.
1. Decreased muscle tone is a symptom of hypokalemia. Hypokalemia is not caused by adrenal insufficiency.
2. A client with adrenal insufficiency is not likely to experience hypertension. Resultant hyponatremia with adrenal insufficiency may be exhibited as postural hypotension.
4. Fever is a symptom of hypernatremia, not hyponatremia. Hypernatremia is not caused by adrenal insufficiency.

518   Test Bank Answer Key

21. 1, p. 1136
Rationale:
1. A calcium level of 3.9 mEq/L should be reported to the physician. A normal calcium level is 4.5 to 5.5 mEq/L.
2. A sodium level of 140 mEq/L is within the normal range of 135 to 145 mEq/L.
3. A potassium level of 3.5 mEq/L is within the normal range of 3.5 to 5.0 mEq/L.
4. A magnesium level of 2.1 mEq/L is within the normal range of 1.5 to 2.5 mEq/L.

22. 3, p. 1144
Rationale:
3. Hypertension is manifested with fluid volume excess.
1. The urine specific gravity would be decreased with fluid volume excess. The nurse would anticipate an increased urine specific gravity with fluid volume deficit.
2. The nurse would anticipate an increase, not a decrease, in body weight with fluid volume excess.
4. The nurse would anticipate an increase, not a decrease, in pulse strength in fluid volume excess.

23. 2, p. 1160
Rationale:
2. Lactated Ringer's is an isotonic solution.
1. 0.45% Saline is a hypotonic solution.
3. 5% Dextrose in normal saline is a hypertonic solution.
4. 5% Dextrose in lactated Ringer's is a hypertonic solution.

24. 4, p. 1192
Rationale:
4. After stopping the blood transfusion the nurse should obtain and send a urine specimen to the lab to determine the presence of hemoglobin as a result of RBC hemolysis.
1. In an acute hemolytic reaction, management of the reaction does not include the administration of an antipyretic.
2. The nurse does not begin an infusion of epinephrine. The nurse should be prepared to administer emergency drugs, such as diuretics, per the physician's order.

3. The nurse should not turn off the blood and simply turn on the normal saline that is connected to the Y-tubing set. This would cause blood remaining in the Y-tubing to infuse into the client. Even a small amount of mismatched blood can cause a major reaction. The nurse should run normal saline directly into the IV line (not through the blood tubing).

Chapter 41

1. 3, p. 1200
Rationale:
3. The ascending reticular activating system (RAS) located in the upper brain stem is believed to contain special cells that maintain alertness and wakefulness.
1. Infradian rhythms, not ultradian rhythms, occur in a cycle longer than 24 hours.
2. Nonrapid eye movement refers to the sleep cycle that most clients experience in a low-stimulus environment.
4. The bulbar synchronizing region is the area of the brain where serotonin is released to produce sleep. It is not responsible for REM sleep.

2. 3, p. 1204
Rationale:
2. Structural abnormalities such as a deviated septum, nasal polyps, certain jaw configurations, or enlarged tonsils predispose a client to obstructive apnea.
1. Individuals with mixed apnea often have signs and symptoms of right-sided heart failure.
3. Respiratory infections do not predispose a client to obstructive sleep apnea.
4. Clients with obstructive apnea are often middle-aged, obese men. Obesity itself does not predispose a client to obstructive sleep apnea.

3. 2, p. 1205
Rationale:
2. Psychological symptoms of sleep deprivation include confusion and irritability.
1. Elevated blood pressure is not a symptom of sleep deprivation.

3. Rapid respirations are not a symptom of sleep deprivation. A decreased ability of reasoning and judgment could lead to inappropriateness.
4. Decreased temperature is not a symptom of sleep deprivation. The client with sleep deprivation is often withdrawn, not talkative.

4. 3, p. 1206
Rationale:
3. Infants usually develop a nighttime pattern of sleep by age 3 months.
1. This is not when infants usually develop a nighttime pattern of sleep.
2. This is not when infants usually develop a nighttime pattern of sleep.
4. This is not when infants usually develop a nighttime pattern of sleep.

5. 4, p. 1219
Rationale:
4. The nurse should advise the parent to maintain a regular bedtime and wake-up schedule and to reinforce patterns of preparing for bedtime. A bedtime routine (e.g., same hour for bedtime, quiet activity) used consistently helps young children avoid delaying sleep.
1. It is most important that the parent maintain a consistent bedtime routine. If a bedtime snack is already part of that routine, then this is allowable. If it is not, then the child may use having a snack only as a measure of procrastination.
2. After age 3 years, the child may give up daytime naps. A bedtime routine used consistently will be more effective in helping the child resist going to sleep.
3. The same regular bedtime and wake-up schedule should be maintained.

6. 1, p. 1207
Rationale:
1. A school-age child will be tired the following day if allowed to stay up later than usual. The nurse should ask a question to assess the child's usual sleep patterns.
2. The nurse should first assess the child's usual sleep pattern. This response is not appropriate because the nurse is assuming the child is not adhering to a bedtime.

3. The nurse should first assess the child's usual sleep pattern. A sleep problem is often the cause of fatigue.
4. The nurse is assuming the child is experiencing insomnia. The nurse should first determine the child's sleep pattern.

7. 4, p. 1207
Rationale:
4. As people age, a progressive decrease occurs in stages 3 and 4 NREM sleep; some older adults have almost no stage 4, or deep sleep.
1. As people age, they do not become more difficult to arouse.
2. The older adult does not require more sleep than the middle-aged adult.
3. An older adult awakens more often during the night, and it may take more time for an older adult to fall asleep.

8. 1, p. 1208
Rationale:
1. For the client who is currently taking a diuretic, the nurse should inform the client that he or she might experience nighttime awakening because of nocturia.
2. Diuretic use does not cause nightmares.
3. Diuretics do not cause increased daytime sleepiness.
4. Diuretics do not reduce REM sleep.

9. 3, p. 1218
Rationale:
3. Infants are usually placed on their backs to prevent suffocation or on their sides to prevent aspiration of stomach contents.
1. To reduce the chance of suffocation, pillows, stuffed toys, or the ends of loose blankets should not be placed in cribs.
2. An infants should not be covered loosely with a blanket, because the infant might pull it over the faces and suffocate.
4. To reduce the chance of suffocation, pillows should not be placed in cribs.

10. 1, p. 1210
Rationale:
1. To assess the client's sleeping problem, the nurse should inquire about predisposing factors, such as by asking, "What do you do just before going to bed?" Assessment is aimed at understanding the characteristics of any sleep problem and the client's usual sleep habits so that ways for promoting sleep can be incorporated into nursing care.
2. Older adults sleep best in softly lit rooms.
3. Napping more during the daytime is often not the best solution. The nurse should first assess the client's sleeping problem.
4. The client does not always have to eat something before going to bed. The nurse should first assess the client's sleeping problem. It may not be difficulty falling asleep.

11. 4, p. 1211
Rationale:
4. Partners of clients with sleep apnea often complain that the client's snoring disturbs their sleep.
1. Restlessness is not most associated with sleep apnea.
2. Sleeptalking is associated with sleep-wake transition disorders, not sleep apnea.
3. Somnambulism is associated with parasomnias (specifically arousal disorders and sleep-wake transition disorders).

12. 1, p. 1219
Rationale:
1. The nurse should explain that if possible, the bedroom should not be used for intensive studying, snacking, TV watching, or other nonsleep activity, besides sex.
2. The nurse should instruct the client to avoid heavy meals for 3 hours before bedtime; a light snack may help.
3. The nurse should instruct the client to try to exercise daily, preferably in morning or afternoon, and to avoid vigorous exercise in the evening within 2 hours of bedtime.
4. The nurse should advise the client to get out of bed and do some quiet activity until feeling sleepy enough to go back to bed if the client does not fall asleep within 30 minutes of going to bed.

13. 2, p. 1219
Rationale:
2. At home a client should not try to finish office work or resolve family problems before bedtime.
1. Noise should be kept to a minimum. Soft music may be used to mask noise if necessary.
3. Reading a light novel, watching an enjoyable television program, or listening to music helps a person to relax. Relaxation exercises can be useful at bedtime.
4. A dairy-product snack such as warm milk or cocoa that contains L-tryptophan may be helpful in promoting sleep.

14. 3, p. 1222
Rationale:
3. The benzodiazepines cause relaxation, antianxiety, and hypnotic effects by facilitating the action of neurons in the CNS that suppress responsiveness to stimulation, therefore decreasing levels of arousal.
1. Withdrawal from CNS depressants such as barbiturates can cause insomnia and must be managed carefully. Barbiturates can cause tolerance and dependence.
2. CNS stimulants, such as amphetamines, should be used sparingly and under medical management. Amphetamine sulfate may be used to treat narcolepsy. Prolonged use may cause drug dependence.
4. Tricyclic antidepressants can cause insomnia when discontinued and should be managed carefully. They are used primarily to treat depression.

15. 4, p. 1212
Rationale:
4. To assess for sleep apnea, the nurse may ask, "Do you snore loudly?" and, "Do you experience headaches after awakening?" A positive response may indicate that the client experiences sleep apnea.
1. This question is directed at assessing the potential presence of insomnia.
2. This question is directed at determining the potential presence of narcolepsy.
3. This question is directed at determining the potential presence of narcolepsy.

16. 3, p. 1219

Rationale:

3. To promote sleep, daytime naps should be eliminated. If naps are used, they should be limited to 20 minutes or less twice a day.

1. Alcohol should be limited in the late afternoon and evening because it has an insomnia-producing effect.

2. The use of nonprescription sleeping medications is not advisable. Over the long term, these drugs can lead to further sleep disruption, even when they initially seemed to be effective.

4. Following a bedtime routine should be consistent, not necessarily going to bed. The client should engage in quiet activities that promote relaxation, and then may go to bed. If the client hasn't fallen asleep in 30 minutes, the client should get up out of bed and do some quiet activity until they feel sleepy enough to go back to bed.

Chapter 42

1. 1, p. 1253

Rationale:

1. The gate-control theory suggests that cutaneous stimulation activates larger, faster-transmitting A-beta sensory nerve fibers. This decreases pain transmission through small-diameter A-delta and C fibers. A back massage is a nursing intervention based on the gate-control theory.

2. Changing the client's position in bed is not a form of cutaneous stimulation used to relieve pain.

3. Giving the client a pain medication is a pharmacological approach to relieving pain. It is not based on the gate-control theory.

4. Limiting the number of visitors may provide a quiet environment conducive to relaxation, but it is not based on the gate-control theory.

2. 3, p. 1261

Rationale:

3. When clients are receiving epidural analgesia, monitoring occurs as often as every 15 minutes, including assessment of respiratory rate, respiratory effort, and skin color. Complications of epidural opioid use include nausea and vomiting, urinary retention, constipation, respiratory depression, and pruritis. A common complication of epidural anesthesia is hypotension. Assessing vital signs is the priority nursing intervention.

1. Because of the catheter location, strict surgical asepsis is needed to prevent a serious and potentially fatal infection.

2. To reduce the risk of accidental epidural injection of drugs intended for IV use, the catheter should be clearly labeled "epidural catheter." However, it is not the priority nursing intervention.

4. Supplemental doses of opioids or sedative/hypnotics are avoided because of possible additive central nervous system adverse effects. However, this is not the priority nursing intervention.

3. 3, p. 1243

Rationale:

3. Deep or visceral pain is diffuse and may radiate in several directions. Visceral pain may be described as a burning sensation.

1. Referred pain is felt in a part of the body separate from the source of pain, such as with myocardial infarction, in which pain may be referred to the jaw, left arm, and left shoulder.

2. Radiating pain feels as though it travels down or along a body part, such as low back pain that is accompanied by pain radiating down the leg from sciatic nerve irritation.

4. Superficial or cutaneous pain is of short duration and is localized, as in a small cut.

4. 3, p. 1243

Rationale:

3. Descriptive scales are a more objective means of measuring pain intensity.

1. Asking the client what precipitates the pain does not assess intensity, but rather is an assessment of the pain pattern.

Asking the client about the location of pain does not assess the intensity of the client's pain.

To determine the quality of the client's pain, the nurse may ask open-ended questions to find out about the sensation experienced.

1, p. 1244
Rationale:

To determine the quality of the client's pain the nurse might say, "What does your discomfort feel like?" It is more accurate to have clients describe the pain in their own words whenever possible.

Inquiring about what activities make the pain worse is a type of question directed at determining the pain pattern.

Having the client rate his or her pain on a pain scale is a method of measuring the intensity of pain.

To determine the client's expectations, the nurse may ask the client, "How much discomfort are you able to tolerate?"

1, p. 1259
Rationale:

With a PCA system, the client controls medication delivery.

The PCA system is designed to deliver no more than a specified number of doses. The client does not choose the dosage.

The physician prescribes the type of medication to be used. The advantage for the client is that he or she may self-administer opioids with minimal risk of overdose.

The client does not control the route for administration. Systemic PCA typically involves IV drug administration, but can also be given subcutaneously.

3, p. 1256
Rationale:

A nonopioid analgesic, such as acetaminophen, is used to treat mild musculoskeletal pain effectively.

Fentanyl is about 100 times more potent than morphine. It is typically used for cancer pain, not mild musculoskeletal pain.

Diazepam is given as an antianxiety agent.

4. Meperidine hydrochloride is an opioid analgesic used to treat moderate to severe acute pain, not mild pain.

8. 3, p. 1254
Rationale:

3. Pain can be prevented by anticipating painful events. Before performing procedures, the nurse considers the client's condition, aspects of the procedure that may be uncomfortable, and techniques to avoid causing pain. The nurse who tells the client that the urinary catheter insertion may feel uncomfortable is an example of anticipatory response.

1. This is not an example of using distraction. Distraction directs a client's attention to something else and thus can reduce the awareness of pain and even increase tolerance.

2. Reducing pain perception means to remove stimuli that are uncomfortable or to prevent stimuli that are painful, such as changing wet linens, or preventing constipation with fluids, diet, and exercise.

4. This is not an example of self-care maintenance. Self-care maintenance implies that the client is able to carry out necessary activities to care for himself or herself. This may include pain-management measures.

9. 2, p. 1257
Rationale:

2. PCA is a safe method for postoperative pain management, such as the client recovering from total hip replacement surgery.

1. PCA would not be the mode of choice for treating psychogenic pain.

3. PCA would not be recommended for the client with renal dysfunction. The client with renal impairment would be at increased risk for drug toxicity due to decreased drug excretion.

4. Clients must be able to understand the use of the equipment and be physically able to locate and press the button to deliver the dose. The client who recently experienced a cerebrovascular accident may have difficulty managing the PCA system.

10. 2, p. 1254
Rationale:
2. When a client feels pain, the TENS unit is turned on, and a buzzing or tingling sensation is created. The tingling sensation can be applied until pain relief occurs.
1. The client may adjust the intensity of skin stimulation. It does not have to remain on high.
3. The electrodes do not have to be removed at bedtime.
4. Medication can be administered with a TENS unit.

11. 3, p. 1261
Rationale:
3. The best choice of treatment often changes as the client's condition and the characteristics of pain change. It is realistic to expect that a terminally ill client's need for pain medication will change over time with disease progression.
1. The goal is not to oversedate the client, but to provide pain control without excessive sedation.
2. It would be unrealistic to expect that the pain of terminal cancer will be completely alleviated.
4. Analgesics should not be withheld, as this would only increase the client's level of pain. The medication regimen may require adaptation to meet the client's needs.

12. 4, p. 1233
Rationale:
4. Acute severe or deep pain, as with kidney stones, will cause a parasympathetic response. The client would likely exhibit nausea and vomiting.
1. Tachycardia is a response of sympathetic stimulation, commonly seen with pain of low to moderate intensity and superficial pain.
2. Diaphoresis is a response of sympathetic stimulation, commonly seen with pain of low to moderate intensity and superficial pain.
3. Pupil dilation is a response of sympathetic stimulation, commonly seen with pain of low to moderate intensity and superficial pain.

13. 1, p. 1241
Rationale:
1. A client's self-report of pain is the single reliable indicator of the existence and intensity of pain and any related discomfort. is individualistic.
2. A misconception about pain is that chronic pain is psychological.
3. The belief that administering analgesics regularly will lead to drug addiction is a misconception.
4. A misconception about pain is that the amount of tissue damage is accurately reflected in the degree of pain perceived.

14. 2, p. 1252
Rationale:
2. Pleasurable stimuli cause the release of endorphins. The nurse assesses activities enjoyed by the client that may act as distraction. Distraction directs a client's attention to something else and thus can reduce the awareness of pain and even increase tolerance.
1. Acupressure does not focus on promoting pleasurable and meaningful stimuli. Acupressure is finger pressure applied therapeutically at selected points of the body.
3. Biofeedback focuses on an individual's physiological responses (e.g., blood pressure or tension) and ways to exercise voluntary control over those responses.
4. Hypnosis does not focus on promoting pleasurable and meaningful stimuli. Hypnosis is a condition resembling sleep in which the mind is susceptible to suggestions.

15. 3, p. 1261
Rationale:
3. To prevent catheter displacement, the catheter should be secured carefully to the outside skin.
1. The infusion tubing should be changed every 24 hours to prevent infection.
2. To prevent infection, the dressing should be routinely changed over the site.
4. A transparent dressing should be used over the site to secure the catheter and aid inspection.

6. 2, p. 1263
Rationale:

The unit should be left intact and not chewed. The unit is placed in the client's mouth and swabbed over the inside of the cheeks and lower gums.
No more than two units should be used per breakthrough pain episode.
The unit needs to be allowed to dissolve and absorb over a 15-minute period.

7. 3, p. 1256
Rationale:

To treat a client who is experiencing continuous severe pain, the nurse should expect the client to receive opioid and nonopioid analgesics for severe pain experiences.
Intramuscular administration of analgesics is not expected because the injection itself is painful, and inconsistent erratic absorption of the drug may occur.
The nurse should administer opioids before the client's pain becomes intense. It is easier to maintain pain control than it is to get intense pain under control.
Large doses of opioids are not given initially to clients who have not taken the medications before as it may cause respiratory depression. The expectation is to begin with lower doses and titrate upward.

8. 3, p. 1233
Rationale:

An expected assessment finding of a client experiencing acute pain would be diaphoresis due to sympathetic nerve stimulation.
An expected assessment finding of a client experiencing acute pain would be an increased heart rate, not bradycardia.
An expected assessment finding of a client experiencing acute pain would be an increased respiratory rate, not bradypnea.
The client experiencing acute pain will have increased muscle tension.

9. 1, p. 1255
Rationale:

The nurse should end the backrub with long firm strokes down the back.

2. The backrub is not finished with light strokes while moving up the back in a circular motion.
3. Kneading movements toward the sacrum are done before ending the backrub with long, firm strokes down the back.
4. The nurse should begin a backrub by massaging in a circular motion upward from buttocks to shoulders.

Chapter 43

1. 4, p. 1296
Rationale:

4. For families on limited budgets, substitutes can be used. For example, bean or cheese dishes can often replace meat in a meal. Peas and lentils also are inexpensive food sources of protein.
1. Oranges and potatoes are not high in protein content.
2. Potatoes and rice are sources of carbohydrates, not protein.
3. Rice and macaroni are carbohydrates and are not high in protein.

2. 1, p. 1275
Rationale:

1. The fat-soluble vitamins are A, D, E, and K. With the exception of vitamin D, which can be obtained through exposure to sunlight, these vitamins are provided through dietary intake, including fortified milk.
2. The B vitamins are not fat soluble; they are water-soluble vitamins.
3. Increasing protein intake will improve (decrease) a negative nitrogen imbalance, not increase it. Furthermore, increasing protein intake does not address the problem of a fat-soluble vitamin deficiency.
4. Although this is a true statement, it does not address the problem of a fat-soluble vitamin deficiency.

3. 4, p. 1316
Rationale:

4. The treatment of malabsorption syndromes, such as celiac disease, includes a gluten-free diet. Gluten is present in wheat, rye, barley, and oats.

1. Citrus fruits do not contain gluten.
2. Vegetables do not contain gluten.
3. Red meats do not contain gluten.

4. 2, p. 1281
Rationale:
2. Anorexia nervosa is characterized by self-imposed starvation.
1. Bulimia nervosa is characterized by a lack of control over eating patterns.
3. Bulimia nervosa is characterized by binge/purge cycles.
4. Clients with bulimia may exercise excessively to prevent weight gain.

5. 4, p. 1282
Rationale:
4. Folic acid intake is particularly important for DNA synthesis and the growth of red blood cells. Inadequate intake may lead to fetal neural tube defects, anencephaly, or maternal megaloblastic anemia. It is now recommended that women planning future pregnancies discuss preconception folic acid supplements.
1. The recommended weight gain for pregnancy is 25 to 35 pounds for the woman of average weight. No need exists for the client to limit her weight gain to a maximum of 25 pounds based on this being her third pregnancy.
2. The client needs to increase her protein intake to 60 g during pregnancy, but she does not need to double it. (This is an increase of approximately 20 g of protein.)
3. Prenatal care usually includes vitamin and mineral supplementation to ensure daily intakes. The recommended intake of vitamin A does not increase over that of the nonpregnant state. Calcium intake increases from 800 to 1200 mg during pregnancy.

6. 2, pp. 1293, 1298
Rationale:
2. The client who has had throat surgery sh first be offered clear liquids. If the client t ates clear liquids, then he or she may advanced to a full liquid diet, and then mechanical soft diet. Because the client throat surgery, excoriating liquids such as c juices should be avoided. To be able to asses bleeding, red or dark liquids should be avo (e.g., apple juice or ginger ale is recommen rather than grape or cranberry juice).
1. The client should begin oral intake with liquids. Chicken noodle soup is not on a liquid diet.
3. The client should begin oral intake with liquids. Oatmeal is not on a clear liquid d
4. Hot tea with lemon would not be rec mended. Liquids should not be hot or con citrus, which could cause pain or excoria and possible bleeding at the surgical site.

7. 4, p. 1317
Rationale:
4. HIV-infected clients typically experience t wasting and severe weight loss. Restora care for these clients focuses on maximi kilocalories and nutrients. Low-fat diets small, frequent, nutrient-dense meals ma better tolerated.
1. No need exists to restrict potassium, p phate, and sodium in the client with infection.
2. The client with HIV infection does not r to reduce carbohydrate intake.
3. The client with HIV infection does not r to decrease protein and folic acid intake.

8. 2, p. 1309
Rationale:
2. Before introducing a feeding through an dwelling gavage tube for enteral nutrition is essential that the nurse check to see that tube is properly placed.
1. It is not necessary to irrigate the tube v normal saline.
3. The client's head should be elevated 30 to degrees to help prevent the chance of asp tion.

4. The tube may be flushed with 30 ml of water before initiating the feeding. However, the nurse should first verify correct tube placement.

9. 2, p. 1312
Rationale:
2. The infusion should be maintained at a consistent rate. If an infusion falls behind schedule, the nurse should not increase the rate in an attempt to catch up, as this could lead to osmotic diuresis and dehydration. An infusion should not be discontinued abruptly as it may cause hypoglycemia.
1. An initial rate of 40 to 60 ml/hr is recommended.
3. To avoid infection, the infusion tubing should be changed every 24 hours with lipids and every 48 hours when lipids are not infused.
4. Protein levels do not need to be monitored daily. The client should be weighed daily until maximal administration rate is reached and maintained for 24 hours; then weigh the client 3 times per week.

10. 1, p. 1300
Rationale:
1. The procedure should be explained to the client, including how to communicate during intubation by raising his or her index finger to indicate gagging or discomfort. This will help reduce anxiety and help the client to assist in insertion. This statement by the nurse is correct.
2. The length of the tube to be inserted is measured from the tip of the nose to the earlobe, to the xiphoid process of the sternum.
3. The client should be told to mouth-breathe and swallow during the procedure. The client should not hold his or her breath.
4. The nurse should instruct the client to flex the head toward the chest after the tube has passed the nasopharynx.

11. 1, p. 1273
Rationale:
1. A complete protein contains all essential amino acids in sufficient quantity to support growth and maintain nitrogen balance. Eggs and meats are examples of complete proteins.

2. Incomplete proteins lack one or more of the nine essential amino acids and include oats (cereals).
3. Incomplete proteins lack one or more of the nine essential amino acids and include legumes (lentils).
4. Incomplete proteins lack one or more of the nine essential amino acids and include legumes (peanuts).

12. 3, p. 1278
Rationale:
3. According to the Food Guide Pyramid, the average adult's diet should include three to five servings of vegetables per day.
1. This is not the recommended number of servings per day for vegetables.
2. According to the Food Guide Pyramid, the average adult's diet should include two to four servings per day of fruit.
4. According to the Food Guide Pyramid, the average adult's diet should include two to four servings per day of grains.

13. 3, p. 1281
Rationale:
3. School-age children's diets should be carefully assessed for adequate protein and vitamins A and C. School-age children frequently fail to eat a proper breakfast and have unsupervised intake at school.
1. An increase in B-complex vitamins is needed to support heightened metabolic activity of the adolescent but not the school-age child.
2. The pregnant woman has a need to increase iron intake significantly, but the school-age child does not.
4. Increased energy needs are expected in the adolescent period, not in the school-age group. Therefore an 8-year-old child does not need to increase carbohydrates to meet increased energy needs.

14. 4, p. 1285
Rationale:
4. Clients who practice Islam or Judaism share an avoidance of pork in their diet.
1. Clients who practice Islam avoid alcohol. Clients who practice Judaism do not restrict alcohol intake.

2. Clients who practice Judaism eat only fish with scales and will avoid shellfish. Seventh-day Adventists also avoid shellfish. Clients who practice Islam will eat shellfish.

3. Clients who practice Islam will avoid caffeine. Mormons also avoid caffeine. Clients who practice Judaism do not restrict caffeine intake.

15. 1, p. 1298
Rationale:
1. Custard is included in a full liquid diet.
2. Pureed meats are allowed in a pureed diet, not a full liquid diet.
3. Soft fresh fruit is not included in a full liquid diet. Fresh fruit is often part of a high-fiber diet. Cooked or canned fruits are allowed on a mechanical soft diet.
4. Canned soup is not part of full liquid diet, as it may contain noodles or rice or vegetables. Soups are allowed on a mechanical soft diet.

16. 4, p. 1314
Rationale:
4. If the client begins to experience abdominal cramping and nausea during an enteral tube feeding, the nurse should decrease the administration rate to increase tolerance.
1. Administration of cold formula may cause abdominal cramping and nausea. The formula is best tolerated at room temperature.
2. The nurse should not remove the tube if the client complains of abdominal cramping and nausea.
3. The formula may require dilution if the client is complaining of abdominal cramping and nausea.

17. 2, p. 1316
Rationale:
2. The client diagnosed with a peptic ulcer may be allowed to add green vegetables to his diet. The client with a peptic ulcer should avoid foods that increase stomach acidity, such as caffeine, decaffeinated coffee, frequent milk intake, citric acid juices, and certain seasonings (hot chili peppers, chili powder, black pepper). Smoking, alcohol, and aspirin also are discouraged.

1. The client diagnosed with a peptic ulcer should avoid citric acid juices.
3. The client diagnosed with a peptic ulcer should avoid frequent milk intake.
4. The client diagnosed with a peptic ulcer should avoid decaffeinated coffee.

18. 3, p. 1281
Rationale:
3. Cheerios are an appropriate finger food for toddler or preschool child.
1. Nuts have been implicated in choking deaths and should be avoided.
2. Popcorn has been implicated in choking deaths and should be avoided.
4. Hot dogs have been implicated in choking deaths and should be avoided. If they are given to this age child, they should be cut into irregularly shaped pieces, such as long strips.

19. 2, p. 1281
Rationale:
2. Adolescent boys require additional iron for muscle development.
1. Daily requirements of protein increase for both adolescent boys and girls.
3. B-complex vitamins are needed to support heightened metabolic activity. Vitamin needs are not decreased during the adolescent period.
4. Energy and caloric needs are increased to meet greater metabolic demands of growth during the adolescent period.

20. 1, p. 1299
Rationale:
1. If the client has unilateral weakness, the nurse should place food in the stronger side of the mouth.
2. The client should be positioned in an upright seated position to prevent aspiration.
3. Clients with unilateral weakness often have difficulty using a straw.
4. Thickened liquids are often tolerated better and will help prevent aspiration, as clients with impaired swallowing often choke more with thin liquids.

1. 3, p. 1304
Rationale:

. After the radiographic confirmation, the next best method involves testing the feeding tube aspirate pH and observing its appearance. A properly obtained pH of 0 to 4 is a good indication of gastric placement.

. Placing the end of the tube in water and observing for bubbling is not an accurate method of checking for tube placement.

. Auscultation is no longer considered a reliable method for verification of tube placement, because a tube inadvertently placed in the lungs, pharynx, or esophagus can transmit a sound similar to that of air entering the stomach.

. Asking the client to speak as a method of checking for tube placement has a high degree of inaccuracy. Cases have been reported in which clients have been able to speak despite placement of feeding tubes in the lung.

22. 4, p. 1312
Rationale:

4. After catheter placement, the catheter is flushed with saline or heparin until the position is radiographically confirmed.

1. Aseptic technique, not sterile technique, is used during the administration of feedings.

2. An initial rate of 40 to 60 ml/hr is recommended, and the rate is gradually increased. The rate of administration is not the priority. The nurse must first confirm correct placement of the catheter.

3. A single container of PN should hang no longer than 24 hours; lipids, no more than 12 hours. The nurse must first confirm correct placement of the catheter before any infusion is begun.

23. 1, p. 1308
Rationale:

1. When a client is tolerating tube feedings well, the nurse should expect the physician to order the feedings be increased by 50 ml/day to achieve needed volume and calories in six to eight feedings.

2. Formula is started at full strength for isotonic formulas.

3. Intermittent feedings are allowed to infuse over at least 20 to 30 minutes.

4. Feedings should be begun with no more than 150 to 250 ml at one time.

24. 1, p. 1283
Rationale:

1. Ampicillin may cause an alteration in taste.

2. Opiates, such as morphine, cause decreased peristalsis and may result in constipation. Morphine does not affect the client's sense of taste.

3. Decreased drug absorption may occur when diuretics, such as furosemide, are administered with food. Furosemide does not affect the client's sense of taste.

4. Decreased acetaminophen absorption may occur if it is administered with food. Overdose of acetaminophen is associated with liver failure. Acetaminophen does not affect the client's sense of taste.

25. 4, p. 1297
Rationale:

4. E. coli may be contracted from undercooked meat, such as ground beef.

1. Sausage is a potential source of trichinosis, not E. coli.

2. Soft cheeses are a potential source of listeriosis, not E. coli.

3. Milk products are a potential source of shigellosis, not E. coli.

Chapter 44

1. 4, pp. 1367, 1368
Rationale:

4. Pelvic floor exercises, also known as Kegel exercises, improve the strength of pelvic floor muscles and consist of repetitive contractions of muscle groups. These exercises have demonstrated effectiveness in treating stress incontinence, overactive bladders, and mixed causes of urinary continence.

1. The client is oriented and therefore could be taught Kegel exercises to improve pelvic floor muscle tone. Applying adult diapers does not improve the client's problem of incontinence and places the client at risk for skin breakdown.
2. Because bladder catheterization carries the risk of urinary tract infection (UTI), it is preferable to rely on other measures for management of incontinence. The nurse can support the use of Kegel exercises as an inexpensive nonpharmacological intervention to reduce the client's stress incontinence.
3. Bethanechol (Urecholine) stimulates the parasympathetic nervous system to promote complete bladder emptying and is used primarily to treat urinary retention and possible overflow incontinence. Nonpharmacological approaches should be attempted before pharmacological approaches are taken.

2. 1, p. 1361
Rationale:
1. The urinary drainage bag should be emptied at least every 8 hours. If large outputs are noted, more frequent emptying will be required.
2. The perineum should be cleansed, and then down the catheter for a length of approximately 10 cm (4 inches).
3. Use sterile technique only to collect specimens from a closed drainage system.
4. Avoid raising the drainage bag above the level of the bladder. If it becomes necessary to raise the bag during transfer of the client to a bed or stretcher, clamp the tubing or empty the tubing contents to the drainage bag first. The drainage bag can be attached to the wheelchair below the level of the client's bladder for transport. It should not be placed on the client's lap.

3. 2, p. 1328
Rationale:
2. Irritation to bladder and urethral mucosa results in blood-tinged urine (hematuria). Hematuria is a sign of a bladder infection.
1. Chills are a more-systemic symptom associated with pyelonephritis.

3. Flank pain is a more-systemic symptom associated with pyelonephritis.
4. Incontinence is not a symptom of a bladder infection.

4. 4, p. 1335
Rationale:
4. A sterile specimen can be obtained through the special port found on the side of the indwelling catheter. The nurse clamps the tubing below the port, allowing fresh, uncontaminated urine to collect in the tube. After the nurse wipes the port with an antimicrobial swab, a sterile syringe needle is inserted and at least 3 to 5 ml of urine is withdrawn. With sterile technique, the nurse transfers the urine to a sterile container.
1. The catheter should not be disconnected from the drainage tubing. The system should remain a closed system to prevent infection.
2. A urinometer is a device used to determine the specific gravity of urine. It is not a sterile device and should not be used for obtaining urine for a sterile urine specimen.
3. Urine should not be obtained from a drainage bag for a specimen, as the urine would not be fresh and would be contaminated from microorganisms in the drainage bag.

5. 2, p. 1341
Rationale:
2. After an intravenous pyelogram (IVP), the nurse should encourage fluid intake to dilute and flush dye from the client and observe the client for late symptoms of allergy (rash, etc.)
1. No increased risk of infection of the urinary bladder occurs from an IVP. This would be more likely with an invasive procedure, such as an endoscopy (cystoscopy).
3. An IVP should not injure tissues of the kidney
4. An IVP does not cause paralysis of the urinary sphincter.

6. 3, p. 1327
Rationale:
3. Alcohol inhibits the release of antidiuretic hormone (ADH), resulting in increased water loss in urine. The client may show signs of decreased fluid volume (dehydration), including dry mucous membranes.

The effects of excessive alcohol intake and reduced ADH will not cause hematuria.

Having decreased ADH will lead to increased urine production. The client may exhibit a decreased blood pressure because of decreased fluid volume.

Having decreased ADH will lead to increased urine production. The client may exhibit an increased serum sodium level with dehydration.

4, p. 1341

Rationale:

Although this procedure may be accomplished by using local anesthesia, it is more commonly performed by using general anesthesia or conscious sedation to avoid unnecessary anxiety and trauma for the client.

A cystoscopy involves direct visualization. No contrast dye is used; therefore the nurse does not need to ask if the client is allergic to iodine.

A signed consent form is obtained.

Fluids are not restricted before or after the procedure. The flushing action helps remove bacteria from the urethra.

3, p. 1343

Rationale:

3. The nurse can pour warm water over the client's perineum and create the urge to urinate.

1. A client with normal renal function who does not have heart or kidney disease should drink 2000 to 2500 ml of fluid daily. Increasing the client's fluid intake to 3500 ml is excessive.

2. Because bladder catheterization carries the risk of UTI, it should be avoided if possible. The nurse should try other noninvasive measures to promote urination before calling the physician for an order to insert a Foley catheter.

4. The nurse should not apply firm pressure over the bladder of a postpartum woman with an intact nervous system. The nurse could create more damage by exerting force on the client's uterus at this time.

9. 4, p. 1328

Rationale:

4. With urinary retention, urine continues to collect in the bladder, stretching its walls and causing feelings of pressure, discomfort, tenderness over the symphysis pubis, restlessness, and diaphoresis. The sphincter temporarily opens to allow a small volume of urine (25 to 60 ml) to escape, with no real relief of discomfort.

1. Severe flank pain and hematuria are supporting data for an upper UTI (pyelonephritis).

2. Pain and burning on urination are symptoms of a lower UTI (such as a bladder infection).

3. Supportive data for reflex incontinence would include a loss of the urge to void.

10. 4, p. 1337

Rationale:

4. To collect a clean-voided specimen, the nurse should collect the specimen (30 to 60 ml) after the initial stream of urine has passed.

1. Nonsterile gloves are adequate.

2. Fluids are encouraged so the client will be more likely to be able to void.

3. The specimen should be collected in a sterile container and then placed into a plastic specimen bag.

11. 2, p. 1324

Rationale:

2. The kidneys play a role in calcium and phosphate regulation by producing a substance that converts vitamin D into its active form. Clients with chronic alterations in kidney function do not make sufficient amounts of the active vitamin D.

1. Clients with chronic alterations in kidney function do not suffer from an insufficient amount of vitamin A.

3. Clients with chronic alterations in kidney function do not suffer from an insufficient amount of vitamin E.

4. Clients with chronic alterations in kidney function do not suffer from an insufficient amount of vitamin K.

12. 3, p. 1349

Rationale:

3. The nurse expects to find the client with reflex incontinence to have no urge to void and an unawareness of bladder filling.
1. A constant dribbling of urine may be seen with overflow incontinence.
2. Stress incontinence occurs when the client is unable to control loss of urine when coughing or sneezing.
4. Functional incontinence is seen when an immediate urge to void is felt, but not enough time to get to the bathroom.

13. 3, p. 1324

Rationale:

3. Although output does depend on intake, the normal adult urine output is 1500 to 1600 ml/day.
1. This is not the urinary output for an average adult.
2. This is not the urinary output for an average adult.
4. This is not the urinary output for an average adult.

14. 1, p. 1335

Rationale:

1. Missed specimens make the whole collection inaccurate. The test must be restarted.
2. The urine specimen is kept in a collection container, which may contain preservatives, or the urine may be kept in a collection container on ice. The urine specimen being kept cold is not a reason to restart a timed urine collection.
3. This is correct. The timed period begins after the client urinates. The first voided urine is discarded, and then the time for collection begins.
4. The urine specimen is kept in a collection container, which may contain preservatives.

15. 4, p. 1329

Rationale:

4. Special skin care is a priority in caring for a client with a urinary diversion. Local irritation and skin breakdown occur when urine comes in contact with the skin for long periods.

1. Special clothing is not necessary for the c with a urinary diversion.
2. The client with a urinary diversion must a stomal pouch continuously because sphincter control exists for regulation of t flow.
3. No need is found to plan for a reductio activity.

16. 3, p. 1353

Rationale:

3. Before inserting the indwelling catheter, balloon should be tested by injecting the f from the prefilled syringe into the ball port.
1. The dominant hand is kept sterile throug the procedure. The nondominant hand is kept sterile, as it touches the client.
2. If the catheter is misplaced, it should be le the vagina as a landmark indicating wh not to insert, and another sterile cath should be inserted into the urethra.
4. The catheter should be advanced 2 to 3 inc in the female client.

17. 1, p. 1365

Rationale:

1. The amount of fluid used to irrigate the b der and catheter should be subtracted fr the total output to determine an accurate nary output. 1725 ml – 950 ml = 775 ml.
2. This is not the correct calculation of client's urinary output.
3. This is not the correct calculation of client's urinary output.
4. This is not the correct calculation of client's urinary output.

18. 3, p. 1368

Rationale:

3. A bladder-retraining program includes init ing a toileting schedule on awakening, at l every 2 hours during the day and eveni before getting into bed, and every 4 hour night.
1. Negative reinforcement should not be u when the client is incontinent. However, p itive reinforcement should be provided wh continence is maintained.

2. The client should be offered protective under-garments to contain urine and reduce the client's embarrassment (not diapers).
4. Tea, coffee, other caffeine drinks, and alcohol should be minimized.

19. 2, p. 1335
Rationale:
2. Offering a young child fluids 30 minutes before requesting a specimen may help.
1. Because bladder catheterization carries the risk of UTI, blockage, and trauma to the urethra, it is preferable to rely on other measures for specimen collection.
3. Applying pressure over the urinary bladder of a child with an intact nervous system will not help and may create more stress in the child.
4. Squeezing urine from a child's diaper is not an accurate method of obtaining a urine specimen to determine whether the child has a UTI.

20. 2, p. 1339
Rationale:
2. The normal specific gravity of urine is 1.010 to 1.025.
1. The normal urine pH is 4.6 to 8.0, with an average of 6.0.
3. Protein is not normally found in the urine. The normal value for urine protein is none, or up to 8 mg/100 ml.
4. The number of WBCs is 0 to 4 per low-power field, and casts should be none in a normal urinalysis.

21. 2, p. 1348
Rationale:
2. Cholinergic drugs, such as bethanechol (Urecholine), increase contraction of the bladder and improve emptying. Bethanechol (Urecholine) stimulates parasympathetic nerves to increase bladder-wall contraction and relax the sphincter.
1. Oxybutynin chloride (Ditropan) is an anti-cholinergic drug that depresses the neuro-transmitter acetylcholine (which normally stimulates the bladder) and thus reduces incontinence.

3. Propantheline (Pro-banthine) is an anti-cholinergic drug that depresses the neuro-transmitter acetylcholine (which normally stimulates the bladder) and thus reduces incontinence.
4. Nystatin (Mycostatin) is an antifungal agent.

22. 3, pp. 1361, 1365
Rationale:
3. The nurse should not cut the catheter to deflate the balloon. The nurse inserts an empty, sterile syringe into the injection port. The nurse slowly withdraws all of the solution to deflate the balloon totally. The nurse then pulls the catheter out smoothly and slowly.
1. The nurse positions the client in the same position as during catheterization. The nurse places a towel between a female client's thighs or over a male client's thighs.
2. Some institutions recommend collecting a sterile urine specimen before removal of the catheter or sending the catheter tip for culture and sensitivity tests.
4. The nurse assesses the client's urinary function by noting the first voiding after catheter removal and documenting the time and amount of voiding for the next 24 hours.

23. 3, p. 1366
Rationale:
3. A 1- to 2-inch space should be left between the tip of the penis and the end of the catheter.
1. Nonsterile gloves are worn to apply a condom catheter.
2. Standard adhesive tape should never be used to secure a condom catheter because it does not expand with change in penis size and is painful to remove.
4. The tubing of a condom catheter is not taped tightly to the thigh. The drainage bag is attached to the lower bed frame.

24. 4, p. 1333
Rationale:
4. An initial urinary symptom of diabetes mellitus is polyuria.

1. Urgency is not a symptom of diabetes mellitus. Urgency may be caused by a full bladder, bladder irritation from infection, incompetent urethral sphincter, or psychological stress.
2. Dysuria is not a symptom of diabetes mellitus. Dysuria may be caused by bladder inflammation, trauma, or inflammation of the urethral sphincter.
3. Hematuria is not a symptom of diabetes mellitus. Hematuria may be a symptom of neoplasms of the bladder or kidney, glomerular disease, infection of the kidney or bladder, trauma to urinary structures, calculi, or bleeding disorders.

Chapter 45

1. 4, p. 1377
Rationale:
4. An expected change in bowel elimination is decreased chewing and decreased salivation, resulting in less efficient mastication.
1. Decreased nutrient absorption of the small intestine occurs in the older adult.
2. Esophageal emptying slows as a result of reduced motility, especially in the lower third of the esophagus.
3. With decreased peristalsis and weakened musculature, the older adult is more prone to constipation. Duller nerve sensations may place the older adult at increased risk for fecal incontinence.

2. 2, p. 1379
Rationale:
2. Excess loss of colonic fluid due to diarrhea can result in serious fluid and electrolyte or acid/base imbalances. Infants and older adults are particularly susceptible to associated complications.
1. Pain from abdominal cramping may occur with diarrhea, but it is not the major problem associated with severe diarrhea.
3. Excessive flatus is not the major problem associated with severe diarrhea.

4. Because repeated passage of diarrhea stool exposes the skin of the perineum and buttocks to irritating intestinal contents, meticulous skin care and containment of fecal drainage is needed to prevent skin breakdown. The greatest danger of severe diarrhea is a fluid and electrolyte or acid/base imbalance.

3. 2, p. 1389
Rationale:
2. Light sedation is required for a colonoscopy.
1. Special preparation is required before colonoscopy. Clear liquids are given the day before, and then some form of bowel cleanse such as GoLytely. Enemas until clear also may be ordered.
3. No restriction of metallic objects is made for colonoscopy.
4. A colonoscopy does not require swallowing an opaque liquid.

4. 4, p. 1386
Rationale:
4. Tests performed by the laboratory for occult blood in the stool and stool cultures require only a small sample. The nurse collects about an inch of formed stool or 15 to 30 ml of liquid stool.
1. Clean technique is used for collection.
2. Tests for measuring the output of fecal fat require a 3- to 5-day collection of stool, not for testing for occult blood.
3. The specimen does not have to be kept warm for an occult blood test. Tests that measure for ova and parasites require the stool to warm.

5. 4, p. 1410
Rationale:
4. During the first weeks after surgery, many physicians recommend low-fiber diets because the bowel requires time to adapt the diversion. Low-fiber foods include bread, noodles, rice, cream cheese, eggs (not fried), strained fruit juices, lean meats, fish, and poultry. Poached eggs and rice would appropriate for this client.

. After the ostomy heals, the client is allowed to eat fruits and vegetables. High-fiber foods such as fresh fruits and vegetables help ensure a more-solid stool needed to achieve success at irrigation. Ostomy clients may benefit from avoiding foods that cause gas and odor, including broccoli, cauliflower, dried beans, and brussels sprouts.

. After the ostomy heals, the client is allowed to eat fruits and vegetables. High-fiber foods such as fresh fruits and vegetables help ensure a more-solid stool needed to achieve success at irrigation.

. Whole-grain breads are high in fiber and are not recommended until the ostomy has had time to heal.

6. 4, p. 1389
Rationale:
4. Stool that is white or clay-colored indicates an absence of bile.
1. Bloody feces are not an indication of biliary disease.
2. Pus-filled feces indicate infection.
3. Black or tarry feces may indicate upper GI bleeding or iron ingestion.

7. 1, p. 1377
Rationale:
1. Bulk-forming foods, such as grains, fruits, and vegetables, absorb fluids and increase stool mass.
2. Fruit juice is not a bulk-forming food.
3. Rare meats are not bulk-forming foods.
4. Milk products are not bulk-forming foods.

8. 3, p. 1397
Rationale:
3. Emollient solutions are stool softeners that may increase the amount of water secreted into the bowel.
1. Laxative overuse can cause serious diarrhea that can lead to dehydration and hypokalemia.
2. Salt tablets should not be taken to increase the solute concentration of extracellular fluid.
4. Bulk-forming additives do not turn the urine pink. Phenolphthalein or danthron stimulant cathartics (e.g., Doxidan, Correctol, Ex-Lax) may cause pink or red urine.

9. 2, p. 1401
Rationale:
2. The nurse should lower the container if the client complains of abdominal cramping. Cramping may prevent the client from retaining all of the fluid, which would alter the effectiveness of the enema.
1. If the nurse stops the infusion, the client will not receive all of the fluid, and the enema will be less effective. The nurse may slow the infusion until the abdominal cramping passes.
3. The enema tubing should not be advanced farther.
4. The tubing may be clamped temporarily if fluid escapes around the rectal tube. The instillation should be slowed in the instance of abdominal cramping.

10. 3, p. 1378
Rationale:
3. Any surgery that involves direct manipulation of the bowel temporarily stops peristalsis. This condition, called paralytic ileus, usually lasts about 24 to 48 hours.
1. Colitis is inflammation of the colon. It is not a result of anesthetic used during surgery.
2. Stomatitis is inflammation of the mouth. It is not caused by anesthetic used during surgery.
4. The gastrocolic reflex is the peristaltic wave in the colon induced by entrance of food into the stomach. It is not a result of anesthetic used during surgery.

11. 3, p. 1376
Rationale:
3. Disorders of calcium metabolism contribute to difficulty with the passage of stools. The nurse should implement measures to prevent constipation in clients with hypocalcemia.
1. Hypocalcemia does not cause gastric upset.
2. Hypocalcemia does not cause malabsorption.
4. Hypocalcemia does not cause fluid secretion.

12. 2, p. 1398
Rationale:
2. Kayexalate is a type of medicated enema used to treat clients with dangerously high serum potassium levels. This drug contains a resin that exchanges sodium ions for potassium ions in the large intestine.

1. Kayexalate enemas are not used to treat or prevent constipation.
3. Neomycin enemas, not kayexalate enemas, may be used to reduce bacteria in the colon before diagnostic testing.
4. Kayexalate is not an antidiarrheal medication.

13. 3, p. 1399
Rationale:
3. The appropriate amount of fluid to prepare for an enema to be given to an average-size school-age child is 300 to 500 ml.
1. This is the appropriate amount of fluid to prepare for an enema to be given to an infant.
2. This is the appropriate amount of fluid to prepare for an enema to be given to a toddler.
4. This is the appropriate amount of fluid to prepare for an enema to be given to an adolescent.

14. 1, p. 1409
Rationale:
1. If a yeast infection occurs, thorough cleansing should be performed, followed by patting the area dry and applying a prescribed topical agent, such as triamcinolone acetonide (Kenalog) spray or nystatin (Mycostatin), to the affected region.
2. The peristomal skin should be cleansed gently with warm tap water by using gauze pads or a clean washcloth.
3. An ostomy deodorant may be placed into the pouch, not around the stoma.
4. Alcohol should not be used to clean the stoma. The area may be cleaned with warm tap water.

15. 3, p. 1407
Rationale:
3. Once placement is confirmed, a mark should be placed, either by making a red mark or using tape, on the tube to indicate where the tube exits the nose. The mark or tube length is to be used as a guide to indicate whether displacement may have occurred.
1. The tube should be taped to the nose, not to the ear.
2. The tubing should be secured to the client's gown, not to the bed.

4. The tubing should not be changed daily; it may be irrigated daily.

16. 1, p. 1387
Rationale:
1. Whole-wheat bread may be eaten before a fecal occult blood test.
2. A lean, T-bone steak may cause false-positive results if eaten before a fecal occult blood test.
3. Veal may cause false-positive results if eaten before a fecal occult blood test.
4. Salmon may cause false-positive results if eaten before a fecal occult blood test.

Chapter 46

1. 4, p. 1427
Rationale:
4. Immobility causes gastrointestinal disturbances such as decreased appetite and slowing of peristalsis.
1. In the immobilized client, decreased circulating fluid volume, pooling of blood in the lower extremities, and decreased autonomic response occur. These factors result in decreased venous return, followed by a decrease in cardiac output, which is reflected by a decline in blood pressure.
2. Recumbency increases cardiac workload and results in an increased pulse rate.
3. Fluid intake can diminish with immobility, and this, combined with other causes, such as fever, increases the risk of dehydration. Urinary output may decline on or about the fifth or sixth day after immobilization, and the urine is often highly concentrated.

2. 2, p. 1442
Rationale:
2. Because edema moves to dependent body regions, assessment of the immobilized client should include the sacrum, legs, and feet. Unilateral increases in calf diameter can be an early indication of thrombosis.
1. The client who has suffered a cerebrovascular accident with left-sided paralysis may not be capable of an even gait.

3. Having the client hold his or her breath frequently is not an appropriate nursing intervention to be implemented by the nurse. To prevent stasis of pulmonary secretions, the client's position should be changed every 2 hours, and fluids should be increased to 2000 ml, if not contraindicated. The client should deep breathe and cough every 1 to 2 hours to promote chest expansion.

4. Two-point crutch technique would not be appropriate for the client with left-sided paralysis. The client would most likely ambulate safely with a walker or a cane. If crutches are used, the client should use a three-point support.

3. 2, p. 1460
Rationale:
2. The nurses should be standing even with the client's shoulders when they prepare to move the client up in bed.
1. This is not the correct position for the nurses.
2. This is not the correct position for the nurses.
4. This is not the correct position for the nurses.

4. 4, p. 1468
Rationale:
4. Before transferring the client from the bed to the stretcher, the nurse should assess the situation for any potentially unsafe complications.
1. The head of the bed should be at the same level as the head of the stretcher. The nurse should first assess the situation before changing the height of the head of the bed.
2. This client has had preoperative sedation, which may impair his or her cognition. The nurse should simplify instructions when explaining the procedure to the client, but this should be done immediately before transferring the client. The nurse should first assess the situation for any potential unsafe complications.
3. The sedated client is transferred most easily in the supine position, unless contraindicated. The nurse should first assess the situation for any potential unsafe complications.

5. 2, p. 1451
Rationale:
2. Inflation pressures average 40 mm Hg.
1. Initial measurement is made around the largest part of the client's thigh.
3. A protective stockinette is placed over the client's leg. Then the stocking is wrapped around the leg, starting at the ankle, with the opening over the patella.
4. Stockings are not removed every hour. For optimal results, SCD/IPCs are used as soon as possible and maintained until the client becomes fully ambulatory. The stockings should be removed periodically to assess the condition of the client's skin.

6. 4, p. 1426
Rationale:
4. Torticollis is inclining of the head to the affected side, in which the sternocleidomastoid muscle is contracted.
1. Lordosis is an exaggeration of the lumbar spine curvature.
2. Kyphosis is an increased convexity in the curvature of the thoracic spine.
3. Kyphoscoliosis is an abnormal anteroposterior and lateral curvature of the spine.

7. 3, pp. 1428, 1441
Rationale:
3. Atelectasis is the collapse of alveoli. In atelectasis, secretions block a bronchiole or a bronchus, and the distal lung tissue (alveoli) collapses as the existing air is absorbed, producing hypoventilation. If the client were suspected of having atelectasis, the nurse would expect diminished breath sounds in the area of hypoventilation.
1. Harsh crackles indicate excessive airway secretion.
2. Wheezing on inspiration indicates narrowing of the lumen of a respiratory passageway.
4. Bronchovesicular sounds are a mixture of bronchial and vesicular sounds. Bronchovesicular whooshing would not be an expected sound indicating atelectasis.

8. 1, p. 1442
Rationale:
1. Calf and thigh circumference should be measured daily. Unilateral increases in calf or thigh diameter can be an early indication of thrombosis.
2. Homan's sign is not always positive in the presence of thrombosis.
3. Assessing the temperature of the feet is not the best approach to determine the presence of thrombosis.
4. Observing for hair loss and skin turgor of the lower legs is not the best approach to determine the presence of thrombosis. A lack of hair may indicate a chronic lack of oxygen. Skin turgor is a measure of hydration.

9. 2, p. 1441
Rationale:
2. When getting the client up for the first time after a period of bed rest, the nurse should document orthostatic changes. The nurse first obtains a baseline blood pressure.
1. Assessing the client's respiratory function is not the nurse's first intervention when getting a client up for the first time after prolonged bed rest.
3. After the nurse assesses the client's blood pressure, the nurse can assist the client to a sitting position at the side of the bed.
4. After the client is in the sitting position at the side of the bed, the nurse should ask the client if he or she feels lightheaded.

10. 2, p. 1451
Rationale:
2. The nurse should actively work with the immobilized client to deep breathe and cough every 1 to 2 hours to promote chest expansion.
1. The client's position should be changed every 2 hours to reduce stagnation of secretions.
3. The physician must order oxygen and nebulizer treatments. These interventions are used primarily to treat the client who is experiencing an impaired air exchange, not to promote respiratory function in the immobilized client.
4. The client should be suctioned as needed, not every hour.

11. 3, pp. 1451, 1452
Rationale:
3. The primary purpose of antiemboli stockings (TEDs) is to maintain external pressure on the muscles of the lower extremities and thus promote venous return.
1. The primary purpose of antiemboli stockings is not to keep the skin warm and dry.
2. Antiemboli stockings are not used to prevent abnormal joint flexion.
4. Antiemboli stockings are not primarily used to prevent bleeding. They are used to prevent clot formation due to venous stasis.

12. 3, p. 1455
Rationale:
3. To meet the psychosocial needs of an immobilized client, the nurse should encourage the client to be involved in his or her care whenever possible. Asking the client if the staff can make changes in routine care is an appropriate question.
1. Visitors should not be limited for the immobilized client. The client needs socialization throughout the day.
2. If possible, the client should be placed in a room with others who are mobile and interactive.
4. Clients should be encouraged to wear their glasses or artificial teeth and to shave or apply makeup. These are activities through which people maintain their body image. The nurse provides for the psychosocial needs of an immobilized client by having the client perform as much self-care as possible.

13. 2, p. 1455
Rationale:
2. A trochanter roll prevents external rotation of the hips when the client is in a supine position.
1. The footboard prevents footdrop by maintaining the feet in dorsiflexion.
3. The trapeze bar allows the client to pull with the upper extremities to raise the trunk off the bed, to assist in transfer from bed to wheelchair, or to perform upper arm exercises.
4. A bed board is used to increase back support and alignment, especially with a soft mattress.

14. 2, p. 1455

Rationale:

2. High-top tennis shoes or an ankle/foot orthotic may be used to help maintain dorsiflexion and prevent footdrop.
1. A trapeze bar is not used to keep the foot in dorsiflexion. A trapeze bar is used to assist the client in mobility.
3. A trochanter roll prevents external rotation of the hips when the client is in a supine position. It is not used to prevent footdrop.
4. Thirty-degree lateral positioning does not prevent plantar flexion. It may be used for clients at risk for pressure ulcers.

15. 4, p. 1434

Rationale:

4. While the client is performing range of motion exercises, support should be provided for the distal joints.
1. The joint should be flexed to the point of resistance, not to the point of discomfort.
2. When performing range-of-motion exercises, begin at distal joints and work toward proximal joints.
3. Joints should be moved slowly through the range of motion. Quick movement could cause injury.

Chapter 47

1. 3, p. 1508

Rationale:

3. To collect an aerobic wound culture, the nurse uses a sterile swab from a culturette tube and sterile technique.
1. The nurse never collects a wound-culture sample from old or superficial drainage. Resident colonies of bacteria from the skin grow in superficial drainage and may not be the true causative organisms of a wound infection.
2. The nurse should clean a wound first with normal saline to remove skin flora before obtaining the culture.
4. The nurse uses different methods of specimen collection for aerobic or anaerobic organisms.

2. 3, p. 1484

Rationale:

3. Pressure is the major cause in pressure ulcer formation. Prolonged, intense pressure affects cellular metabolism by decreasing or obliterating blood flow, resulting in tissue ischemia and ultimately tissue death.
1. Nitrogen build-up is not the primary cause of pressure ulcer formation.
2. Prolonged illness or disease may place a client at risk for pressure ulcer development, but it is not the primary cause of pressure ulcers.
4. Poor nutrition may place a client at risk for pressure ulcer development, but it is not the primary cause of pressure ulcers.

3. 2, p. 1487

Rationale:

2. This description is consistent with a stage II pressure ulcer. A stage II pressure ulcer is defined as partial-thickness skin loss involving the epidermis and/or dermis. The ulcer is superficial and appears as an abrasion, blister, or shallow crater.
1. A stage I pressure ulcer is an observable pressure-related alteration of intact skin whose indicators may include changes in one or more of the following: skin temperature, tissue consistency, and/or sensation. The description is not consistent with a stage I pressure ulcer.
3. A stage III pressure ulcer has full-thickness skin loss involving damage or necrosis of subcutaneous tissue that may extend down to, but not through, underlying fascia. The description is not consistent with a stage III pressure ulcer.
4. A stage IV pressure ulcer has full-thickness skin loss with extensive destruction, tissue necrosis, or damage to muscle, bone, or supporting structures. The description is not consistent with a stage IV pressure ulcer.

4. 3, p. 1515

Rationale:

3. The frequency of repositioning should be individualized for the client; however, clients should be repositioned at least every 2 hours. The AHCPR guidelines recommend that a written turning and positioning schedule be used.

1. Clients able to sit in a chair should be limited to sitting for 2 hours or less.
2. Elevating the head of the bed to 30 degrees or less will decrease the chance of pressure ulcer development from shearing forces.
4. Pelvic muscle training may help prevent incontinence, but is not the best intervention for maintaining the client's skin integrity.

5. 1, p. 1518
Rationale:
1. Pressure ulcers should be cleansed only with wound cleansers that are not cytotoxic, such as normal saline. Normal saline will not damage or kill cells such as fibroblasts and healing tissue.
2. Hydrogen peroxide is cytotoxic and therefore should not be used to clean a wound that is granulating.
3. Povidone-iodine (Betadine) is cytotoxic and therefore should not be used to clean a wound that is granulating.
4. Sodium hypochlorite (Dakin's solution) is cytotoxic and therefore should not be used to clean a wound that is granulating.

6. 2, pp. 1518, 1521
Rationale:
1. Removal of necrotic tissue is necessary to rid the ulcer of a source of infection, to allow visualization of the wound bed, and to provide a clean base necessary for healthy tissue to regenerate.
2. Autolytic debridement uses synthetic dressings over a wound to allow the eschar to be self-digested by the action of enzymes that are present in wound fluids. The wound is not irrigated.
3. Mechanical methods include wet-to-dry dressings, wound irrigation, and whirlpool treatments. Surgical debridement involves direct surgical removal of the eschar layer of the wound.
4. Enzymatic debridement requires a physician's order.

7. 2, p. 1543
Rationale:
2. The gentle washing action of the irrigatio cleanses a wound of exudate and debris.
1. The primary purpose of wound irrigation not to decrease scar formation.
3. The primary reason for irrigating a clien wound is not to improve circulation, but remove debris from the wound.
4. The primary reason for irrigating a clien wound is not to decrease irritation fro wound drainage, but to remove debris fro the wound.

8. 1, p. 1514
Rationale:
1. The skin should be cleansed and complete dried, and a protective moisturizer applied keep the epidermis well lubricated.
2. Hydrogen peroxide is cytotoxic and shou not be used. A heat lamp is not necessary ar would increase the client's risk of an accide tal burn.
3. The area should not be soaked, as this ma lead to maceration of the skin.
4. The area should not be cleansed with a astringent and painted with povidone-iodin An astringent may cause excessive drying the tissue, and povidone-iodine is cytotoxic

9. 4, p. 1528
Rationale:
4. A dressing should support a moist woun environment if the wound is healing by se ondary intention, such as with a large abdom inal wound. A moist wound base facilitat the movement of epithelialization, thu allowing the wound to resurface as quickly possible.
1. Only mild soap or saline may be use Antiseptics may be damaging to granulatio tissue.
2. A heat lamp should not be used, as it will dr the wound and impair the movement c epithelialization.
3. Clean dressings may be used in the home se ting.

10. 1, p. 1533
Rationale:
1. A foam dressing absorbs exudate and debris while maintaining a moist environment. Topical agents, such as antibiotic ointment, also may be used with a foam dressing. This would be the most appropriate type of dressing for this wound.
2. A hydrogel dressing provides moisture to a clean granular wound. A hydrogel dressing would not be appropriate for a wound with a large amount of exudate.
3. A hydrocolloid dressing interacts with the wound fluid to provide a moist environment. Hydrocolloid dressings may stay in place until the seal is broken. It would not be appropriate for a wound with a large amount of exudate that appears infected.
4. Transparent film protects from friction injury and may be left in place up to 7 days. It would not be appropriate for a wound with a large amount of exudate that appears infected.

11. 3, p. 1493
Rationale:
3. During the proliferative phase, the wound fills with granulation tissue (including collagen formation), the wound contracts, and the wound is resurfaced by epithelialization.
1. Primary intention is not a phase of wound healing. Wounds that heal by primary intention have minimal tissue loss, such as a surgical wound. The edges are approximated, and the risk of infection is low.
2. During the inflammatory phase, platelets gather to stop bleeding, a fibrin matrix forms, and white blood cells reach the wound, clearing it of debris.
4. Secondary intention is not a phase of wound healing. Wounds that heal by secondary intention have loss of tissue, such as a pressure ulcer. The wound is left open until it becomes filled by scar tissue.

12. 2, p. 1527
Rationale:
2. If a client is bleeding, the nurse applies direct pressure and elevates the affected part.

1. When a penetrating object is present, it is not removed. Removal could cause massive, uncontrolled bleeding.
3. Vigorous cleaning can cause bleeding or further injury. Abrasions and minor lacerations should be rinsed with normal saline and lightly covered with a dressing.
4. Puncture wounds are allowed to bleed to remove dirt and other contaminates.

13. 4, p. 1494
Rationale:
4. A strategy to prevent dehiscence is to use a folded thin blanket or pillow placed over an abdominal wound when the client is coughing. This provides a splint to the area, supporting the healing tissue when coughing increases the intra-abdominal pressure.
1. A client who has an infection is at risk for poor wound healing and dehiscence. However, prophylactic use of antibiotics is not the best intervention to prevent dehiscence.
2. Using appropriate sterile technique is always important to prevent the development of infection. It is not the best intervention to prevent dehiscence.
3. Keeping sterile towels and extra dressings at the client's bedside will not prevent wound dehiscence.

14. 1, p. 1494
Rationale:
1. Serous drainage is clear, watery plasma.
2. Purulent drainage is thick, yellow, green, tan, or brown.
3. The nurse does not know that this drainage is cerebrospinal fluid without further testing. The nurse should describe the drainage by its appearance (i.e., serous).
4. Serosanguineous drainage is pale, red, and watery: a mixture of clear and red fluid.

15. 4, p. 1507
Rationale:
4. This is the most complete description of the client's wound. It describes the wound according to characteristics observed and the dressing that covers it.

1. This nursing entry does not provide objective data. It is the nurse's impression that it is "healing well." It does not describe what type of dressing is present.
2. This nursing entry is incomplete. It does not describe the type of drainage or if any dressing is present.
3. Wounds should be measured by using the metric system; not described as the size of objects. This entry does not indicate the type of drainage present or how many 4 × 4s were applied.

16. 3, p. 1503
Rationale:
3. Exposure to gastric and pancreatic drainage has the highest risk for skin breakdown.
1. Exposure to urine, bile, stool, acidic fluid, and purulent wound exudates carries a moderate risk for skin breakdown.
2. Exposure to urine, bile, stool, acidic fluid, and purulent wound exudates carries a moderate risk for skin breakdown.
4. Serosanguinous drainage is not caustic to the skin, and the risk of skin breakdown from exposure to this fluid is low.

17. 4, p. 1537
Rationale:
4. To remove tape safely, the nurse loosens the tape ends and gently pulls the outer end parallel with the skin surface toward the wound.
1. Tape should not be pulled in a direction away from the wound, as this may cause the wound edges to separate.
2. Holding the tape at a right angle to the skin surface may pull on the wound bed, causing separation of wound layers, or may damage the underlying skin.
3. Holding the tape at a right angle to the skin surface may pull on the wound bed, causing separation of wound layers, or may damage the underlying skin. Tape should not be pulled in a direction away from the wound, as this may cause the wound edges to separate.

18. 3, p. 1543
Rationale:
3. To cleanse the area of an isolated drain si the nurse cleans around the drain, moving circular rotations outward from a point close to the drain.
1. The nurse never uses the same piece of gau or swab to cleanse across an incision wound twice.
2. The wound should be cleansed in a directic from the least contaminated area, such from the wound to the surrounding skin. T wound is cleaned from the center region the outer region.
4. An antiseptic solution is not used to clean wound, as it may be cytotoxic.

19. 4, p. 1536
Rationale:
4. The wound should be packed only until th packing material reaches the surface of th wound. Wound packing that overlaps on the wound edges can cause maceration of th tissue surrounding the wound. It also ca impede the proper healing and closing of th wound.
1. The wound should be packed to the upp edge of the wound to prevent dead space ar the formation of abscesses.
2. The gauze should be saturated with the pr scribed solution, wrung out, unfolded, ar lightly packed into the wound.
3. The wound should not be packed too tightl Overpacking the wound may cause pressu on the tissue in the wound bed.

20. 3, p. 1555
Rationale:
3. Direct trauma such as fractures or sprains ma be treated with cold. The application of col can initially diminish swelling and pain.
1. Application of heat to reduce muscle tensio and pain would be more appropriate for th client with menstrual cramping.
2. The application of cold is not indicated fc the client with an infected wound, as reduces the blood flow to the area. This woul limit the number of macrophages to clear th area of bacteria and would lessen the nutrier supply to the already impaired tissue.

4. The effects of heat application would be more beneficial to the client with degenerative joint disease.

21. 2, p. 1516
Rationale:
2. Air-fluidized beds are recommended for clients with burns or multiple stage III or stage IV pressure ulcers.
1. A foam mattress is recommended for pressure reduction in clients at high risk for developing a pressure ulcer.
3. A rotokinetic bed is recommended for clients who are at risk for or have developed atelectasis and/or pneumonia.
4. A static support surface is not recommended for a client with a stage IV ulcer. It is used for clients at high risk for developing a pressure ulcer.

22. 1, p. 1495
Rationale:
1. According to the Norton Scale, a lower score indicates a higher risk for pressure ulcer development. The total score ranges from 5 to **20**. The client at highest risk would be the client with a score of 6.
2. According to the Norton Scale and these scores, this would not be the client at highest risk for pressure ulcer development.
3. According to the Norton Scale and these scores, this would not be the client at highest risk for pressure ulcer development.
4. According to the Norton Scale and these scores, this would not be the client at highest risk for pressure ulcer development.

23. 4, p. 1551
Rationale:
4. After applying the binder, the nurse should assess the client's ability to ventilate properly, including deep breathing and coughing.
1. Wounds should be entirely covered with dressings; the binder is applied over the dressing.
2. The binder should not be loose, or it will be ineffective in providing support.

3. The client should be lying supine with head slightly elevated and knees slightly flexed for application of the abdominal binder.

24. 3, p. 1489
Rationale:
3. A client with a knife wound is an example of an acute wound. An acute wound is caused by trauma from a sharp object.
1. A contusion is a closed wound caused by a blow to the body by a blunt object, resulting in a bruise.
2. A clean wound is a wound that contains no pathogenic organisms, such as a closed surgical wound that does not enter the GI, respiratory, or genitourinary (GU) system.
4. An intentional wound is a wound resulting from therapy, such as a surgical incision.

25. 4, p. 1498
Rationale:
4. Smoking reduces the amount of functional hemoglobin in the blood, thus decreasing tissue oxygenation.
1. Antiinflammatory drugs suppress protein synthesis.
2. Radiation creates tissue fragility.
3. Chemotherapeutic drugs can depress bone marrow function.

26. 3, p. 1515
Rationale:
3. Elevating the head of the bed to 30 degrees or less will decrease the chance of pressure ulcer development from shearing forces.
1. The client should not be positioned directly on the trochanter, as this can create pressure over the bony prominence.
2. Donut-shaped cushions are contraindicated because they reduce blood supply to the area, resulting in wider areas of ischemia.
4. Bony prominences should not be massaged. Massaging reddened areas increases breaks in the capillaries in the underlying tissues and increases the risk of injury to underlying tissue and pressure ulcer formation.

27. 1, p. 1559
Rationale:
1. An application should last only 20 to 30 minutes. Providing a timer for the client will help prevent injury to the tissue.
2. The temperature setting is fixed by inserting a plastic key into the temperature regulator. In many institutions, the central supply room sets the regulators to the recommended temperature.
3. The nurse does not place the pad directly on the client's skin. To prevent injury, it should be covered with a thin towel or pillowcase.
4. The recommended temperature is 105°F to 110°F. It should not be used at the highest temperature that is tolerated by the client.

28. 4, p. 1499
Rationale:
4. Citrus fruits contain vitamin C, which is important in collagen synthesis, capillary wall integrity, and fibroblast function.
1. Fish contains protein and vitamin E. Protein plays a role in neogenesis, collagen formation, and wound remodeling.
2. Eggs contain protein and vitamin E. Protein plays a role in neogenesis, collagen formation, and wound remodeling.
3. Liver contains vitamin A, which is important in epithelialization and wound closure.

29. 3, p. 1499
Rationale:
3. Vitamin A can reverse steroid effects on skin and delayed healing.
1. Iron does not reverse the effects of steroids. It is important in the transport of oxygen.
2. Folic acid does not reverse the effects of steroids. It is a B-complex vitamin needed for DNA synthesis.
4. The B-complex vitamins do not reverse the effects of steroids. The B vitamins affect growth and stimulate appetite, lactation, and the gastrointestinal, neurological, and endocrine systems.

Chapter 48

1. 3, p. 1581
Rationale:
3. Clients between the ages of 40 and 64 year should have an eye examination every 1 to 2 years if there is a family history of glaucoma or if the client is of African ancestry.
1. This is not the recommended frequency of eye examinations for this age group.
2. This is not the recommended frequency of eye examinations for this age group.
4. This is not the recommended frequency of eye examinations for this age group.

2. 4, p. 1570
Rationale:
4. Older adults experience tactile changes including declining sensitivity to pain, pressure, and temperature.
1. Older adults have an increased sensitivity to glare.
2. Older adults have a decreased number of taste buds.
3. Older adults have difficulty discriminating the consonants (z, t, f, g) and high-frequency sounds (s, sh, ph, k).

3. 1, p. 1576
Rationale:
1. Some antibiotics, such as streptomycin, gentamicin, and tobramycin, are ototoxic and can permanently damage the auditory nerve.
2. Narcotic analgesics, sedatives, and antidepressant medications can alter the perception of stimuli.
3. Chloramphenicol can irritate the optic nerve.
4. Prolonged use of streptomycin does not result in a loss of taste.

4. 1, p. 1571
Rationale:
1. The waiter is at least risk for sensory alterations.
2. A welder is at risk for visual alterations.
3. A computer programmer is at risk for peripheral nerve injury.
4. A construction worker is at risk for hearing alterations.

5. 2, p. 1585
Rationale:
2. To promote communication with the client who has a hearing impairment, the nurse should use visible expressions, such as speaking with the hands, face, or eyes.
1. A normal tone of voice and inflections of speech should be used when communicating with a client with a hearing impairment.
3. The nurse should get the client's attention and not startle the client when entering a room. The nurse should not approach a client from behind.
4. It is best to select a quiet environment without background noise to facilitate communication when a client is hearing impaired.

6. 2, p. 1583
Rationale:
2. If a client is overly sensitive to tactile stimuli (hyperesthesia), the nurse must minimize irritating stimuli. Keeping bed linens loose to minimize direct contact with the client and protecting the skin form exposure to irritants are helpful measures.
1. Frequent tactile contact is not an appropriate intervention for the client with hyperesthesia.
3. Allowing the client to lie motionless is not an appropriate intervention for the client with hyperesthesia.
4. Using touch as a form of therapy would not be an appropriate nursing intervention for the client with hyperesthesia.

7. 3, p. 1585
Rationale:
3. For the client with aphasia, the nurse can communicate by using a picture chart or communication board for the client's responses.
1. The nurse should not speak loudly and slowly to the client with expressive aphasia. The client is able to understand; this may seem patronizing to the client.
2. The nurse should not speak to the client on the unaffected side, as this will not improve communication.

4. Using hand gestures to convey information to the client may be helpful for the client with receptive aphasia, not expressive aphasia.

8. 3, o, 1588
Rationale:
3. A meal tray can be set up as a clock. The visually impaired client can easily become oriented to the items after the nurse or family member explains each item's location. This enables the client to perform self-care (feeding), which is essential for self-esteem.
1. The client should be allowed to feed himself or herself to maintain self-esteem.
2. Allowing the client to experiment with foods is not assisting the client in performing self-care.
4. The client should be allowed to feed himself or herself to maintain self-esteem.

9. 4, p. 1584
Rationale:
4. Sometimes settings on electrical appliances and equipment are highlighted only in black and white or shades of gray. Color contrasts help to distinguish settings. The greatest concern for safety for the client with sensory impairment is the gray/black setting on the stove handles.
1. Low-pile carpeting helps to prevent falls.
2. A handrail on the stairs that extends the full length is beneficial for preventing falls.
3. Higher-wattage iridescent lighting helps prevent glare and is an appropriate adaptation for visual loss.

10. 3, p. 1587
Rationale:
3. To assist the client who is legally blind, the nurse should warn the client when approaching doorways or narrow spaces, including upcoming curbs or stairs.
1. To assist the client who is legally blind, the nurse should walk one-half step ahead and slightly to the side of the visually impaired person. The client can place his or her hand on the nurse's forearm.

2. This is not the most appropriate response. The client may need orientation to the environment and extra time but should not be made to feel dependent on the nurse. Often sensorially impaired clients can help themselves, and it is essential that they do so for self-esteem.
4. Placing the client in a wheelchair is not the best response. The client who is able should be encouraged to ambulate.

11. 3, p. 1584
Rationale:
3. A safety tip the nurse can share with this client is to keep the car in good working condition.
1. The nurse should advise the client to go slowly, but not too slowly, for safety.
2. The nurse can offer the driving tip to drive in familiar areas, not on long road trips by themselves.
4. The client should be advised to avoid driving at dusk or at night.

12. 3, p. 1569
Rationale:
3. Altered spatial perception is a sign of sensory deprivation.
1. Increased anxiety is a sign of sensory deprivation.
2. Poor task performance is a sign of sensory deprivation.
4. An increased need for physical stimulation is a sign of sensory deprivation.

13. 1, p. 1585
Rationale:
1. Clients with impaired tactile sensation, such as the client with diabetic neuropathy, should be cautioned to have the setting on the water heater no higher than 120°F.
2. The greatest risk for the client with diabetic peripheral neuropathy is an improper water-heater setting, as the client would not be able to feel a setting that is too hot, and could therefore experience injury.
3. An absence of smoke detectors is not the greatest risk for the client with diabetic peripheral neuropathy. It would be of greater risk for the client who has an olfactory impairment.

4. Although a lack of bathroom grab bars may place a client at risk for falls, it is not the greatest risk for the client with diabetic peripheral neuropathy.

14. 4, p. 1574
Rationale:
4. To assess basic visual acuity, the nurse should ask the client to identify crayon colors.
1. The Snellen chart may be used for the adult client, but would be less appropriate for the 4-year-old child.
2. The 4-year-old client may not be able to read. This would be an inaccurate assessment of visual acuity of a 4-year-old.
3. A 4-year-old client may have difficulty understanding following the movement of an object by using his or her peripheral vision.

15. 2, p. 1585
Rationale:
2. If the client has problems with comprehension, as in receptive aphasia, the nurse should use simple short questions, facial gestures, and repeated behaviors to communicate.
1. Providing a client with a letter chart would be more appropriate for the client with expressive aphasia. Questions should be simple, not complex, to aid comprehension.
3. A notepad would be appropriate for the client with expressive aphasia, not receptive aphasia.
4. Clients with expressive aphasia but not clients with receptive aphasia often require a speech therapist.

16. 4, p. 1581
Rationale:
4. Children at risk for hearing impairment include those who were exposed to rubella in utero.
1. Children at risk for visual impairment include those who received excessive oxygen as newborns.
2. Follow-up auditory testing is not necessary for a child who was exposed in utero to diabetes.
3. Follow-up auditory testing is not necessary for a child who was exposed in utero to a respiratory infection.

17. 1, p. 1583

Rationale:

1. Brighter colors such as red, orange, and yellow are easier for the older adult to see.
2. Black and white colors are not the best recommendation for promoting safety in the older adult.
3. Perception of the colors blue, violet, and green usually declines with age.
4. Perception of the colors blue, violet, and green usually declines with age.

18. 2, p. 1583

Rationale:

2. Good oral hygiene keeps the taste buds well hydrated and will enhance the client's gustatory sense.
1. Taste perception is heightened if foods are eaten separately.
3. Taste perception is heightened if foods are differently textured.
4. Taste perception is heightened if foods are well seasoned, but not necessarily extremely spicy.

19. 1, p. 1585

Rationale:

1. A reduced sensitivity to odors means that the client may be unable to smell a smoldering fire. The client should use smoke detectors as a safety measure.
2. A home safety measure specific for a client with diminished vision is the use of extra lighting in hallways.
3. A home safety measure specific for a client with diminished hearing is the use of amplified telephone receivers.
4. A home safety measure specific for a client with reduced tactile sensation is having mild water heater temperatures.

20. 2, p. 1580

Rationale:

2. Safety is always a top priority.
1. The nursing diagnosis of *Social isolation* is not the highest priority.
3. The nursing diagnosis of *Adjustment, impaired* is not the highest priority.
4. The nursing diagnosis of *Communication, impaired verbal* is not the highest priority.

21. 1, p. 1571

Rationale:

1. Whites have more hearing impairment problems than do African-Americans and Asian-Americans.
2. Hearing impairment is not more common in Asian-Americans.
3. African-Americans are at greater risk for glaucoma, not for hearing impairment.
4. Otitis media is more prevalent among Native Americans than among whites.

22. 3, p. 1574

Rationale:

3. Behaviors of children indicating a possible visual deficit include self-stimulation such as eye rubbing, body rocking, sniffing or smelling, and arm twirling.
1. Poor balance and gait may indicate an impairment of position sense in the adult.
2. A weight change may indicate a deficit in taste in the adult.
4. Failure to respond to touch may indicate a touch deficit in the adult.

Chapter 49

1. 2, p. 1602

Rationale:

2. The client who smokes is at greater risk for postoperative pulmonary complications than is a client who does not.
1. This does not place the client at risk for surgery.
3. The presence of an IV infusion does not place the client at risk for surgery. An IV should be in place for surgery, so access is available to administer medications, fluids, or blood products if necessary. Keeping the client well hydrated will help prevent postoperative thrombophlebitis.
4. A history of employment as a computer programmer does not make the client a surgical risk.

2. 3, p. 1596

Rationale:

3. Ablative surgery is the excision or removal of a diseased body part, such as an appendectomy.
1. Diagnostic surgery is surgical exploration that allows the physician to confirm a diagnosis. This type of surgery may involve removal of tissue for further diagnostic testing. An example would be a breast-mass biopsy.
2. Palliative surgery relieves or reduces the intensity of disease symptoms. It will not produce a cure. An example is resection of nerve roots.
4. Reconstructive surgery restores function or appearance to traumatized or malfunctioning tissues. An example is internal fixation of a hip fracture.

3. 4, p. 1601

Rationale:

4. An obese client is susceptible to poor wound healing and wound infection because of the structure of fatty tissue, which contains a poor blood supply. This increases the risk for dehiscence.
1. An obese client is not at greater risk for anemia. A client who is malnourished is more susceptible to being anemic.
2. An obese client is not more susceptible to seizures.
3. An obese client is not more susceptible to protein loss. A client with liver disease may have altered protein metabolism.

4. 3, p. 1602

Rationale:

3. Anticoagulants alter normal clotting factors and thus increase the risk of hemorrhaging during surgery.
1. This client would not be at the greatest risk during surgery.
2. This client would not be at greatest risk during surgery.
4. Aminoglycosides (a type of antibiotic) may cause mild respiratory depression from depressed neuromuscular transmission. However, the client who has been taking anticoagulants is at greater risk during surgery.

5. 4, p. 1600

Rationale:

4. An older adult is likely to have a reduce glomerular filtration rate. This limits th body's ability to eliminate drugs or toxic su stances.
1. An older adult has reduced tactile sens which decreases the client's ability to respon to early warning signs of surgical complica tions, including sensing pressure over bon prominences.
2. An older adult has a lower basal metabol rate, reducing total oxygen consumption. Th nurse should ensure that the client obtain adequate nutritional intake when diet resumed, but avoids intake of excess calories

6. 4, p. 1606

Rationale:

4. The normal serum creatinine in women is 0. to 1.1 mg/100 ml. A serum creatinine of 3. mg/100 ml should be reported to the phys cian, as it can be an indication of renal failur
1. A Hgb of 14 g/100 ml is within the norma limits of 12 to 16 g/100 ml for women.
2. A BUN of 15 mg/100 ml is within the norma limits of 10 to 20 mg/100 ml.
3. A platelet count of 300,000/mm^3 is within th normal limits of 150,000 to 400,000/mm^3.

7. 4, p. 1611

Rationale:

4. When the client has little or no understand ing about the surgery, the physician will nee to be notified to reinform the client.
1. If the client did not understand the surgica procedure, the client would not be givin informed consent. It is the surgeon's respons bility to explain the procedure and obtain th informed consent.
2. The nurse can augment the physician's expla nations, but it is the physician's responsibilit to teach the client about the procedure. Thi teaching includes the need for the procedure steps involved, risks, expected results, an alternative treatments.
3. It is not the unit manager's responsibility t inform the client about the procedure an obtain consent. That is the responsibility c the surgeon.

8. 2, p. 1625
Rationale:

2. The scrub nurse counts the sponges and instruments, and the circulating nurse verifies the counts. This statement by the nurse reflects accountability in the intraoperative phase.
1. This statement does not reflect nursing accountability in the intraoperative phase. The nurse is not accountable for the choice of anesthetic the client receives.
3. This statement reflects nursing accountability in the preoperative phase, not the intraoperative phase.
4. This statement reflects nursing accountability in the postoperative phase, not the intraoperative phase.

9. 1, pp. 1616, 1639
Rationale:

1. Deep-breathing and coughing exercises place additional stress on the suture line and cause discomfort. Splinting the incision with hands or a pillow provides firm support and reduces incisional pulling.
2. Keeping the client flat will not decrease discomfort in the incisional area when the client coughs. Having the knees bent slightly will aid in relaxing the abdominal muscles, causing less discomfort.
3. Turning the client onto the right side will not decrease discomfort in the incisional area when the client coughs. The client should turn from side to side at least every 2 hours and may splint the incision to decrease discomfort when doing so.
4. Splinting should be done directly over the incision to provide firm support and reduce incisional pulling as the client coughs postoperatively.

10. 2, p.1629
Rationale:

2. The client must receive a composite Aldrete score of 8 to 10 before being discharged from the PACU. The nurse may anticipate that the client with an Aldrete score of 8 will be discharged back to his room on the nursing unit.

1. If the client's condition is still poor after 2 to 3 hours, (an Aldrete score below 8), the physician may transfer the client to an intensive care unit.
3. If the client's condition is still poor after 2 to 3 hours (an Aldrete score below 8), the physician may lengthen the client's stay in the PACU until the score improves.
4. A client with an Aldrete score of 8 is unlikely to return to the operating room for surgical evaluation.

11. 4, p. 1633
Rationale:

4. In the PACU, the client is often drowsy. The effects of anesthetic agents subdue the client's level of consciousness and neurological function.
1. Normally during the immediate recovery phase in the PACU, faint or absent bowel sounds are auscultated in all four quadrants. Clients who have had abdominal surgery may develop paralytic ileus, with a return of bowel sounds 24 to 48 hours later.
2. The acute incisional pain experienced in this stage of recovery is usually not relieved with noninvasive comfort measures, but will recover with pharmacological measures of pain relief.
3. Depending on the surgery, a client may not regain voluntary control over urinary function for 6 to 8 hours after anesthesia.

12. 4, p. 1622
Rationale:

4. After administering preoperative medications, the nurse should raise the side rails on the bed or stretcher and keep the bed or stretcher in low position.
1. Keeping the client quiet is not a safety priority. Preanesthetic medications will help reduce the client's anxiety.
2. Consent must be obtained before preoperative medications are administered or the consent is invalid.
3. Preparing the skin at the surgical site is often done in the operating room. It is not a safety priority after the administration of preoperative medications.

Test Bank Answer Key   549

13. 1, p. 1605

Rationale:

1. An elevated temperature before surgery is a cause for concern. If the client has an underlying infection, the surgeon may choose to postpone surgery until the infection has been treated. An elevated body temperature increases the risk of fluid and electrolyte imbalance after surgery.
2. Anxiety and fear commonly cause elevations in heart rate and blood pressure. A pulse rate of 90 is not a concern.
3. A respiratory rate of 20 is normal for an adult.
4. Anxiety and fear commonly cause elevations in heart rate and blood pressure. A blood pressure of 130/74 is not excessively elevated.

14. 2, p. 1639

Rationale:

2. Malignant hyperthermia should be suspected when unexpected tachycardia and tachypnea, jaw muscle rigidity, body rigidity of limbs, abdomen and chest, or hyperkalemia is found.
1. Temperature elevation is a late sign of malignant hyperthermia.
3. Muscle rigidity, not relaxation, is an early sign of malignant hyperthermia.
4. Skin pallor is not an early sign of malignant hyperthermia. Skin pallor may be seen in the immediate postoperative period, as the body is cool.

15. 3, p. 1638

Rationale:

3. The primary purpose of using an incentive spirometer is to promote lung expansion.
1. Coughing exercises are used to remove excess secretions from the lungs.
2. The specific purpose of using an incentive spirometer is not to increase pulmonary circulation. Ambulation helps increase pulmonary circulation as the respiratory rate increases.
4. The primary purpose of incentive spirometry is not to stimulate the cough reflex, but to promote lung expansion.

16. 3, p. 1621

Rationale:

3. All makeup, including nail polish, should b removed to expose normal skin and nail col to determine the client's level of oxygenatic and circulation during and after surgery.
1. Jewelry and other valuables should be give to family members or secured for safekeepin A wedding band can be taped in place unle the client might experience swelling of tl hand or fingers. For safety, metal items, suc as for pierced areas, should be removed.
2. The client should be NPO before surgery prevent vomiting and aspiration with gener anesthesia.
4. Clients may be allowed to keep personal iten such as a hearing aid until they reach the pr operative area.

17. 4, p. 1622

Rationale:

4. Preoperative medications such as meperidir (Demerol) and hydroxyzine pamoate Vistai help reduce the client's anxiety, the amour of general anesthesia required, the risk of na sea and vomiting and resultant aspiratior and respiratory secretions.
1. Meperidine (Demerol) and hydroxyzir pamoate (Vistaril) may help the client fe drowsy and lessen his or her anxiety assoc ated with fear. The purpose is to ease th induction of anesthesia, which include reducing the client's anxiety.
2. Meperidine (Demerol) and hydroxyzir pamoate (Vistaril) will not promote emptyir of the stomach, but may reduce the risk nausea and vomiting. Hydroxyzine pamoat is often given to control nausea and vomitir by suppressing the CNS.
3. Hydroxycodone pamoate (Vistaril) will hav an anticholinergic affect, reducing body secr tions. These medications given together wi ease the induction of anesthesia.

18. 1, p. 1631

Rationale:

1. Ambulatory surgical clients are discharged t home when they meet certain criteria.

550   Test Bank Answer Key

. With new anesthetic agents and techniques, many ambulatory surgery clients are able to bypass phase I. However, if the client is in need of close monitoring, the client is assessed and cared for in the same fashion as inpatient clients in phase I.

. Whether the client will be able to ambulate as soon as being admitted to the recovery area depends on the ambulatory client's condition, type of surgery, and anesthesia.

. This is not a true statement for all ambulatory surgery clients. The administration of fluids is dependent on the client's condition and type of surgery. The excretion of anesthetic depends on many factors, including the route of administration (e.g., fluids will not promote the excretion of anesthetic gases). Oral fluids cannot be given until it is determined that the client has a gag reflex and bowel sounds. Fluids are often given to prevent circulatory complications.

9. 3, p. 1632
Rationale:

. Signs of internal bleeding after abdominal surgery may include abdominal distention; swelling or bruising around the incision; increased pain; a decrease in blood pressure; elevated heart and respiratory rate; thready pulse; cool, clammy, pale skin; and restlessness.

. The client who is hemorrhaging will have a decreased blood pressure.

. Incisional pain may occur as a result of surgery. A continuous increase in pain in conjunction with other symptoms of bleeding may indicate internal hemorrhaging.

. A client who is bleeding will have a decreased urinary output.

20. 3, pp. 1631, 1632
Rationale:

. Vital sign monitoring on the postoperative nursing unit should initially be hourly for 4 hours and then every 4 hours. As the client's condition stabilizes, frequency of assessment will usually decrease to once a shift until discharge.

1. On the client's arrival in recovery, the nurse repeats vital signs every 15 minutes, but not for the client who is stable on the surgical nursing unit.
2. The client who is not experiencing any complications or difficulties does not require vital sign measurement every 30 minutes.
4. After the client's vital signs are obtained hourly for 4 hours and remain stable, the client may have his or her vital signs measured every 4 hours.

21. 4, p. 1632
Rationale:
4. The nurse should assess peripheral pulses and capillary refill distal to the site of surgery. After surgery to the femoral artery, the nurse assesses posterior tibial and dorsalis pedis pulses. The nurse also compares pulses in the affected extremity with those in the nonaffected extremity.
1. The radial pulse is not distal to the femoral artery.
2. The ulnar pulse is not distal to the femoral artery.
3. The brachial artery is not distal to the femoral artery.

22. 3, pp. 1635, 1638
Rationale:
3. To promote a patent airway, the head of the bed may be slightly elevated and the client's neck slightly extended, with the head turned to the side.
1. This position would not best facilitate a patent airway.
2. The client's head should not be flexed, as this may occlude the airway.
4. This is not the best position to promote respirations. The client's arms should never be positioned over or across the chest, because this reduces maximal chest expansion.

23. 1, p. 1599
Rationale:
1. A client with thrombocytopenia is at risk for hemorrhaging during and after surgery.

2. Clients with immunological disorders or diabetes mellitus have an increased risk of wound infection after surgery.
3. A client who has a fever is at risk for fluid imbalance.

4. A client who has chronic respiratory diseas[e] may be at increased risk for respirator[y] depression, but not the client with thrombo[cyto]cytopenia.